# Supportive care for the renal patient

Edited by

## E. Joanna Chambers
Consultant in Palliative Medicine
Southmead Hospital
Bristol
UK

## Michael Germain
Associate Professor of Medicine
Tufts University School of Medicine
Springfield, Massachusetts
USA

## Edwina Brown
Consultant Nephrologist
Charing Cross Hospital
London
UK

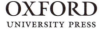

OXFORD
UNIVERSITY PRESS

# OXFORD

UNIVERSITY PRESS

Great Clarendon Street, Oxford OX2 6DP

Oxford University Press is a department of the University of Oxford.
It furthers the University's objective of excellence in research, scholarship,
and education by publishing worldwide in

Oxford  New York

Auckland  Bangkok  Buenos Aires  Cape Town  Chennai
Dar es Salaam  Delhi  Hong Kong  Istanbul  Karachi  Kolkata
Kuala Lumpur  Madrid  Melbourne  Mexico City  Mumbai  Nairobi
São Paulo  Shanghai  Taipèi  Tokyo  Toronto

Oxford is a registered trade mark of Oxford University Press
in the UK and in certain other countries

Published in the United States
by Oxford University Press Inc., New York

A catalogue record for this title is available from the British Library

ISBN 0 19 851616 9

10 9 8 7 6 5 4 3 2 1

Typeset by Integra Software Services Pvt Ltd., Pondicherry, India
Printed in Great Britain
on acid-free paper by Biddles Ltd., King's Lynn, UK

# Dedication

This book is dedicated to our patients and their families, they teach us so much by their continued courage and resilience in adversity. Also to Dr Gary Reiter, a pioneer of renal palliative care and a key collaborator in the Renal Palliative Care Initiative whose untimely death is a loss to both his patients and colleagues.

# Foreword

This book comes at a very timely moment, more so since there have been dramatic changes in the demography and long-term management of patients with end-stage renal disease (ESRD). It represents an excellent and practical compilation in the management and care of ESRD patients in a difficult area of nephrology, that of withdrawal of treatment or conservative palliative care for those in whom dialysis is thought to be inappropriate. Patients with renal failure require lifelong care, which entails not only management of the clinical issues but other related factors that impact in a major way on the quality of life and its continuance. Such life and death matters are difficult and raise enormous ethical problems for the multidisciplinary team looking after the patient.

The demography of ESRD has changed dramatically in the last decade or so. Patient numbers are increasing, with the major increase being in the elderly (especially over the age of 75), diabetic patients, and those with increased cardiovascular co-morbidity and immobility. Gone are the days in the 70s and 80s when only the fittest and the young were treated – here the survival was good, with an acceptable quality of life. End of life decisions were no less difficult but not as overt as now. Indeed, nephrologists probably did not have to make decisions denying therapy as it was 'understood' that such high-risk patients would not receive treatment and hence not be referred. Most patients now have ready access to renal units, and because of the current demography and increasing number of patients, life and death situations in everyday renal failure practice are encountered more frequently. It is also recognised that, for a significant proportion of patients in the high-risk group, dialysis is a palliative therapy where survival is at most a few years.

The key ethical issues are when is dialysis therapy inappropriate in those who have started dialysis and is it appropriate to start dialysis therapy at all? These are critical questions, at times extremely difficult to handle and hitherto not 'openly' debated or discussed. There is still pressure to dialyse patients for whom benefit of dialysis may be very marginal. Medical teams find it difficult to face up to this 'responsibility'. It is not inherent in their training which focuses so much on curative aspects of care. What has changed quite dramatically over the last 2 decades is the involvement of the patient in the decision making process. Shared decision making is now an essential part of the patient-physician relationship. We, as a multidisciplinary team looking after the patient, need to be aware of the pressures upon them. We should be cognisant of the consequences of our decisions and their impact on patient and family, but we should also be brave enough to make the right decision for the patient, with the patient.

This book is therefore timely, and clearly sets out the various issues involved in the supportive care of the renal patient, especially as it applies to end of life decisions. It covers a diverse range of topics, supported by some excellent case scenarios that illustrate the dilemmas present in these situations and shows how to arrive at the right decision. Chapters centre on recommendations for decision making concerning withholding or withdrawing dialysis, and the care of the patients who forego dialysis. An important principle is that of provision of palliative care. All patients should be treated with palliative care throughout their chronic illness, which includes pain and symptom management, attention to psychosocial and spiritual concerns, and identifying what matters most to the dying patient. Other topics covered are patient selection (and therefore denying treatment), spiritual care, and ethical issues.

It is obvious that a multidisciplinary team approach is essential, that patient involvement in the decision is absolutely vital, and that care of the terminally ill patient is to be undertaken with dignity and compassion. This needs to become part of the 'culture' of the multidisciplinary renal team, recognising the various diverse cultural, religious, and ethnic backgrounds that now comprise dialysis populations in many parts of the world but especially in the UK. This is a challenging and relevant area of care and it is going to be even more important in years to come, as more patients in the elderly age group with comorbdity will require dialysis therapy. This has never been an easy aspect of care for nephrologists and the multidisciplinary teams looking after these patients.

We in this profession have been in a privileged position given the opportunity to take care of these patients. We need to recognise this responsibility and exercise it with due care and consideration. At the end of the day it is compassion and caring that matters at all times during the life of the patient with ESRD but especially at the time of dying when all else has failed. There has to be dignity in dying. My plea in writing this foreword is that we should not lose sight of this compassionate approach.

It has been an enlightening experience to read this book and learn from the authoritative text. I very much hope that readers will find it equally inspiring and that it will be a positive help in the care of these patients.

Professor Ram Gokal
Consultant Nephrologist, Manchester Royal Infirmary
Honorary Professor of Medicine, University of Manchester

# Preface

Renal repacelemnt therapy (RRT) with dialysis or transplantation is one of the miracles of modern medicine. First introduced in the 1960s, RRT was only available for a few selected patients. RRT is now established treatment and the number of patients treated continues to grow exponentially, not only because of an increasing number of patients starting on treatment, but also because patients are living longer. We are now aware, though, that dialysis and transplantation are associated with significant morbidity which together with the considerable co-morbidity of patients now accepted or RRT leads to an increasing group of patients with sinificant co-morbidity.

Extending life is not enough. This book looks at how the quality of that extended life can be enhanced by providing appropriate supportive care. It recognizes that care for the patient with ESRD is more than RRT. Dialysis affects all aspects of a person's life and where that effect is detrimental to its quality, the team caring for the patient must attempt to ameliorate the situation and support the patient and his/her family.

Extending life, because we can, is not acceptable. Not starting dialysis is a legitimate option, and where the burden of co-morbid disease or dialysis is too great, then the option to stop dialysis should always be open. Discussions of these options should be held early in the planning of treatment, and are addressed in chapters on withdrawing and withholding treatment and advance care planning. The latter by Jean Holley demonstrates how advance care planning can strengthen relationships and help patients maintain control, important both for quality of life and in dying.

Authors from the UK and US set the scene with respect to the changing pattern of RRT before guiding us through the concept of supportive care and a model for planning a renal palliative care program. The difficulties of measuring quality of life and choosing those for whom dialysis provides good quality extension of life are discussed before a detailed look at pain and other symptom management.

Chapters on the psychological and spiritual care of patients guide us towards a more holistic approach while we journey with the patient and his or her family through renal disease and kidney failure. These journeys may be long and the importance of a multidisciplinary approach is stressed throughout, with particualr reference to relationships between team members themselves as well as between them and renal patients and their families. A well functioning team not only enhances patient care but also the health and well being of team members, itself contributing to patient and family care.

For one editor (EJC) it was meeting and journeying with JJ and his wife (chap 2) in the last year of his life that set her on the path to learn more about the supportive care for the renal patient. She is grateful to his wife for allowing us to tell a small part of his story from which we hope we will continue to learn; resulting in improved care for many.

As the care of patients with ESRD becomes more complex and patients with it, who either receive RRT or choose not to, have greater morbidity, so the importance of supportive care throughout the patient's journey will grow. Team members of all disciplines learn from each other and their patients with benefit to future patients. Bringing together the disciplines of renal and palliative medicine in this book provides practical guidance for all members of both multidisciplinary teams which can enhance the care of our patients and their families

Joanna Chambers
Michael Germain
Edwina Brown

# Contents

# List of Contributors

**Dr David Ansell**
UK Renal Registry
Southmead Hospital
Bristol
UK

**Dr Ira Byock**
Director
The Palliative Care Service
Missoula
USA

**Dr E. Joanna Chambers**
Consultant in Palliative Medicine
Southmead Hospital
Bristol
UK

**Dr Lewis M. Cohen**
Co-Medical Director
Bay State Medical Center
Massachusetts
USA

**Canon Chris Davies**
North Bristol Hospital Chaplains
    Department
Southmead Hospital
Bristol
UK

**Dr Sara N. Davison**
Assistant Professor (Nephrology)
University of Alberta
Canada

**Professor Terry Feest**
Professor of Clinical Nephrology
Department of Renal Medicine
Southmead Hospital
Bristol
UK

**Dr Charles J. Ferro**
Consultant Nephrologist
University Hospital NHS Trust
Edgbaston
Birmingham
UK

**Dr Frederic O. Finkelstein**
Clinical Professor of Medicine
Yale University and Chief of Nephrology
Hospital of St Raphael
USA

**Dr Michael Germain**
Associate Professor of Medicine
Tufts University School of Medicine
Massachusetts
USA

**Helen Hirst**
Peritoneal Dialysis Nurse Specialist
Renal Department
Manchester Royal Infirmary
Manchester
UK

**Dr Jean L. Holley**
Professor of Medicine
University of Rochester
USA

**Dr Jean Hooper**
Clinical Psychologist
Gloucestershire Partnership NHS Trust
UK

**Dr Alastair Hutchison**
Consultant Nephrologist and
    Clinical Director
Renal Department
Manchester Royal Infirmary
Manchester
UK

**George Kelly**
National Kidney Foundation of Michigan Inc
Ann Arbor
Michigan
USA

**Dr Donna L. Lamping**
Department of Public Health and Policy
London School of Hygiene and Tropical
    Medicine
London
UK

**Dr Jeremy Levy**
Consultant Nephrologist and Physician
Imperial College School of Medicine
London
UK

**Dr Lionel U. Mailloux**
Associate Professor of Medicine
NYU School of Medicine
New York
USA

**Sharon McCarthy**
Nurse Practitioner
Western New England Renal and Transplant
    Association
Massachusetts
USA

**Dr Alvin Moss**
Professor of Medicine and
Director for Health Ethics and Law
Section of Nephrology
Robert C Byrd Health Science Center
West Virginia University
USA

**Dr Erica Perry**
Nephrology Social Worker
University of Michigan
USA

**Dr Gary S. Reiter** (deceased)
Assistant Professor of Medicine
University of Massachusetts
USA

**Julie Gumban Roberts**
Clinical Social Worker
Renal and Pancreas Transplant
    Program
University of Michigan Health System
USA

**Dr Paul Roderick**
Health Care Research Unit
University of Southampton
Southampton
UK

**Dr Mohamed Abed Sekkarie**
Clinical Associate Professor
Department of Medicine
West Virginia University
USA

**Dr Shirin Shirani**
Fellow in Nephrology
Hospital of St Raphael
Yale University
USA

**Professor Richard Swartz**
Professor of Internal Medicine
(Nephrology)
University of Michigan
USA

# Abbreviations

| | |
|---|---|
| AIDS | acquired immune deficiency syndrome |
| APD | ambulatory peritoneal dialysis |
| APKD | adult polycystic kidney disease |
| ARF | acute renal failure |
| ASA | acetylsalicylic acid |
| ASN | American Society of Nephrology |
| B3G | buprenorphine-3-glucuronide |
| b.d. | twice a day |
| BDI | Beck Depression Inventory |
| BUN | blood urea nitrogen |
| CAPD | continuous ambulatory peritoneal dialysis |
| CCPD | continuous cycling peritoneal dialysis |
| CKD | chronic kidney disease |
| CMV | cytomegalovirus |
| CPAP | continuous positive airway pressure |
| CPR | cardiopulmonary resuscitation |
| CRF | chronic renal failure |
| CRN | community renal nurse |
| CVD | cardiovascular disease |
| GAS | general adaptation syndrome |
| ED | erectile dysfunction |
| ERA | European Renal Association |
| ESF | established renal failure |
| ESRD | end-stage renal disease |
| ESRF | end-stage renal failure |
| FSH | follicle-stimulating hormone |
| GABA | gamma aminobutyric acid |
| GFR | glomerular filtration rate |
| GHRH | gonadotrophin-releasing hormone |
| GI | gastrointestinal |
| GM | glomerulonephritis |
| h | hour(s) |
| H3G | hydromorphone-3-glucuronide |
| HAART | highly active antiretroviral therapy |
| Hb | haemoglobin |
| HCG | human chorionic gonadotrophin |
| HD | haemodialysis |

| | |
|---|---|
| HIV | human immunodeficiency virus |
| HRQL | health-related quality of life |
| 5-HT$_3$ | 5-hydroxytryptamine 3 |
| ICD | International Classification of Diseases |
| IDDM | insulin-dependent diabetes mellitus |
| IM | intramuscular(ly) |
| IOM | Institute of Medicine |
| IV | intravenous(ly) |
| KDOQI | Kidney Disease Outcomes Quality Initiative |
| KDQOL | Kidney Disease Quality of Life Questionnaire |
| LH | luteinizing hormone |
| LVEF | left ventricular ejection fraction |
| M&M | morbidity and mortality |
| M3G | morphine-3-glucuronide |
| M6G | morphine-6-glucuronide |
| MOAIs | monoamine oxidase inhibitors |
| NCHSPCS | National Council for Hospice and Specialist Palliative Care Services |
| NECOSAD | Netherlands Cooperative Study on Adequacy of Dialysis |
| NHP | Nottingham Health Profile |
| NHS | [UK] National Health Service |
| NICE | National Institute for Clinical Excellence |
| NMDA | N-methyl-D-aspartate |
| NNT | number needed to treat |
| NPT | nocturnal penile tumescence |
| NTDS | North Thames Dialysis Study |
| PD | peritoneal dialysis |
| pmp | per million population |
| PMTs | pain measurement tools |
| PO | by mouth (*per os*) |
| PR | rectally (*per rectum*) |
| prn | as needed |
| PTH | parathyroid hormone |
| PVD | peripheral vascular disease |
| QALY | quality adjusted life year |

| | |
|---|---|
| q.h.s. | at bedtime |
| q.o.d. | every other day |
| q.i.d. | four times a day |
| RBC | red blood cell |
| rHuEpo | recombinant human erythropoietin |
| RLS | restless legs syndrome |
| RPA | Renal Physicians Association [of the USA] |
| RPCI | Renal Palliative Care Initiative |
| RRT | renal replacement therapy |
| SC | subcutaneous(ly) |
| SCr | serum creatinine |
| SF-36 | Medical Outcomes Study Short Form-36 |
| SIP | Sickness Impact Profile |
| SSRIs | selective serotonin re-uptake inhibitors |
| STAI | State Trait Anxiety Inventory |
| stat | immediately |
| TCA | tricyclic antidepressants |
| TENS | transcutaneous electric nerve stimulation |
| t.i.d. | three times a day |
| UK | United Kingdom |
| USA | United States of America |
| USRDS | US Renal Data System |
| WHO | World Health Organization |
| WHOQOL | World Health Organization Quality of Life [Assessment] |
| WNERTA | Western New England Renal and Transplantation Associates |

# Introduction to ethical case analysis

Alvin Moss

Since 1991 the nephrology community has recognized the need for a clinical practice guideline to address ethical issues in starting and stopping dialysis. In 1998 the leadership of the Renal Physicians Association and the American Society of Nephrology gave this topic the highest priority for guideline development because the renal professional community recognized that the end-stage renal disease (ESRD) population had changed substantially. Nephrologists reported being increasingly asked to dialyse patients for whom they perceived dialysis to be of marginal benefit. The Renal Physicians Association and the American Society of Nephrology convened a multidisciplinary work group to develop the clinical practice guideline. The guideline addresses withholding and withdrawing from dialysis in adult patients with either acute renal failure or ESRD. It represents a consensus of expert opinion informed by ethical principles, case and statutory law, and a systematic review of research evidence from the medical literature. The guideline provides nine recommendations with regard to decision-making about withholding or withdrawing dialysis and the care of patients who forgo dialysis. These guideline recommendations (see text below) and the process for ethical decision-making described in the guideline (see Box) provide the basis for the ethics case analyses presented throughout this book. For further information, readers are referred to the Renal Physicians Association and the American Society of Nephrology clinical practice guideline *Shared Decision-Making in the Appropriate Initiation of and Withdrawal from Dialysis* (Washington, DC: Renal Physicians Association, February 2000). Throughout the ethical case analyses it is referred to as the RPA/ASN guideline.

## The patient as person history

(from Center for Health Ethics and Law, Robert C. Byrd Health Sciences Center of West Virginia University, Morgantown, WV, USA)

1. As you understand it, what is your medical problem?
2. How serious is your illness? What will happen if you are not treated?
3. What do you think caused your illness, and why did it start when it did?
4. Why are you being tested and treated as you are? Are there other choices for treatment beside the one you are receiving?
5. How has your illness affected you?
6. What is most important to you in receiving treatment for your illness?
7. What would you want to avoid in the treatment of your illness?
8. What is your understanding of the meaning of your illness? Is God or religion important to you as you face your illness?
9. What are your sources of strength? What role does faith play in your life?

10. How does faith influence your thinking about your illness?

11. Are there religious practices that are particularly meaningful to you?

12. Are there issues in your spiritual life that are troubling you now?

13. Would you like to talk with someone about these issues?

14. Help me understand how you see your family (and/or other significant social relationship)? What are your thoughts about their concerns or your concerns about them?

These questions are helpful in learning the patient's goals for treatment, in advance care planning, and in dealing with disruptive patients to learn their perspective.

# Recommendation summary

The following recommendations are based on the expert consensus opinion of the RPA/ASN Working Group. They developed *a priori* analytic frameworks regarding decisions to withhold or withdraw dialysis in patients with acute renal failure and end-stage renal disease. Systematic literature reviews were conducted to address pre-specified questions derived from the frameworks. In most instances, the relevant evidence that was identified was contextual in nature and only provided indirect support to the recommendations. The research evidence, case and statutory law, and ethical principles were used by the Working Group in the formulation of their recommendations.

## Recommendation 1: shared decision-making

A patient–physician relationship that promotes shared decision-making is recommended for all patients with either ARF or ESRD. Participants in shared decision-making should involve at a minimum the patient and the physician. If a patient lacks decision-making capacity, decisions should involve the legal agent. With the patient's consent, shared decision-making may include family members or friends and other members of the renal care team.

## Recommendation 2: informed consent or refusal

Physicians should fully inform patients about their diagnosis, prognosis, and all treatment options, including: (1) available dialysis modalities, (2) not starting dialysis and continuing conservative management which should include end-of-life care, (3) a time-limited trial of dialysis, and (4) stopping dialysis and receiving end-of-life care. Choices among options should be made by patients or, if patients lack decision-making capacity, their designated legal agents. Their decisions should be informed and voluntary. The renal care team, in conjunction with the primary care physician, should insure that the patient or legal agent understands the consequences of the decision.

## Recommendation 3: estimating prognosis

To facilitate informed decisions about starting dialysis for either ARF or ESRD, discussions should occur with the patient or legal agent about life expectancy and quality of life. Depending upon the circumstances (e.g. availability of nephrologists), a primary care physician or nephrologist who is familiar with prognostic data should conduct these discussions. These discussions should be documented and dated. All patients requiring dialysis should have their chances for survival estimated, with the realization that the ability to predict survival in the individual patient is difficult and imprecise. The estimates should be discussed with the patient or legal agent, the patient's family, and among the medical team. For patients with ESRD, these discussions should occur as early as possible in the course of the patient's renal disease and continue as the renal disease progresses. For patients who experience major complications that may substantially reduce survival or quality of life, it is appropriate to discuss and/or reassess treatment goals, including consideration of withdrawing dialysis.

## Recommendation 4: conflict resolution

A systematic approach for conflict resolution is recommended if there is disagreement regarding the benefits of dialysis between the patient or legal agent (and those supporting the patient's position) and a member(s) of the renal care team. Conflicts may also occur within the renal care team or between the renal care team and other healthcare providers. This approach should review the shared decision-making process for the following potential sources of conflict: (1) miscommunication or misunderstanding about prognosis, (2) intra-personal or interpersonal issues, or (3) values. If dialysis is indicated emergently, it should be provided while pursuing conflict resolution, provided the patient or legal agent requests it.

## Recommendation 5: advance directives

The renal care team should attempt to obtain written advance directives from all dialysis patients. These advance directives should be honoured.

## Recommendation 6: withholding or withdrawing dialysis

It is appropriate to withhold or withdraw dialysis for patients with either ARF or ESRD in the following situations:

1. Patients with decision-making capacity, who being fully informed and making voluntary choices, refuse dialysis or request dialysis be discontinued.
2. Patients who no longer possess decision-making capacity who have previously indicated refusal of dialysis in an oral or written advance directive.
3. Patients who no longer possess decision-making capacity and whose properly appointed legal agents refuse dialysis or request that it be discontinued.
4. Patients with irreversible, profound neurological impairment such that they lack signs of thought, sensation, purposeful behaviour, and awareness of self and environment.

## Recommendation 7: special patient groups

It is reasonable to consider not initiating or withdrawing dialysis for patients with ARF or ESRD who have a terminal illness from a non-renal cause or whose medical condition precludes the technical process of dialysis.

## Recommendation 8: time-limited trial of dialysis

For patients requiring dialysis, but who have an uncertain prognosis, or for whom a consensus cannot be reached about providing dialysis, nephrologists should consider offering a time-limited trial of dialysis.

## Recommendation 9: palliative care

All patients who decide to forgo dialysis or for whom such a decision is made should be treated with continued palliative care. With the patient's consent, persons with expertise in such care, such as hospice healthcare professionals, should be involved in managing the medical, psychosocial, and spiritual aspects of end-of-life care for these patients. Patients should be offered the option of dying where they prefer including at home with hospice care. Bereavement support should be offered to patients' families.

## Systematic evaluation of a patient or family request to stop dialysis

1. Determine the reasons or conditions underlying the patient/surrogate desires regarding withdrawal of dialysis. Such assessment should include specific medical, physical, spiritual, and psychological issues, as well as interventions that could be appropriate. Some of the potentially treatable factors that might be included in the assessment are as follows:

    (a) Underlying medical disorders, including the prognosis for short- or long-term survival on dialysis.

    (b) Difficulties with dialysis treatments.

    (c) The patient's assessment of his/her quality of life and ability to function.

    (d) The patient's short- and long-terms goals.

    (e) The burden that costs of continued treatment/medications/diet/transportation may have on the patient/family/others.

    (f) The patient's psychological condition, including conditions/symptoms that may be caused by uraemia.

    (g) Undue influence or pressure from outside sources, including the patient's family.

    (h) Conflict between the patient and others.

    (i) Dissatisfaction with the dialysis modality, the time or the setting of treatment.

2. If the patient wishes to withdraw from dialysis, did he/she consent to referral to a counselling professional (e.g. social worker, pastoral care, psychologist, or psychiatrist)?

3. If the patient wishes to withdraw from dialysis, are there interventions that could alter the patient's circumstances which might result in him/her considering it reasonable to continue dialysis?

    (a) Describe possible interventions.

    (b) Does the patient desire the proposed intervention(s)?

4. In cases where the surrogate has made the decision to either continue or withdraw dialysis, has it been determined that the judgement of the surrogate is consistent with the stated desires of the patient?

5. Questions to consider when a patient asks to stop dialysis.

    (a) Is the patient's decision-making capacity diminished by depression, encephalopathy, or other disorder?

    (b) Why does the patient want to stop dialysis?

    (c) Are the patient's perceptions about the technical or quality-of-life aspects of dialysis accurate?

(d) Does the patient really mean what he/she says or is the decision to stop dialysis made to get attention, help, or control?

(e) Can any changes be made that might improve life on dialysis for the patient?

(f) Would the patient be willing to continue dialysis while the factors responsible for the patient's request are addressed?

(g) Has the patient discussed his/her desire to stop dialysis with significant others such as family, friends, or spiritual advisors? What do they think about the patient's request?

## The process of ethical decision-making in patient care

1. Identify the ethical question(s).

2. Gather the medical, social, and all other relevant facts of the case.

3. Identify all relevant guidelines and values. Be sure to consider any distinctive values of the patient, family, physician, nurse, other healthcare professionals, or the healthcare institution.

4. Determine if there is a solution that respects all the relevant guidelines and values in the case; if there is, use it. If not, proceed to step 5.

5. Propose possible solutions to resolve the conflict(s) in values, or in other words, answer the question, 'What could you do?'.

6. Evaluate the possible solutions for the particular case, determine which one is better, justify your choice, and respond to possible criticisms. In other words, answer the questions, 'What should you do?' and 'Why?'.

7. Determine what changes in policy, procedure, or practice could prevent such conflicts in the future.

## Supportive Care Series

**Volumes in the series:**

*Surgical Palliative Care*
G. Dunn and A. Johnson

*Supportive Care in Respiratory Disease*
S. Ahmedzai and M. Muers

Chapter 1

# Changing patterns of renal replacement therapy

Paul Roderick and David Ansell

## 1.1 Introduction

End-stage renal disease (ESRD) is inevitably fatal unless treated by renal replacement therapy (RRT). In the decades after the Second World War thousands of people died of this condition as there was no treatment available. It was not until the introduction of haemodialysis (HD), first for acute renal failure and then long-term for chronic renal failure, with the development of the arteriovenous shunt in the early 1960s that the outlook changed.

Renal transplantation was started in the late 1960s and it became much more successful once graft rejection could be effectively countered with the introduction of the effective immunosuppressant cyclosporin in the late 1970s. In the 1980s peritoneal dialysis (PD) was also established in some countries as an important mode of therapy, particularly because of its lower cost and as there is no requirement for major infrastructure. In the decades up to 1990s there was considerable debate about the equity of provision of this high-cost technology, which at population level only benefits a relatively small number of patients. Treatment in some countries, particularly those with tax-based systems such as the UK's National Health Service (NHS), was rationed, with care being restricted to younger, fitter patients. However, as technology and clinical expertise advanced it became possible to treat older, sicker patients successfully. In consequence provision of RRT expanded and the debate has widened to developing humane alternative palliative models of care to dialysis for those likely to have a poor outcome on RRT. The great success of RRT has generated the new problem of caring for a very large and growing pool of patients on RRT and emphasized the public health importance of ESRD. Moreover the significant and rising cost of RRT programmes make it a crucial issue for all healthcare systems.

This chapter outlines the scale of this growth in RRT and considers the implications for the provision of renal services.

## 1.2 Sources of information on the epidemiology of RRT

Data on RRT have come from renal registries, which were established in most developing countries to monitor the patterns of this emerging technology. There are two widely used measures: acceptance and prevalence rates. Acceptance (or take-on) rates of renal replacement therapy (RRT) are 'new' cases started on RRT per year per million population. These rates are influenced not only by the underlying incidence of end-stage renal disease (ESRD) in the population, but also by levels of detection, referral, and acceptance onto RRT. Comparison of crude rates does not take account of different population demographics. There are variations in the definition of a new case. For example, in the USA a new case is not included until after 90 days of treatment; this clearly excludes patients with established ESRD who die in the first 90 days and it underestimates incidence and workload for healthcare providers. However, ascertaining patients at day 0 is difficult. If those that die early are included as an acceptance then this may inflate estimates of mortality, as some patients may have had acute renal failure and therefore recovered renal function and not needed chronic HD. Some countries also include patients restarting dialysis after a failed transplant as 'new' patients. Such differences in definition need to be borne in mind when comparing rates.

Prevalence rates, also called 'stock' rates, are measures of the total number of patients on RRT at any time (usually at the year end) in a defined population. They indicate the healthcare burden and costs of an RRT programme.

RRT rates are not true epidemiological measures of underlying renal disease in the population, but as they are widely available they have been used as proxy measures. Mortality data are unreliable because of significant under ascertainment of renal disease on death certificates.[1] Moreover, International Classification of Diseases (ICD) coding does not reliably distinguish between acute and chronic forms of renal failure. Hospital utilization data are an invalid measure of incidence or prevalence as they only relate to known treated cases, most RRT is delivered to outpatients or to patients at home, and as mentioned ICD coding lacks precision.

The incidence of 'diagnosed' chronic kidney disease (CKD) in the population has been investigated in some countries using the results of raised serum creatinine (SCr) concentration from chemical pathology laboratories.[2,3] SCr is a specific, though insensitive, marker and is widely measured in routine clinical practice. Such studies, however, exclude a proportion of people with CRF such as those who are asymptomatic and who have not had a urea and electrolyte test, and high-risk groups such as diabetics who have not had regular blood tests.[4] However, such population studies of laboratory results are more likely to be representative than nephrology clinic studies where selection factors apply.[5] A more accurate measure of the burden of CKD can be ascertained from the measurement of SCr in population health surveys, as has been carried out in some countries[6] especially when SCr is converted into an estimated Glomerular Filtration Rate (GFR).

This chapter utilizes renal registry data based on the authors' experience in the UK and contrasted where appropriate with data from other developed countries.

## 1.3 Trends in acceptance rates

In the UK the number and rate of patients accepted onto RRT has steadily increased over the last two decades from 20 per million population (pmp) in 1982 to 96 pmp in 1998 (Fig. 1.1). The type of patient being treated has changed dramatically. In the late 1970s RRT was restricted almost exclusively to those under 65 and patients with diabetic ESRD were rarely treated. Figure 1.2 shows that in several European countries the median age was 45 in 1980 and 20 years later nearly half of the cases being treated were over 65.[7] In the UK, diabetes accounted for only 2% of patients starting RRT in 1980, but it is now the commonest single cause of ESRD amongst those accepted.[8]

The main growth has been due to an increase in the acceptance rates in patients over the age of 65 years, especially since the early 1990s. Age-specific patterns of acceptance rates in 2000 are shown in Fig. 1.3 for European countries, again demonstrating the higher rates in older ages.

However, there is still substantial variation in the most recent acceptance rates with the USA having the highest rate closely followed by Japan (Table 1.1). In Europe the highest rate is seen in Germany (175 pmp in 2000). In Eastern Europe RRT programmes are developing fast although rates are generally below those of Western Europe.[9]

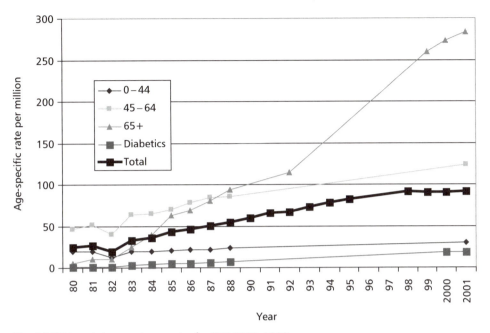

**Fig. 1.1** UK trends in acceptance rates for RRT, 1982–2000.

Establishing the cause of ESRD can be difficult, and coding systems vary between registries. Nevertheless it is possible to discern that the pattern of renal disease has also changed. Figure 1.4 shows that the rate of primary renal diseases such as glomerulonephritis (GN), polycystic kidney disease, and pyelonephritis has remained fairly constant over the last two decades.[7] The biggest increases have been in patients with diabetic ESRD, hypertensive ESRD, renovascular disease, and

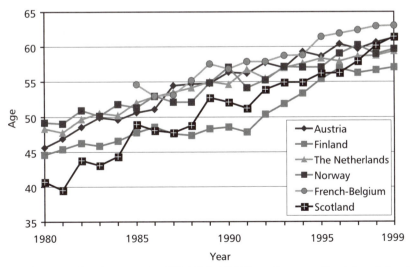

**Fig. 1.2** Median age of patients starting RRT, 1980–1999 (from European Renal Association (ERA) Registry).

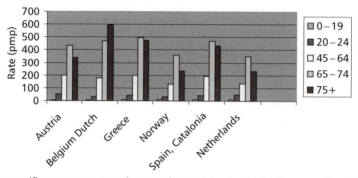

**Fig. 1.3** Age-specific acceptance rates in countries participating in the European Renal Association Registry, 2000.

also unknown causes. These changes reflect the different age distributions of causes of ESRD. In particular renovascular and Type 2 diabetes are more commonly found in the elderly. For example in Spain in 2000, rates of GN, diabetes mellitus, and renovascular disease were 33, 39 and 23 pmp in the age group 45–64 and 22, 43 and 83 pmp in those over 75. Jungers showed that the mean age

**Table 1.1** Patterns of RRT in different countries[7,8,11,18,26,28]

| Country | Year | Mean age | Median age | Acc. rate (pmp) | % with diabetes | Diabetic ESRD rate (pmp) | Prevalence rate (pmp) | % ESRD on dialysis |
|---|---|---|---|---|---|---|---|---|
| Australia | 2000 | 58 | 61 | 91 | 22 | 20 | 605 | 55 |
| Austria | 2000 | 62 | 64 | 129 | 33 | 43 | 714 | 52 |
| Belgium—Dutch | 2000 | 66 | 69 | 144 | 20 | 30 | 806 | 55 |
| Canada | 2000 | | | 143 | 32 | 46 | 609 | 58 |
| Czech Republic | 1998 | | | 136 | 37 | 50 | 563 | |
| Greece | 2000 | 64 | 67 | 154 | 26 | 39 | 798 | 83 |
| Japan | 2000 | | | 253 | 37 | 94 | 1630 | |
| Norway | 2000 | 62 | 65 | 89 | 15 | 13 | 577 | 25 |
| Poland | 1998 | | | 66 | 18 | 12 | 252 | |
| Spain, Catalonia | 2000 | 63 | 67 | 145 | 20 | 29 | 993 | |
| Spain | 2000 | | | 132 | 18 | 23 | 848 | 57 |
| Sweden | 2000 | | | 125 | 25 | 31 | 712 | 47 |
| Netherlands | 2000 | 58 | 62 | 94 | 16 | 15 | 624 | 49 |
| New Zealand | 2000 | 55 | 58 | 107 | 36 | 39 | 610 | 57 |
| Basque region | 2000 | 61 | 65 | 117 | 14 | 17 | 777 | |
| Germany | 2000 | 64 | 66 | 175 | 36 | 63 | 870 | 74 |
| Croatia | 2000 | 59 | 62 | 106 | 28 | 30 | 620 | |
| USA | 2000 | | 64 | 333 | 43 | 142 | 1309 | 73 |
| UK | 2000 | 61 | 64 | 95 | 18 | 17 | 554 | 53 |

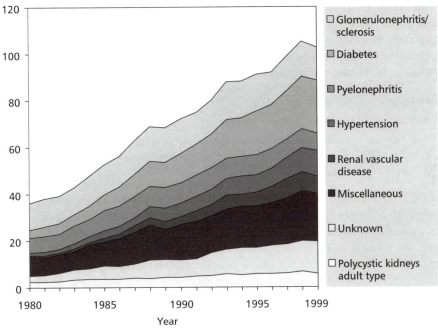

**Fig. 1.4** Trends in incidence rates of new acceptances by cause of end-stage renal disease from European Renal Association Registry, 1980–1999.

at start was 50 for GN patients and 56 for polycystic kidney disease, compared with 66 for Type 2 diabetes and 71 for renovascular disease.[10] Over the same period the co-morbidity associated with new patients has been rising. The most complete data come from Canada (Table 1.2).[11]

Table 1.1 demonstrates the large intercountry variation in diabetic ESRD. Whilst this can be partly explained by variation in ascription (i.e. to what extent the presence of proteinuria, other microvascular disease, or biopsy changes are required for the diagnosis), it is also due to patterns of diabetes, especially Type 2, the effectiveness of preventive health measures, and referral patterns for diabetics with renal disease. As an example, in the UK, while 19% of patients accepted onto RRT have diabetes listed as the primary cause of ESRD, collection of co-morbidity data by the UK Registry indicates that an additional 7% of patients starting RRT are diabetic. Analysis of survival

**Table 1.2** Trends in co-morbidity in new patients starting RRT in Canada. Percentage reported with condition

|  | MI | PVD | CVA | Diabetes |
|---|---|---|---|---|
| 1988 | 16.1 | 18.5 | 7.5 | 29.6 |
| 1992 | 17.6 | 15.4 | 8.2 | 31.5 |
| 1996 | 19.9 | 18.5 | 11.0 | 38.5 |
| 2000 | 21.8 | 19.6 | 12.8 | 44.4 |

Abbreviations: MI, myocardial infarction; PVD, peripheral vascular disease; CVA, cerebrovascular accident.

of these two patient groups indicates that they have a similar prognosis. Many countries do not specify whether or not 'diabetes' is limited to those that have diabetes as the cause of ESRD.

Important questions are why have rates increased so much and what rate would equate with population need (i.e. the rate of cases of ESRD who would benefit from RRT). The factors contributing to the increase in acceptance rates can be summarized as:[12]

1. greater referral/acceptance;
2. increased incidence in ESRD due to demographic change;
3. true increased incidence of ESRD due to change in underlying risk (this can be due to increased incidence of underlying disease and/or a reduction in competing risk such as cardiovascular mortality).

Some of the increase in acceptance rates can be ascribed to greater awareness of ESRD, a lower threshold for referral of older, sicker patients with ESRD to nephrologists, and a greater acceptance by nephrologists of such patients. This has partly been due to technical advances in dialysis therapy allowing for safe and long-term care of such patients. Studies of physicians' and nephrologists' attitudes over the last decade demonstrate this liberalization of attitudes.[13–15] In relation to the decision to accept patients onto RRT, whilst there is a greater propensity for American nephrologists to dialyse certain patients compared with British or Canadian nephrologists, this is not thought to be a major reason for intercountry variation in rates.

The key factors at a population level determining ESRD rates are the age structure and presence of certain ethnic minority groups. Feest and colleagues demonstrated the almost exponential rise of ESRD by age in a population-based study of patients with SCr over 500 $\mu$mol/1.[2] In the UK and elsewhere indigenous and migrant ethnic minority groups have high rates of Type 2 diabetes and ESRD.[16] In the UK and USA, for example, Blacks have RRT acceptance rates four times higher than Whites.[17,18] There are similar findings for Hispanics and Native Americans in the USA and Indo-Asians in the UK. In the UK, ethnic minority populations have a lower median age than Whites, and as these populations mature over the next two decades this will lead to a significant increase in demand for renal replacement therapy.[16] The median age of the ethnic minority population in the UK accepted on to renal replacement therapy in 2000 was 57 compared with an age of 64 from the White population.[8]

The underlying incidence of ESRD has probably also risen over the last two decades due to the ageing of the population and increased rates of Type 2 diabetes (which are age related) especially in ethnic minority groups. These changes have predominantly affected older age groups and are set to continue. In contrast, the incidence of ESRD has probably been unchanged in younger age groups as shown by a relatively constant rate of acceptance and the presumed nearly complete acceptance on to RRT.[19] Giuseppe reviewed the 'epidemic of elderly patients on dialysis' and suggested that the principal cause was the increased incidence of ESRD, particularly due to diabetes and renovascular disease (which often coexist), and that this maybe consequent on a reduction in the competing risk of cardiovascular mortality in patients with vascular disease/diabetes.[20] Lippert considered that population ageing, increased prevalence of Type 2 diabetes, and improved survival of diabetics were the three important factors responsible for the 'rising tide' of ESRD from Type 2 diabetic nephropathy.[21]

Even now current acceptance rates are probably too low in most countries given the intercountry variation in rates, and as such they are likely to continue to rise considerably to meet both this current unmet population need and future increases in need. It is important to recognize that it is unethical to use chronological age as a bar to treatment, and in the UK the Department of

Health has stated this to all Health Commissioners.[22] Although older patients are likely to have more co-morbidity and medical and social problems, their standardized quality of life (compared with the age- and gender-matched general population) is better than that of younger HD patients.[23,24] One study even found that the mental health component score of the SF36 was almost the same in elderly dialysis patients as the general age-specific population norm.[25]

## 1.4 Prevalence rates

In the UK the prevalence rate increased from only 27 pmp in 1981 to 529 pmp in 1998, with over 30 000 patients being treated.[26] Throughout the 1990s there was a 4% annual increase in these numbers. In 1998, 49% had a functioning renal transplant; for dialysis, HD was the modality for 33% of patients, followed by PD (19%) and home HD (2%). Since the 1980s the major absolute growth has been in the numbers of HD patients. The increase in PD patients has slowed down after the initial rapid rise since its introduction in the early 1980s. However, the proportion of dialysis patients in the UK on PD is still much higher when compared with other developed countries except New Zealand, which is known to have constraints on HD due to lack of resources. These patterns have arisen due to shortages of organs for transplantation and recognition that HD is an appropriate mode for many elderly patients.

Organ donor rates in the UK have fallen slightly in recent years, and although there has been an increase in live donor transplantation, the overall renal transplant rate has marginally declined. The numbers with a functioning renal transplant have fallen below 50% for the first time in recent years in the UK. The percentage of patients with a functioning transplant is a reflection of the total numbers on ESRD programme, the historical and current transplant rate (cadaveric and live), and the failure rate. In the USA only 29% of ESRD patients have a functioning transplant, although this is a prevalence rate of 370 pmp for transplants with a transplant incidence rate of 47 pmp. This compares with the UK where 48% of ESRD patients have a functioning transplant, but the transplant prevalence rate is only 260 pmp and the transplant incidence rate 29 pmp.

The comparable recent prevalence rates and modality patterns in selected developed countries are shown in Table 1.1. Figure 1.5 shows the steep growth in HD rates in Canada in the 1990s, and the flat PD rates, so that as in the UK, HD has become by far the most common form of dialysis and has overtaken the stock share of transplantation.[11] This pattern is seen in all countries, even those with high PD rates.

As with acceptance rates there is huge variation between countries in the overall stock but also in the patterns of modes of RRT. This reflects a variety of factors including the cultural

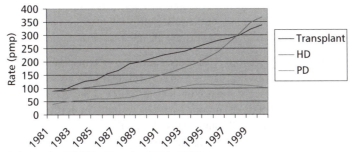

**Fig. 1.5** Trends in mode of RRT in Canada, 1981–2000.

acceptance of and legal structure for organ donation, the organization of cadaver and live donation programmes, financial incentives for HD in certain healthcare systems and conversely for PD in others, clinician preferences, and historical precedent. Most countries have experienced a falling proportion of patients with transplants due to a falling supply of cadaver organ donors being outstripped by demand for such therapy from the growing stock on RRT. Two exceptions are Spain, which has instituted a systematic approach to cadaver organ donation, and Norway which has the most active live donation programme. Spain has actually increased the proportion of stock with a functioning graft from 39% in 1996 to 43% in 2000.[27]

Due to the shortage of kidneys for transplantation in most countries transplantation is most commonly given to younger patients. Consequently the elderly on RRT are mainly treated with dialysis, particularly HD.[28] As these elderly patients may have additional medical problems and lack social support, hospital HD has been the mainstay. In some countries such as the UK and Australia, there has been a shift to open satellite units both to cope with demand for HD and to provide more accessible dialysis for patients. In UK these units are largely run by nurses with visiting medical input but are linked to larger renal units.[26] They are an important and growing type of care for the elderly.

The rise in the number of stock RRT patients in all countries is due to two factors—the increase in acceptance rates as outlined in the section above and improvements in patient survival which are discussed below.

## 1.5 Patient survival on RRT

The key factors that affect patient survival on RRT are listed below.

1. **Sociodemographic**: age—poorer survival in older ages. Ethnic minority—Blacks in the USA have better survival than Whites. There is no evidence for gender or socioeconomic status.

2. **Co-morbidity**: any cardiovascular disease, diabetes, malignancy, major organ system (e.g. respiratory) disease worsens survival. It can be measured by various scoring systems (Khan, Charlson, Lister). The degree of independence as measured by the Karnofsky Performance Score is also predictive of outcome.

3. **Primary renal disease**: primary renal disease, e.g. GN, polycystic kidney disease, has better survival than systemic causes, e.g. diabetic nephropathy, renovascular disease.

4. **Morbidity at start of RRT**: poor nutritional status, e.g. low serum albumin, symptomatic with complications of ESRD, e.g. fluid overload, and the need for temporary access all worsen survival. Patients who are referred late are more likely to have these factors.

5. **Care on RRT**: mode—dialysis has a poorer survival than transplantation (though large selection factors apply), adequacy of dialysis, control of anaemia, control of serum phosphate, management of cardiovascular disease all affect survival.

Comparisons of mortality between renal units, countries, or time periods can be misleading without adjustment for case mix. Registry data on survival are usually presented in combinations by mode, age group, and presence/absence of diabetic ESRD. Several countries calculate their first-year survival starting from day 90 onwards. As 46% of deaths in the first year occur between days 0 and 90 this may account for the apparent wide variations in quoted 1-year survival data. Table 1.3 shows Canadian data for 1991–2000. This highlights the impact of age and diabetic status on survival and that survival is better after transplantation.[11] The improved survival

**Table 1.3** Patient survival in Canada, 1991–2000

| | Age (years) | Haemodialysis | | | Transplantation | | |
|---|---|---|---|---|---|---|---|
| | | 1 year | 3 years | 5 years | 1 year | 3 years | 5 years |
| Non-diabetic | 20–44 | 89 | 76 | 65 | 99.8 | 98 | 97 |
| | 45–64 | 81 | 60 | 45 | 99 | 96 | 91 |
| | 65+ | 71 | 44 | 27 | 98 | 92 | 86 |
| Diabetic | 20–44 | 85 | 57 | 38 | 99.5 | 97 | 91 |
| | 45–64 | 83 | 53 | 31 | 99 | 92 | 83 |
| | 65+ | 72 | 41 | 21 | – | – | – |

on transplantation should not be wholly attributed to transplantation as there is an element of selection bias in that fitter patients with less co-morbidity are more likely to receive a transplant. European Renal Association (ERA) Registry data for six countries show a similar pattern of mortality from day 1.[7]

In Australia the annual death rates of all patients/100 patient years was 15.7 for dialysis (equivalent to a loss of 12% of all patients on dialysis per year) and 3.2 for transplants.[29] In the UK 1-year survival on dialysis is currently 77%, but it is age related, being higher in those under 65 (88%) and 65% in those over 65%. Two-year survival is of the order of 67%.[8]

## 1.6 Causes of death

Compared with the general population, death rates are higher in RRT patients.[8] Table 1.4 shows the increased risk of death for non-diabetic dialysis patients compared with people of the same age in the general population. These data are similar to those published by Mignon and colleagues in 1993.[22]

Cardiovascular causes predominate in all countries[12] which reflects the complex interrelationship of renal failure and risk of cardiovascular disease (CVD).[30] Renal impairment leads to secondary hypertension, abnormal lipid profiles, arterial wall damage, and adversely alters other CVD risk factors (e.g. homocysteine and fibrinogen levels). Some factors such as smoking, and diseases such as diabetes, are important risk factors for both conditions.

With the increasing acceptance of older patients with more co-morbid disease there will inevitably be a rise in the proportion of patients who are ultimately withdrawn from dialysis due to deteriorating quality of life, sometimes triggered by an acute event.[31] Such data are not

**Table 1.4** Increased risk of death for non-diabetic dialysis patients compared with people of the same age in the general population

| Age band | Increased risk of death |
|---|---|
| 45–54 | 18.5 |
| 55–64 | 14.6 |
| 65–74 | 9.1 |
| >75 | 4.5 |

**Table 1.5** Cause of death on RRT in Canada, 2000. Proportions by age band

|                | 15–44 (*n* = 164) | 45–64 (*n* = 663) | 65–74 (*n* = 815) | 75 + (*n* = 881) |
|----------------|:---:|:---:|:---:|:---:|
| Cardiovascular | 33 | 39 | 42 | 35 |
| Social         | 12 | 12 | 13 | 21 |
| Infection      | 15 | 11 | 9  | 9  |
| Other          | 19 | 19 | 20 | 17 |
| Uncertain      | 21 | 19 | 16 | 18 |

reliably collected by all registries. The UK registry has found that 12% of deaths on dialysis are ascribed to withdrawal.[8] Withdrawal as a cause of death was significantly higher in the first year of starting RRT, at 14%. There was also a difference by age, with withdrawal accounting for 6.7% of deaths in those aged under 65 on dialysis compared with 15% in the over 65s. In Canada the category, 'social causes', which includes refusal or discontinuation of treatment and suicide, is most common in the over 75s (see Table 1.5).[11]

Likewise in Australia 21% of deaths overall in 2000 were ascribed to withdrawal, 74% of which were in over the 65s and most were initiated by the patients not the clinical team. This contrasts with the 14% of deaths due to withdrawal from RRT in Australia for the period 1983–1992.[32]

In the European Renal Association Registry withdrawal was coded less frequently at under 5%; it is not clear whether this represents a true difference or underrecording.[12] A single-centre study in the UK showed that withdrawal was the commonest cause of death in the over 75s particularly in later deaths.[23]

As it impossible to predict the survival of individual patients and how they will adapt to treatment, some have suggested the use of a trial of dialysis for all patients except in cases with obvious poor prognosis such as severe dementia or advanced malignancy.[22] Withdrawal from RRT will remain an important and probably increasing cause of death which has considerable implications for supportive terminal care of such patients and their families.[23] However, some patients who are referred for RRT may be considered unsuitable for RRT due to poor prognosis and/or associated problems, and this number is likely to increase over time. There is then a challenge to develop models of palliative care to support such patients and their families.

## 1.7 Late referral for RRT

A major and enduring problem is that up to 40% of patients requiring RRT are only referred to the renal unit within 4 months of commencement of treatment.[33–35] This reduces opportunities for interventions to reduce cardiovascular risk[36] or the complications of CKD, to establish permanent access for dialysis and to assess suitability for dialysis, and to allow patients a choice of modality. Patients presenting late generally fare less well since they are often in a poorer clinical state (e.g. lower albumin) and they need temporary access to start dialysis, they have longer initial hospitalization, and a higher early mortality.[37] One study showed that whilst a proportion are unavoidable (e.g. late presenters with no prior symptoms or signs of chronic renal failure (CRF), or irreversible acute renal failure) around 50% are potentially avoidable, the commonest reason being documented rising creatinine levels for several years.[33]

## 1.8 Future demand for RRT

Demand for RRT will continue rise for the following reasons:

1. Demographic change with an ageing population, which is most marked in ethnic minority and indigenous populations.
2. Type 2 diabetes epidemic leading to increased ESRD rates.
3. Increased referral of patients to meet population need.
4. In all countries a steady state has not been reached at which input (acceptances per year and transfers in) is equal to the annual death rate and transfers out. Previous modelling suggested that this would not occur for over 20 years.[38]
5. Improvements in the management of patients on RRT by implementation of national guidelines will improve survival and hence increase the stock of patients.

A simulation model developed for England has shown that prevalence will increase from the current level of about 30 000 patients (600 pmp) to over 900 pmp by 2010 and to 60 000 by 2025.[39] Even with assumptions of increased transplant supply the largest absolute growth is predicted to be in elderly patients receiving hospital HD. There have been other projections of RRT demand. Schaubel *et al.* predicted an 85% increase in the prevalence of RRT in Canada from 1996 to 2005, a mean annual increase of 5.8%.[40] Projection of current trends in RRT in Australia from 1998–2007 predicted a more than doubling of dialysis requirements if the transplant supply remained at 23 pmp, falling to an 80% increase (8% per annum) if it rose to 35 pmp and only 50% if it achieved Spanish levels of 47 pmp.[41] Xue *et al.* forecast future growth in the USA based on extrapolation of US Renal Data System (USRDS) data from 1982–1997.[42] They predicted linear growth in the acceptance rate but an exponential increase with a quadratic component for prevalence, with an annual (geometric) rate of 6.4% for all patients and 7.1% for dialysis patients.

## 1.9 Conclusion

There has been a continuing and substantial growth in the incidence and prevalence of RRT in all developed countries, though there are substantial intercountry variations, particularly in comparison with rates in the USA and Japan. Such growth will continue for the foreseeable future, particularly in the elderly and in patients with diabetes and/or vascular disease, highlighting the importance of prevention of ESRD.

The predominant mode of therapy will be HD, even if efforts to enhance live and cadaver donation programmes are successful. An increasing proportion of patients will be elderly with the attendant medical problems and general frailty. Even if such problems are not present when they start RRT they are inevitable as patients age on dialysis. There are considerable challenges to nephrology services to supporting this increasing pool of elderly patients undergoing complex RRT.

## References

1. Goldacre, M.J. (1993). Cause-specific mortality: understanding uncertain tips of the disease iceberg. *J. Epidemiol. Community Health*, **47**: 491–6.
2. Feest, T.G., Mistry, C.D., Grimes, D.S., Mallick, N.P. (1990). Incidence of advanced chronic renal failure and the need for end stage renal replacement treatment. *Br. Med., J.* **301**: 897–900.

3. Khan, I.H., Catto, G.R., Edward, N., MacLeod, A.M. (1994). Chronic renal failure: factors influencing nephrological referral. *Q. J. Med.,* **87**: 559–64.

4. Kissmeyer, L., Kong, C., Cohen, J., Unwin, R., Woolfson, R., Neild, G. (1999). Community nephrology: audit of screening for renal insufficiency in a high risk population. *Nephrol. Dial. Transpl.,* **14**: 2150–5.

5. Jungers, P., Chauveau, P., Descamps, L.B., Labrunie, M., Giraud, E., Man, N.K., *et al.* (1996). Age and gender-related incidence of chronic renal failure in a French urban area: a prospective epidemiologic study. *Nephrol. Dial. Transpl.,* **11**: 1542–6.

6. Jones, C.A., McQuillan, G.M., Kusek, J.W. (1998). Serum creatinine levels in the US population: Third National Health and Nutrition Examination Survey. *Am. J. Kidney Dis.,* **32**: 992–9.

7. European Renal Association/European Dialysis and Transplantation Association Registry (ERA-EDTA) (2002). www.era-edta-reg.org

8. Ansell, D., Feest, T. (2002). *The UK Renal Registry Fourth Annual Report.* Bristol: UKRR.

9. Rutkowski, B. (2000). Changing pattern of end-stage renal disease in central and eastern Europe. *Nephrol. Dial. Transpl.,* **15**: 156–60.

10. Jungers, P., Choukroun, G., Robino, C., Massy, Z.A., Taupin, P., Labrunie, M., *et al.* (2000). Epidemiology of end-stage renal disease in the Ile-de-France area: a prospective study in 1998. *Nephrol. Dial. Transpl.,* **15**: 2000–6.

11. Canadian Organ Replacement Register (2000). www.cihi.ca

12. van Dijk, P.C., Jager, K.J., de Charro, F., Collart, F., Cornet, R., Dekker, F.W., *et al.* (2001). Renal replacement therapy in Europe: the results of a collaborative effort by the ERA-EDTA registry and six national or regional registries. *Nephrol. Dial. Transpl.,* **16**: 1120–9.

13. Challah, S., Wing, A.J., Bauer, R., Morris, R.W., Schroeder, S.A. (1984). Negative selection of patients for dialysis and transplantation in the United Kingdom. *Br. Med., J.* **288**: 1119–22.

14. Parry, R.G., Crowe, A., Stevens, J.M., Mason, J.C., Roderick, P. (1996). Referral of elderly patients with severe renal failure: a questionnaire survey of physicians. *Br. Med., J.* **313**: 466.

15. McKenzie, J.K., Moss, A.H., Feest, T.G., Stocking, C.B., Siegler, M. (1998). Dialysis decision making in Canada, the United Kingdom, and the United States. *Am. J. Kidney Dis.,* **31**: 12–18.

16. Raleigh, V.S. (1997). Diabetes and hypertension in Britain's ethnic minorities: implications for the future of renal services. *Br. Med., J.* **314**: 209–13.

17. Roderick, P.J., Raleigh, V.S., Hallam, L., Mallick, N.P. (1996). The need and demand for renal replacement therapy in ethnic minorities in England. *J. Epidemiol. Community Health,* **50**: 334–9.

18. United States Renal Data System (USRDS) (2002). www.usrds.org

19. Stewart, J.H., Disney, A.P., Mathew, T.H. (1994). Trends in the incidence of end-stage renal failure due to hypertension and vascular disease in Australia, 1972–1991. *Aust. N.Z. J. Med.,* **24**: 696–700.

20. Giuseppe, P., Mario, S., Barbara, P.G., Paola, M., Pacitti, A., Antonio, M., *et al.* (1996). Elderly patients on dialysis: epidemiology of an epidemic. *Nephrol. Dial. Transpl.,* **11**(S9): 26–30.

21. Lippert, J., Ritz, E., Schwarzbeck, A., Schneider, P. (1995). The rising tide of endstage renal failure from diabetic nephropathy type II—an epidemiological analysis. *Nephrol. Dial. Transpl.,* **10**: 462–7.

22. Mignon, F., Michel, C., Mentre, F., Viron, B. (1993). Worldwide demographics and future trends of the management of renal failure in the elderly. *Kidney Int.* **Suppl.,** **41**: S18–S26.

23. Munshi, S.K., Vijayakumar, N., Taub, N.A., Bhullar, H., Nelson Lo, T.C., Warwick, G. (2001). Outcome of renal replacement therapy in the very elderly. *Nephrol. Dial. Transpl.,* **16**: 128–33.

24. Rabello, P., Ortgea, F., Baltar, J.M., Alvarez-Ude, F., Navascues, R.A., Alvarez-Grande, J. (2001). Is the loss of health-related quality of life during renal replacement therapy lower in elderly patients than in younger patients. *Nephrol. Dial. Transpl.,* **16**: 1675–80.

25. Lamping, D., Constantinovici, N., Roderick, P., Normand, C., Henderson, L., Harris, S., *et al.* (2000). Clinical outcomes, quality of life, and costs in the North Thames Dialysis Study of elderly people on dialysis: a prospective cohort study. *The Lancet,* **356**: 1543–50.

26. Roderick, P.J., Ferris, G., Feest, T.G. (1998). The provision of renal replacement therapy for adults in England and Wales: recent trends and future directions. *Q. J. Med.,* **91**: 581–7.

27. Sociedad Espanola de Nefrologia (2002). www.senefro.org

28. Krishnan, M., Lok, C.E., Jassal, S.V. (2002). Epidemiology and demographic aspects of treated end-stage renal disease in the elderly. *Semin. Nephrol.,* **15**: 79–83.

29. ANZData (Australian and New Zealand Dialysis and Trensplant Register) (2002). www.anzdata.org.au

30. Baigent, C., Burbury, K., Wheeler, D. (2000). Premature cardiovascular disease in chronic renal failure. *The Lancet,* **356**: 147–52.

31. Neu, S., Kjellstrand, M. (1986). An empirical study of withdrawal of life-supporting treatment. *New Engl. J. Med.,* **314**: 14–20.

32. Disney, A.P. (1995). Demography and survival of patients receiving treatment for chronic renal failure in Australia and New Zealand: report on dialysis and renal transplantation treatment from the Australia and New Zealand Dialysis and Transplant Registry. *Am. J. Kidney Dis.,* **25**: 165–75.

33. Eadington, D.W., Craig, K.J., Winney, R.J. (1994). Late referral for RRT: still a common cause of avoidable morbidity. *Nephrol. Dial. Transpl.,* **9**: 1686.

34. Roderick, P., Jones, C., Tomson, C., Mason, J. (2002). Late referral for dialysis: improving the management of chronic renal disease. *Q. J. Med.,* **95**: 363–70.

35. Sesso, R., Belasco, A.G. (1996). Late diagnosis of chronic renal failure and mortality on maintenance dialysis. *Nephrol. Dial. Transpl.,* **11**: 2417–20.

36. Jungers, P., Zingraff, J., Albouze, G., Chauveau, P., Page, B., Hannedouche, T., *et al.* (1993). Late referral to maintenance dialysis: detrimental consequences. *Nephrol. Dial. Transpl.,* **8**: 1089–93.

37. Metcalfe, W., Khan, I.H., Prescott, G.J., Simpson, K., MacLeod, A.M. (2000). Can we improve early mortality in patients receiving renal replacement therapy? *Kidney Int.,* **57**: 2539–45.

38. Davies, R., Roderick, P. (1997). Predicting the future demand for renal replacement therapy in England using simulation modelling. *Nephrol. Dial. Transpl.,* **12**: 2512–16.

39. Roderick, P., Davies, R., Jones, C., Feest, T., Smith, S., Farrington, K. (2003). Predicting future demand in England, a simulation model of renal replacement therapy. In: *The UK Renal Registry Fifth Annual Report*, ch., 6. Bristol:UKRR.

40. Schaubel, D.E., Morrison, H.I., Desmeules, M., Parsons, D.A., Fenton, S.S. (1999). End-stage renal disease in Canada: prevalence projections to 2005. *Can. Med. Assoc., J.* **160**: 1557–63.

41. Branley, P., McNeil, J.J., Stephenson, D.H., Evans, S.M., Brigant, E.M. (2000). Modelling the future dialysis requirements under various scenarios of organ availability in Australia. *Nephrology,* **5**: 243–9.

42. Xue, J.L., Jennie, Z., Louis, T.A., Collins, A.J. (2001). Forecast of the number of patients with end-stage renal disease in the United States to the year 2010. *J. Am. Soc. Nephrol.,* **12**: 2753–8.

Chapter 2

# The concept of supportive care for the renal patient

Gary S. Reiter and Joanna Chambers

The utility of living consists not in the length of days, but in the use of time: a man may have lived long, and yet lived but little.

Montaigne, 1533–92

## 2.1 Introduction

End-stage renal disease (ESRD) presents many challenges to the patients who experience and suffer from it and the healthcare professionals who care for them. Its chronicity and the morbidity associated with it, which often includes difficult and intractable symptoms, make palliative and supportive care natural accompaniments to its management. The team-based approach to the care of patients with ESRD makes it ideally suited to incorporate palliative and supportive care. Programmes for the management of ESRD should include a supportive care plan as well as routine prevention, diagnosis, renal replacement therapy, and transplantation.

## 2.2 The development of palliative care

In 1990 the World Health Organization (WHO) defined palliative care (see Appendix 1) as:

> The active total care of patients whose disease is not responsive to curative treatment. Control of pain, of other symptoms, and of psychological, social and spiritual problems is paramount. The goal of palliative care is achievement of the best quality of life for patients and their families. Many aspects of palliative care are also applicable earlier in the course of the illness in conjunction with anticancer treatment.[1]

Although this definition applied primarily to patients with cancer it is equally appropriate for people with other chronic diseases and echoes many of the ideas embedded in the more recent WHO definition (Appendix 2). It importantly highlights that palliative care has applications early in the course of an illness and looks at the needs of the whole person in the context of his or her social situation.

Many subsequent definitions have built on this concept of addressing patients' symptoms as well as psychosocial and spiritual needs in addition to disease-directed therapy in chronic and life-limiting illnesses. This distinction regarding the broad clinical applicability and appropriateness of palliative care is important, because until the mid 1980s palliative care was seen as end-of-life care. In both the USA and the UK it was synonymous with hospice care. Palliative care, often felt to be 'terminal care', was then seen as separate from 'aggressive care' which

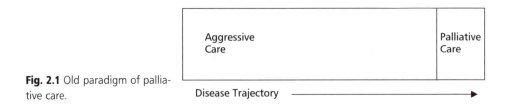

**Fig. 2.1** Old paradigm of palliative care.

people were to receive throughout the majority of their illness (Fig. 2.1). Just as palliative care should not be reserved only for the end of life, referring to all treatment short of palliative care as aggressive is inaccurate.

Hospice care in the UK was developed for the care of the dying, almost exclusively for those dying of cancer, because of the visible suffering of people with cancer and the low importance given to symptom control and psychosocial support for those who were terminally ill. Even as early as 1967 Dame Cicely Saunders, the founder of the first modern hospice, St Christopher's, had the vision to include a multiprofessional approach and to integrate research into its structure.

Since then hospice care has become part of palliative care, and that in turn has become part of the broader concept of supportive care. The role of the hospice has changed from a place where people die, to being part of a larger supportive care strategy. Its role includes refuge for good symptom control or respite care, outreach and support to people in their own homes, as well as excellent terminal care within the hospice or at home through 'Hospice at Home' programmes and bereavement support. In the US there can be barriers to Hospice care particularly for the patient who choses to continue dialysis.

## 2.3 Supportive care

A more accurate description of what has traditionally been referred to as 'aggressive care' is 'restorative care'. Restorative care is disease-specific therapy that seeks to reverse, halt, or minimize the underlying pathophysiological processes of disease. Its goal is to return the patient to as normal a baseline as possible by correcting those pathophysiological processes where it can. Both restorative care and palliative care may be aggressive. Any clinician who has struggled with treating severe pain or intractable nausea is aware of just how vigorous palliative care can be.

A broader view of supportive care has evolved that embraces both restorative disease-specific treatment and palliative care to maximize disease control and quality of life. Supportive care integrates the two concepts of restorative and palliative care. This model of supportive care (Fig. 2.2) envisages a continuous overlap of the two disease management

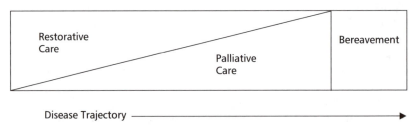

**Fig. 2.2** Model of supportive care.

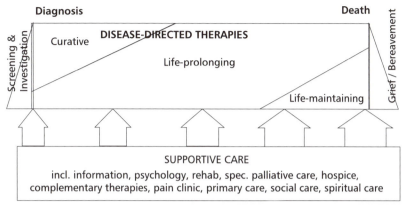

**Fig. 2.3** Ahmedazi and Walsh's development of the model of supportive care[2]

strategies. It seeks to minimize the disease pathophysiology, the toxicity of treatment, and the many symptoms associated with chronic illness and its co-morbidities. It includes psychosocial support and attention to spiritual issues. Fewer restorative options may be available as the disease progresses, necessitating a greater reliance on palliative interventions and an increase in psychosocial support. Palliative and supportive care should continue through bereavement.

Ahmedzai and Walsh[2] have further developed this model in relation to cancer (Fig. 2.3). Their model integrates the three parallel strands of care: 'cancer-directed care', 'patient-directed care', and 'family-directed care'. It is applicable to most chronic diseases including ESRD, where it demonstrates the importance of dialysis or transplantation while recognizing that many other specialties and modalities are needed to support the patient and family through an illness that will last for the rest of their lives.

In describing the integration of palliative care with cancer treatment, Ahmedzai and Walsh define the needs of that population as 'effective communication, good decision-making, aggressive management of complications, first rate symptom control, and sensitivity to psychosocial distress. Most important is a positive proactive approach.' This could equally well describe the care of patients with ESRD. Restorative therapy in ESRD is associated with significant morbidity and may at times be a considerable burden for the patient. It can impair functioning in a social role as an earner/breadwinner, spouse, parent, or friend. Failure to address these issues will lead to technical treatment without healing.

When offering and discussing any treatment there is always a balance to be achieved between the potential of the treatment offered and its associated side-effects and risks. In the case of ESRD, treatment has the potential to prolong life considerably, at a cost in terms of morbidity that is initially uncertain though often severe. There is also the near certainty of death if treatment once started is stopped. Good initial communication, with sensitively delivered accurate information, enables patients to make informed choices.

## 2.4 Palliative treatment modalities

Any treatment which relieves symptoms but is not aimed at cure is palliative and extends beyond the dictionary definition of the word which means to cloak or hide. It can encompass all modalities of medical and nursing care which are used to enhance quality of life, including surgery. Some palliative treatments will be life extending, while others, such as pain relief, will be life enhancing. In the USA there is growing recognition that palliative medicine should be available to all patients with chronic illness who experience physical or psychosocial distress. The lessons that have been learned in palliating the discomforts of acquired immune deficiency syndrome (AIDS) and cancer can be broadly applied to all disciplines in modern medicine. Patients should not have to have a terminal illness, or be in the terminal phase of an illness, to benefit from excellent pain and symptom management or to have psychosocial issues addressed.

Ideal palliative therapies are patient centred, effective in alleviating the distressing symptoms of disease, easy to administer, and have a minimum of side-effects.[3] For many years clinicians have thought of palliative therapies as being composed primarily of analgesics, sedatives, and other non-specific treatments. However, more recently, it has been recognized that some disease-modifying therapies provide excellent palliation.

## 2.5 Disease-specific treatment as palliative care

The evolution of treatment for people with human immunodeficiency virus (HIV)/AIDS that took place in the 1990s provided much of the impetus for the changing paradigm of palliative and supportive care as well as the use of disease-specific therapies for palliative purposes. Examining how new treatment modalities evolved for HIV, and how that evolution changed the way that clinicians thought of palliative and restorative care, is illuminating for other disease states.

From the discovery of the AIDS epidemic in 1981 until the development of highly active antiretroviral therapy (HAART) in 1996, AIDS was nearly uniformly fatal.[4] While disease-specific therapies for many of the co-morbidities of AIDS, such as *Pneumocystis carinii* pneumonia, *Mycobacterium avium intracellulari* infection, and toxoplasmic encephalitis, were available, they were minimally effective. Until effective therapies directed at reversing the underlying immunodeficiency were developed, treating the co-morbidities simply delayed death.

Because of the relative ineffectiveness of these disease-specific therapies, and the fact that numerous treatable symptoms were present, many HIV clinicians became familiar with the use of palliative therapies. Symptoms such as painful peripheral neuropathy, somatic pain, diarrhoea, anorexia, nausea, vomiting, dysphagia, and a host of others required conventional and novel palliative approaches to maximize quality of life for AIDS patients. In the pre-HAART era, the best HIV clinicians were also good palliative care clinicians, prolonging life when they could, treating a multitude of symptoms, and addressing the myriad psychosocial, spiritual, and existential issues that arose in very young patients dying of AIDS.

Many hospice programmes in the USA in the 1980s and early 1990s were caring for patients dying of AIDS. As the AIDS census grew in these programmes, many hospice professionals began to realize that certain AIDS-associated illnesses were best palliated or prevented with disease-specific treatments. One example of this is cytomegalovirus (CMV) retinitis. CMV retinitis was a common complication in patients with advanced AIDS. In the pre-HAART era, untreated patients would typically progress from minimal vision loss to blindness within 14 days of the first symptoms of CMV retinitis. Even in hospice patients, the use of disease-specific antiviral agents such as ganciclovir or foscarnet, was the only way to prevent blindness. CMV retinitis is a classic example where disease-specific agents provide the very best palliative treatments available.[3,5] Recognition of this fact caused many hospice programmes to reconsider a myriad of agents previously felt to be inappropriate in terminally ill patients.

In a similar way, chemotherapy for cancer is used for palliation as well as with the intent of cure. In the context of cancer, disease-specific therapy may be used when the median increase in survival is only a few months.[6] The aim of treatment is not cure but palliation. This additional time may allow the patient and family to come to terms with the reality of their situation and to use that time in a way that is most helpful to them. It is now recognized that broader palliative and supportive care throughout such treatment is also needed to minimize the severe toxicity that may accompany it. In order to optimize quality of life proactive management of the toxicity of the treatment and attention to the physical and psychological distress caused by the illness is essential.

For patients with ESRD, both dialysis and transplantation are non-curative, disease-specific palliative therapies. They prolong life and reduce the symptoms of renal failure, yet do not alter the pathophysiological basis of ESRD. Unfortunately the fundamental cause and the resultant effects of the underlying disease process continue to progress in addition to those that develop as a consequence of dialysis or immunosuppression after transplantation. Renal replacement therapy does, however, provide many patients with the opportunity to live an extended life despite this continuation of the underlying pathophysiological processes. Erythropoietin is a similar palliative therapy, introduced initially to treat the disabling symptoms of anaemia in patients with chronic renal disease. It was seen primarily as a symptom control or palliative measure, since it has been clearly shown[7] to improve quality of life for patients and possibly to contribute to prolongation of life through reduction in left ventricular hypertrophy.

## 2.6 The supportive care model and ESRD

The palliative care philosophy, which is patient centred and focuses on the wishes and goals of the individual, should permeate all medical care. Shared decision-making, characterized by full sharing of information and mutual understanding, is helpful when disease trajectories and future care options are complex, such as for the patient with deteriorating renal function. It involves the acknowledgement of uncertainty and of mortality, often with a redefinition of goals. The nature of ESRD makes it possible for the principles and practices of palliative and supportive care to complement its management. A team of healthcare professionals including physicians, nurses, social workers, and, at times, clergy sees most patients with ESRD. The incidence of symptomatic complications and the frequent downhill course of ESRD mean that the balance of good from dialysis needs to be interwoven with psychosocial support and pain and symptom management as well as effective advance care planning.

Patients with ESRD experience a marked decrease in survival compared with their peers. The annual mortality rate for patients on haemodialysis in the USA is 25%. This is higher than the mortality rate for individuals with AIDS or most cancers. The risk of death for a 45-year-old on haemodialysis is 20 times that of a person of the same age who is not. Overall the 5-year survival rate for individuals on haemodialysis aged 55–64 is 33% while for those aged 65–74 it is only 21%.[8,9] These mortality data are complicated by the reality that two-thirds of these patients consider their quality of life to be 'less than good'.[10,11] These facts of life, which all patients with ESRD experience, either first hand or by observing other patients, bring a degree of existential, psychological, and spiritual stress to life that most individuals without chronic disease do not often face.

Most patients with ESRD have significant associated illnesses that have an impact on their quality of life.[10,12,13] Some of these pre-date and may be the cause of renal failure, such as diabetes mellitus, and will continue to contribute to ongoing morbidity. Others are consequent upon renal failure and its management, such as the significant bone and joint problems experienced by patients on maintenance dialysis.[14]

Patients with ESRD experience a myriad of symptoms relating to renal failure:[15] these include insomnia, lethargy, pruritus, constipation, gastritis, depression, sexual dysfunction, and existential symptoms specific for and related to loss of control with dialysis. Between a third and a half of patients on dialysis experience pain[16] which itself contributes to reduced quality of life and is associated with depression. Towards the end of life patients often experience peripheral vascular disease causing ischaemia of the lower limbs, which can lead to the necessity for amputations. Heart failure and associated shortness of breath with exhaustion are also common as disease progresses. Vigorous management of co-morbidities, such as diabetes mellitus, and early and detailed attention to the management of ongoing symptoms will enhance current and future quality of life. The management of many of these symptoms is addressed in later chapters of this book, while recognition of their importance is given in the chapter by Cohen et al.[17] in Palliative Care for Non-cancer Patients.

## 2.7 Interdisciplinary care

In the USA many teams that treat patients with ESRD don't see themselves as true interdisciplinary teams in the same way that hospice/palliative care teams do: the transition to interdisciplinary care is more cognitive than structural. The ESRD care teams are often ideally staffed to address the medical, psychosocial, and existential problems associated with ESRD and haemodialysis. With the supportive care model; nephrologists educated in palliative care can call on psychologists, palliative medicine multidisciplinary teams, and others to complement their management by providing excellent symptom control and strengthening psychosocial and spiritual support. As disease progresses and complications accumulate, referral to a hospice or a palliative medicine specialist service may enhance the already holistic care by making available expert palliative care and opening doors for services, but more importantly by opening the minds of patients, their loved ones, and the professionals caring for them. It can be a transforming moment when it becomes possible to stop the struggle against the impossible and to redefine goals according to the individual's beliefs and wishes. When the burden of treatment outweighs the benefits it can assist and allow the letting go.

Another advantage of early palliative care interventions and advance care planning is that it allows for a smoother transition to hospice care at the end of life. ESRD treatment programmes should maintain close links with local hospice and palliative care organizations, both for palliative care consultation and to facilitate admission to a hospice when appropriate. The need for good symptom control in a patient with ESRD often presages the beginning of the final stages of their illness, though death may be many months or years away. Introduction to the palliative medicine interdisciplinary team when appropriate ensures that there is the extra support and expertise needed to manage difficult symptoms.

If a decision to stop dialysis is made then a rapid transition to terminal care can be made with support available where the patient chooses to die, either at home, in hospital, or a hospice. If there is no primary decision to stop dialysis, but the patient dies of his or her co-morbid conditions then the proper emphasis on maintaining as good a quality of life as is possible has occurred through continued provision of symptom control and psychosocial support to patient and family. The treatment for ESRD affects not just the patient but the whole family, and by holding the patient at the centre of care those others who are significant come into focus and there is a strengthening of the total care. Remembering and providing support for a patient's loved ones also supports the patient.

## 2.8 Supportive care in practice

In the USA it is widely recommended that the palliative care approach be available concomitantly with renal replacement therapy for all patients with ESRD. It is likewise recommended that all healthcare professionals who treat patients with ESRD become proficient in palliative care. This is to both treat the symptoms associated with ESRD effectively and to begin the process of advance care planning. Alvin Moss, one of the authors of the Renal Physicians Association and American Society of Nephrology Guidelines for Initiation and Withdrawal from Dialysis noted that: 'The working group (that developed the guidelines) believed that all ESRD patients should be treated with palliative care throughout their chronic illness. Palliative care includes pain and symptom management, attention to psychosocial and spiritual concerns, and identification of what matters most to the dying patient. The working group's expectation was that nephrologists would become expert at palliative care with their chronically ill patients.'[18,19]

While the only certainty is that all people will die, and therefore should engage in advance care planning, the reality of a limited life expectancy is present for all patients with ESRD. This reality presents patients and healthcare professionals with an opportunity to consider what type of care they would want as their illness advances, who should make decisions for them should they become non-autonomous, and what other goals and aspirations they would like to achieve or address in their lives.

An example of integrated, interdisciplinary ESRD and palliative care is the Renal Palliative Care Initiative in Springfield, Massachusetts. This project, which was funded by the Robert Wood Johnson Foundation, involved the collaboration of healthcare professionals with expertise in nephrology, psychiatry, palliative medicine, nursing, social work, and spirituality. During the 3 years that this project was developed, the team was able to reach several important goals which continue to be met after the initial funding of the project. These goals included:

- Palliative medicine education for the staff working with ESRD patients. Education was provided to physicians, nurses, and social workers.
- Regular assessment of pain and non-pain symptoms and their appropriate management.
- Remedy of the denial of death that is common in dialysis patients and staff. Advance care planning was actively encouraged. Post-death conferences assessed the adequacy of palliative interventions before the patient died. A yearly memorial service was instituted at all treatment sites.
- An increase in healthcare institution and community support for ESRD palliative care services.

The Renal Palliative Care Initiative is recognized in the USA as a model programme of palliative care for patients with ESRD.

Less widespread detailed palliative care guidelines are available in the UK; however, recommendations that units should develop guidelines for palliative care of those patients who choose not to dialyse are incorporated in the standards from the Renal Association of the UK.[20] Similar guidance concerning the provision of both the physical and psychosocial components of palliative care are likely to be included in the UK Department of Health National Service Framework for Renal Disease, currently being developed. Some individual renal units have begun to work more closely with palliative care services with the setting of standards of palliative care in at least one unit.[21] Currently most units have a psychologist as a regular member of the multidisciplinary team and many have links with their hospital palliative care teams.

In Canada, the Northern Alberta Renal Program and the Regional Palliative Care Program based at Edmonton have proposed developing a supportive care service.[22] This is in response to clear evidence of symptom burden in their dialysis population. They found significant symptom distress reported by over 25% of 531 dialysis patients for pain, reduced activity, and pruritus, while 50%, 42%, and 40% respectively reported moderate to severe distress for sense of well-being, appetite, and drowsiness.

Recently the National Council for Hospice and Specialist Palliative Care Services in the UK (NCHSPCS) has put forward the following definition for consultation regarding supportive care for patients with cancer:[23] it is equally applicable to ESRD

> Good supportive care is that which is designed to help the patient and their family to cope with cancer and treatment of it—from pre diagnosis, through the process of diagnosis and treatment, to cure, continuing illness or death and into bereavement. It helps the patient to maximise the benefits of treatment and to live as well as possible with the effects of the disease. It is given equal priority alongside diagnosis and treatment.

The UK Department of Health is developing a supportive care strategy for cancer and at the same time developing National Service Frameworks for other chronic diseases, including renal disease. Each of these will contain a supportive and palliative care section, as the need for people with chronic diseases to receive the best professional support as well as the right treatment is recognized. The key domains for supportive care, derived from patient surveys (Cancerlink) (Appendix 3) are described by the NCHSPCS as: 'Information needs, integrated support services, being treated as a human being, empowerment, physical needs, continuity of care, psychological needs, social needs and spiritual needs'. ESRD patients will have similar needs and others that are specific to their disease.

## 2.9 Conclusion

Nephrologists, like all healthcare professionals who treat patients with chronic disease, have an unprecedented opportunity to bring palliative care skills and philosophy to the management of their patients. It is no longer necessary or wise to wait until a patient has a terminal illness, or is in the terminal phase of their illness, to benefit from state of the art palliative care. Symptom management and psychosocial evaluation are an essential component of medical care. In addition, the existential issues that all patients with chronic disease experience provide a rich background from which healthcare professionals can explore what is most important in the lives of their patients. Frequently, the insights gleaned from these conversations will enrich the lives of the healthcare professional as well as those of their patients.

## Case study

JJ was first noted to have impaired renal function as an incidental finding after an accident at the age of 19. During the following 12 years he developed severe hypertension and needed to dialyse by the time he was 31. At 32 he had reimplantation of his ureters for bilateral pelviureteric junction obstruction, without improvement in his renal function.

His first transplant was at age 33 but lasted only 21/2 years; a second transplant at 37 failed immediately. In total he spent 19 years on haemodialysis, including home haemodialysis for 14 years. In addition JJ spent 3 years on continuous ambulatory peritoneal dialysis (CAPD) following the failure of the first transplant.

**Case study** *(continued)*

Complications of renal failure included: tertiary hyperparathyroidism requiring parathyroidectomy at age 35; aluminium overload requiring chelation therapy; mitral and aortic valve calcification; calcific uraemic arteriolopathy (calciphylaxis) resulting in painful skin necrosis; and dialysis-related amyloidosis, causing bilateral carpal tunnel syndrome requiring surgical release; worsening shoulder stiffness; and uraemic pruritus refractory to emollients, antihistamines, activated charcoal, ultraviolet light, and naltrexone. At age 46 JJ underwent right hemicolectomy for ischaemic ulceration of the caecum. Ischaemic heart disease developed and required angioplasty to a heavily calcified left anterior descending coronary artery. Psoriasis caused severe fissuring of the soles of the feet and required additional treatment. Erective impotence developed. Severe agitated depression was an intermittent problem.

In the last year of his life JJ developed discitis with severe pain managed by an implanted intrathecal morphine pump. At the same time, the first ischaemic ulcer appeared on his foot. Following an unsuccessful attempt to perform an arterial bypass, he had a right below-knee amputation, followed 3 weeks later by a left below-knee amputation. Additionally he had infected necrotic ulceration in his groin and sacral area. JJ had a period of rehabilitation near his home following the second amputation but had to return when further ischaemic problems developed in the right stump and 6 days later he had an above-knee amputation on that side. An extensive sacral sore kept him in hospital for the next 3 months, towards the end of which he developed gangrene of his fourth finger which had to be amputated, followed by gangrene of the right stump. At this point, after protracted discussions with his nephrologist about the limited options available JJ chose to stop dialysis and return home to die.

Until the last year of his life, most of which was spent in hospital, JJ continued to contribute to the running of the family business. In that year he experienced an increasing burden of losses both social and physical. He had experienced unpleasant symptoms for many years and severe pain from many sources in the last year. He experienced moments of sheer hell such as when he experienced major hallucinations from opioid toxicity or contemplated never leaving hospital again. At other times he demonstrated extraordinary resilience and spirit, illustrated by seeing him after both legs had been amputated, sitting in the sun, lifting his head from a Harry Potter book and smiling wryly.

JJ's nephrologist coordinated his care throughout but many others supported him and his wife, including the palliative care team. He also spent two valuable periods of care in the hospice, which gave him and his team respite while he had the opportunity to explore some of his feelings of hopelessness. Pain control in the last year was complex needing frequent review with contributions to his renal team from both a pain anaesthetist and the palliative care team. When the decision to stop dialysis and go home was taken, the palliative care nurse who had known him for the last year was able to liaise and set up the necessary services to enable this to happen rapidly.

## Ethical analysis

JJ's dialysis-related amyloidosis, uraemic pruritus, premature atherosclerosis, and resultant depression are all tragic markers of our inadequacies in managing dialysis patients in previous decades. JJ 'experienced unpleasant symptoms for many years and severe pain from many sources in the last year'. Nonetheless, JJ was a long-term survivor on renal replacement therapy. The 2001 Annual Data Report of the United States Renal Data System documents that fewer than 10% of dialysis patients survive 10 years.

**Ethical analysis** *(continued)*

This case demonstrates the best of dialysis patient management in several areas. First, JJ was able to continue working and contribute to the running of his family business up until the last year of his life. Only a small percentage of dialysis patients continue to work. Being able to dialyse at home for 17 of his 19 years on dialysis facilitated his continued employment. Second, JJ was cared for by a team. We now understand that a team approach is the best way to care for patients who are chronically ill. Third, a palliative care approach, including the involvement of a pain specialist, was instituted in the final year of JJ's life. He had the opportunity to explore the meaning of his life and to deal with his feelings of hopelessness. Because of the involvement of the palliative care team, a smooth transition to hospice care at home occurred. The patient and his wife received the psychosocial and spiritual support that they needed in the patient's final weeks.

This case applies a number of the recommendations in the Renal Physicians Association and the American Society of Nephrology's clinical practice guideline, *Shared Decision-making in the Appropriate Initiation of and Withdrawal from Dialysis*.[18] The case described shared decision-making between the nephrologist, the patient, and his wife. The decision to withdraw from dialysis was made by JJ, who had decision-making capacity and who was fully informed and making a voluntary decision (recommendations 1 and 2). The patient received palliative care that included pain and symptom management and psychosocial and spiritual support (recommendation 9). In this case there is no mention of advance care planning. It was foreseeable that he might lose decision-making capacity and that medical decisions might need to be made for him by someone else. Advance care planning to identify the person that JJ would have preferred to make decisions for him when he lost decision-making capacity and his preferences for end-of-life care should have been conducted (recommendation 5). One of the fortunate aspects of this case is that our thinking with regard to withdrawal from dialysis has progressed. When JJ started dialysis, decisions to stop dialysis were problematic. Now we have an understanding of the ethical and legal principles that should govern a decision to stop dialysis. Ethically and legally, patients with decision-making capacity have a right to accept or refuse life-sustaining treatment such as dialysis. In cases where patients request to stop dialysis, nephrologists have found it helpful to consider a number of issues in responding to patients' requests (see the Introduction). In JJ's case, as in others, if no reversible factors are found to improve the patient's satisfaction with life on dialysis and if the patient is making an informed and voluntary decision that is not hindered by a major depression, encephalopathy, or other major mental disorder, the nephrologist is obligated to honour the patient's informed refusal of continued dialysis (recommendation 2).

# Appendices

## Appendix 1: Completion of WHO definition of 1990[1]

Palliative care:

- ◆ Affirms life and regards dying as a normal process.
- ◆ Neither hastens nor postpones death.
- ◆ Provides relief from pain and other symptoms.
- ◆ Integrates the psychological and spiritual aspects of patient care.
- ◆ Offers a support system to help patients live as actively as possible until death.
- ◆ Offers a support system to help the family cope during the patient's illness and in their own environment.

# Appendix 2: WHO 2002 definition of palliative care[24]

Palliative care is an approach that improves the quality of life of patients and their families facing the problem associated with life-threatening illness, through the prevention and relief of suffering by means of early identification and impeccable assessment and treatment of pain and other problems, physical, psychosocial and spiritual.

Palliative care:

- Provides relief from pain and other distressing symptoms.
- Affirms life and regards dying as a normal process.
- Intends neither to hasten nor postpone death.
- Integrates the psychosocial and spiritual aspects of patient care.
- Offers a support system to help the families cope during the patient's illness and in their own bereavement.
- Uses a team approach to address the needs of patients and their families, including bereavement counselling if indicated.
- Will enhance quality of life, and may also positively influence the course of illness.
- Is applicable early in the course of illness, in conjunction with other therapies that are intended to prolong life, such as chemotherapy, and includes those investigations needed to better understand and manage distressing symptoms.

# Appendix 3: Domains from supportive care for cancer patients— patient generated (Cancerlink)

- **Information**: patients should receive all the information they want concerning their condition and possible treatment and care options. That information should be up to date, honest, timely, and sensitively given.
- **Being treated as a human being**: patients should be treated with dignity and respect as an individual whole person (not just as a disease or as a numbered patient).
- **Empowerment**: patients need to have their voice heard, directly or through advocacy, and to be valued for the knowledge and skills that they can bring to their individual situations. They need to be able to exercise real choice about their care and treatment and where it takes place.
- **Physical needs**: patients need to have their physical symptoms managed, to a degree that is acceptable to them and achievable within current knowledge.
- **Continuity of care**: patients need well-informed health and social care professionals who work in the community and good communication between professionals working within and across the NHS and voluntary sector service providers.
- **Psychological needs**: emotional support for the patient and those caring for them and giving time to listen and understand concerns.
- **Social needs**: patients need support for their carers and family, advice on financial and employment matters, and provision of transport.
- **Spiritual needs**: support for patients to be able to explore the spiritual issues that are important to them.

## References

1. World Health Organization (1990). *Cancer Pain Relief and Palliative Care*, Technical Report Series 804. Geneva: World Health Organization.
2. Ahmedzai, S., Walsh, D. (2000). Palliative medicine and modern cancer care. *Semin. Oncol.*, **27**: 1–6.
3. Reiter, G., Kudler, N. (1996).HIV and palliative care: part I. *AIDS Clin. Care*, **8**(3): 21–6.
4. Palella, F.J., Jr., Delaney, K.M., Moorman, A.C., *et al.* (1998). Declining morbidity and mortality among patients with advanced human immunodeficiency virus infection *New Engl. J. Med.*, **338**: 853–60.
5. Reiter, G., Kudler, N. (1996). HIV and palliative care: part II. *AIDS Clin. Care*, **8**(4): 27–34.
6. Colorectal Cancer Collaborative Group (2000). Palliative chemotherapy for advanced colorectal cancer: systematic review and meta-analysis. *Br. Med., J.* **321**: 531–5.
7. Eschbach, J.W. (1989). The anaemia of chronic renal failure: pathophysiology and effect of recombinant erythropoietin. *Kidney Int.*, **35**: 134–48.
8. United States Renal Data System (1998). Annual report, the excerpts. *Am. J. Kidney Dis.*, **32**: S1–S213.
9. United States Renal Data System (1997). Annual report, the excerpts. *Am. J. Kidney Dis.*, **30**: S1–S213.
10. Levy, W.B., Wynbrant, G.D. (1975). The quality of life on maintenance haemodialysis. *The Lancet* **1**: 1328–30.
11. Roberts, J.C., Kjellstrand, C.M. (1988). Choosing death: withdrawal from chronic dialysis without medical reason. *Acta Med. Scand.*, **223**: 81–6.
12. Harnett, J.D., Foley, R.N., Kent, G.M., Barre, P.E., Murray, D., Parfrey, P.S. (1995). Congestive heart failure in dialysis patients: prevalence, incidence, prognosis and risk factors. *Kidney Int.*, **47**: 884–90.
13. Nelson, C.B., Port, F.K., Wolfe, R.A., Guire, K.E. (1994). The association of diabetic status, age, and race to withdrawal from dialysis. *J. Am. Soc. Nephrol.*, **4**: 1608–14.
14. Brown, E., Gower, P.E. (1982). Joint problems in patients on maintenance haemodialysis. *Clin. Nephrol.*, **18**: 247–50.
15. Parfrey, P.S., Vavasour, H.M., Henry, S., Bullock, M., Gault, M.H. (1988). Clinical features and severity of nonspecific symptoms in dialysis patients. *Nephron* **50**: 121–8.
16. Binik, Y.M., Baker, A.G., Kalogeropoulos, D., *et al.* (1982). Pain, control over treatment, and compliance in dialysis and transplant patients. *Kidney Int.*, **21**: 840–8.
17. Cohen, L.M., Reiter, G.S., Poppel, D.M., Germain, M.J. (2001). Renal palliative care. In: *Palliative Care for Non-cancer Patients*, ed., JM Addington-Hall and IJ Higginson, pp. 103–13. Oxford: Oxford University Press.
18. Renal Physicians Association and American Society of Nephrology (2000). *Shared Decision-making in the Appropriate Initiation of and Withdrawal from Dialysis*, Clinical Practice Guideline number 2. Rockville, MD: RPA.
19. Moss, A.H. (2001). Shared decision making in dialysis: the new RPA/ASN guideline on appropriate initiation and withdrawal of treatment. *Am. J. Kidney Dis.*, **37**: 1081–91.
20. Renal Association (2003). *Treatment of Patients with Renal Failure: Recommended Standards and Audit Measures*. London: Renal Association and Royal College of Physicians.
21. Hine, J. (1998). Standards of palliative care in a renal care setting. *EDTNA/ERCA J.* **24**(4): 27–9, 35.
22. Fainsinger, R.L., Davison, S.N., Brenneis, C. (2003). A supportive care model for dialysis patients. *Palliative Med.*, **17**: 81–2.
23. National Council for Hospice and Specialist Palliative Care Services (2002). *Definitions of Supportive and Palliative Care*. National Council for Hospice and Specialist Palliative Care Services, London.
24. World Health Organization (2002). *National Cancer Control Programmes. Policies and Managerial Guidelines*, 2nd edn., pp. 83–91. Geneva: World Health Organization.

Chapter 3

# Planning a renal palliative care programme and its components

Lewis M. Cohen

## 3.1 Introduction

This chapter intends to describe a demonstration project in which the overarching goal is to integrate palliative medicine and supportive care into the practice of renal dialysis and transplantation.[1,2] It is written with an appreciation that the ordinary treatment of end-stage renal disease (ESRD) in the USA differs in a number of notable respects from that of other countries.[3] Furthermore, the experience of the American clinicians in this project should be viewed as representing their ambitious attempt to change the field, and certainly not taken as the final word on how to create an ideal programme.

Those involved in palliative medicine are becoming progressively more aware that most deaths are caused by 'chronic' disease in the elderly.[4,5] While advanced illness is not restricted to those individuals who are aged 65 years or older, this segment of the American population consumes one-third of the total healthcare expenditure, occupies half of physician time, and constitutes nearly three-quarters of the deaths that occur each year.[5] ESRD is rapidly becoming a geriatric disorder, and its demography reveals a steady increase in numbers, severity of co-morbid illnesses, and patient age. Consequently, it should be no surprise that the annual mortality rate is 23%.[6]

In 1998, Baystate Health System and the Western New England Renal and Transplant Associates began the Renal Palliative Care Initiative (RPCI)[7]. The collaborators in this demonstration project believe that end-of-life care should not be limited to cancer, acquired immune deficiency syndrome (AIDS), and hospice populations, but that the focus should be broadened to include the numerous, chronic, end-stage organ disorders. As will be described, the programme has been remarkably successful in developing multiple, innovative practice interventions, it is garnering considerable attention, and it appears to be catalysing significant change.[8]

Baystate Health System is a not-for-profit provider of a broad range of regional health services in the Connecticut River Valley region of the USA. It includes Baystate Medical Center, a tertiary care and teaching hospital of Tufts University School of Medicine, as well as several small community hospitals. The RPCI consists of the dialysis and transplantation services that are based at those hospitals, as well as at seven free-standing dialysis clinics in the region. The RPCI dialysis facilities are chiefly situated in western Massachusetts, but are also located in Connecticut and New Hampshire. They are owned by Fresenius Medical Care, Inc., the largest proprietary chain of dialysis clinics in the USA. Clinical care is directed by the physicians of the Western New England Renal and Transplantation Associates (WNERTA). This is a large nephrology practice that includes nine nephrologists, four surgeons, one physician assistant, and three nurse practitioners. The practice has a tradition of combining solid clinical care with innovative academic endeavours.

For the past 10 years, an interdisciplinary group of Baystate and WNERTA clinicians has conducted a series of studies examining end-of-life care. The group performed the first prospective research of patients who discontinue dialysis and thereby hasten death.[9] Led by a psychiatrist, the investigators have been interested in the psychosocial aspects of terminal care, its bioethics,[10] and the family perspective.[11] The research is responsible for describing the terminal symptoms in this patient population, as well as underscoring the need for improved management.[12,13] Having defined the problem, the group turned its attention to a solution, namely the need to integrate the recent advances of palliative care into the treatment of all patients with ESRD.[15]

The RPCI team consists of nine dialysis staff members (nephrologists, nurses, and social workers) who have undergone extensive training in palliative medicine. A palliative care physician and nurse designed the didactic course, and subsequently became available for consultations with difficult cases.

## 3.2 Interventions

The RPCI teams developed and implemented a number of interventions, including:

1. **Treatment protocols**: these address common ESRD symptoms and terminal care situations, e.g. facilitating referral to a hospice. This is a highly symptomatic population, and after a literature review, guidelines now address such extremely common symptoms as pruritus and pain. Likewise, although hospices have not traditionally cared for patients with ESRD, they are an important but underutilized resource. Consequently, a protocol now addresses referral procedures. The protocols are present at each clinic nursing station, and are available to physicians and nurse practitioners.

2. **Morbidity and mortality (M&M) conferences**: these are held at each dialysis clinic and provide opportunities to review the circumstances of all deaths. In preparation for these conferences, the RPCI data collector reviews medical records at the hospitals and nursing homes where patients died. This information is combined with data from post-death family questionnaires. These are completed by loved ones four to six weeks after the patient's death, and describe the terminal circumstances, symptoms, and treatment. The tool includes questions as to whether people died in preferred locations, and whether deaths were peaceful. Families are instructed that the team is particularly interested in identifying problems that ought to be addressed. At the M&M conferences, quality of dying scores[16] are completed by staff, along with the successes and failures in palliative care, and whether dialysis should have been terminated.

3. **Bereavement care**: this is a major focus of the RPCI. It has been forestalled in ESRD by a tendency towards 'denying the dying'.[17] The teams have helped each dialysis clinic to develop a means to notify patients and staff when deaths occur. This takes various forms, including posting obituaries in the waiting room, having a message board at the nursing station, or a vase in which a floral tribute is labeled with the name of the deceased. Staff are encouraged to attend funerals and masses.

4. **Annual renal memorial services**: these have been especially well received, and they are attended each year by increasing numbers of families, loved ones, staff, and active patients. Baystate is not unique in offering these services to dialysis facilities, and at least one UK facility has described a programme organized by nursing staff.[18] An RPCI physician survey (see Fig. 3.1 below) finds this intervention to be extremely helpful in changing practice, resulting in physicians attending more to end-of-life issues. The services are an opportunity

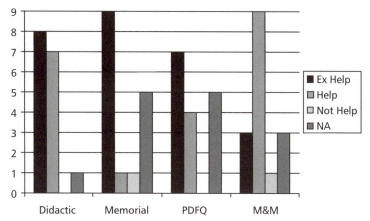

**Fig. 3.1** Renal palliative care interventions: Didactic = lecture series; Memorial = memorial service; PDFQ = post-death family questionnaire; M&M = morbidity and mortality conference; Ex Help = extremely helpful; Help = helpful; Not Help = not helpful; NA = no answer or did not participate.

for the community to demonstrate its spiritual and artistic generosity. Local people offer ecumenical readings and poetry, while musicians include an accomplished soprano, a harpist, and a children's choir. Evidence is accumulating that these moving events have the potential to change the culture of dialysis and transplantation, and to make staff more appreciative of end-of-life issues. Consequently, the RPCI has produced an educational manual and videotape, and it intends to disseminate this intervention to programmes throughout the country. A list has been easily generated of more than 20 dialysis and transplant facilities that will soon institute their own services of remembrance.

## 3.3 Outcomes

### 3.3.1 Well-being and quality of care

A core group of dialysis staff are now trained to work with the renal patients and family members. More attention is being accorded to awareness of symptoms, and patients receive symptom checklists to complete during dialysis sessions. The nephrologists and nurses are better prepared to deal with pain and other problems, and have symptom guidelines and protocols to follow. The palliative care physician and nurse are available to participate in particularly difficult cases.

The dialysis and transplantation social workers are key members of the RPCI, and have shaped its interventions. They are particularly sensitive to the psychosocial end-of-life issues and the bereavement care. The RPCI psychiatrist sees many of the difficult cases in consultation, and has described the group's approach towards evaluating psychiatric factors in discontinuation of dialysis.[19]

### 3.3.2 Bereavement support for loved ones and staff

As previously described, the RPCI is developing a number of interventions to provide support to bereaved family, friends, and staff. Several different approaches to notify people from the dialysis clinics about the deaths are being tried, and letters of condolence are being sent out by the nephrologists to families.

Meticulous attention to a myriad of details is required for successful services of remembrance. The renal memorial service organizing committee consists of social workers, nurses, chaplains, and families, and it meets regularly throughout the year. The services require the participation and contributions of the greater community, and they epitomize the post-death care that should be essential to the practice of dialysis.

In the most recent memorial service feedback survey, one family member wrote, 'I had a hard time containing myself during the service. I was overwhelmed to see all the fine people who came together to honor my husband's struggle with his life and death, and to recognize my pain. ... I cried on the shoulder of his nurse, and I am grateful.'

Many participants commented on the lighting of candles. A son concluded, 'Seeing the doctors and nurses crying, and knowing that you guys care and think about our loved ones was the most meaningful aspect.'

Although the post-death family questionnaire (see section 3.4) endorses the sensitivity of staff to cultural and spiritual concerns, team members are actively discussing new ways to address these matters. Chaplains participate in the regular RPCI meetings, they are available to see hospitalized patients, and also take part in the committees. A programme to introduce chaplains to the dialysis clinics is also being considered.

## 3.4 Quality improvement and research

The RPCI has evolved from a series of end-of-life research studies and is extremely committed to measuring its impact. A number of direct and indirect outcome measures are being followed:

1. **Advance care planning**: in 1995, we found that only 6% ($n = 121$) of our dialysis clinic population had completed an advance directive.[17] In an interview study performed in 2002, 32% of RPCI patients now report having healthcare proxies, and 21% living wills ($n = 618$).[7]

2. **Physician survey**: the 16 nephrologists and surgeons in the programme have been surveyed about the effect of the various RPCI interventions on their practices. As illustrated in Fig. 3.1, they highly endorse the didactic course and the bereavement memorial service.

3. **Memorial service feedback surveys**: participants at the renal memorial services regularly complete these. Attendance has been increasing annually over the past 3 years, and information from the surveys is of considerable practical value.

4. **Hospice referrals**: less than 10% of ESRD patients from the dialysis clinics are usually referred to a hospice. A recent RPCI effort resulted in seven patients being referred to the Visiting Nurse Association & Hospice of Western New England over a 3-month period and equalling the total for the previous year. Further steps are being taken by the RPCI to continue this trend.

5. **Mortality and discontinuation rates**: with the cooperation of the ESRD Network of New England, the population's mortality figures are being compared with those of the geographical region. There appear to be no significant deviations.

6. **Quality of life**: the RPCI interventions are mainly directed at improving terminal care and should not alter the factors measured by quality of life tools. A baseline quality of life battery (including the Medical Outcomes Study Short Form 36 (SF-36)[20] and the Missoula Vitas Quality of Life)[21] has been completed by 618 patients, and shows no significant differences between the programme population and patients treated at a control facility. With the

cooperation of Fresenius Medical Care, SF-36 scores are being obtained on patients' birth-days and 6 months later, and changes can be monitored.

7. **Quality of dying**: forms have been completed for 319 deaths, and are reviewed at M&M meetings. The measure has been described,[16] and data are currently being analysed.

8. **Post-death family questionnaires**: 86 families have completed these, in order to elicit their perspective on end-of-life care. The resulting information is of considerable practical value to clinicians. Half of the respondents are spouses, and the questionnaires are completed about 6 weeks after the death. They indicate that the healthcare team is sensitive to spiritual/religious (73%) and cultural/ethnic (74%) concerns. Two-thirds of the sample believe that patients had a peaceful death. On the other hand, patients frequently appear to have pain in the last week of life (73%), and it is often extremely severe (36%).

## 3.5 Patient goals and preferences

The RPCI is very respectful of patient preferences and choices, and encourages the completion of formal advance directives through the use of the instrument called the 'Five Wishes' (www.agingwithdignity.org). Nephrologists are provided with personalized copies to review with patients, and both Spanish and English versions are available. A companion video is shown during the dialysis session.

The RPCI is interested in identifying patients' goals and preferences for terminal care, and uses questions derived from the SUPPORT study,[22] which asked, 'If you had to make a choice at this time, would you prefer a course of treatment that focuses on extending life as much as possible, even if it means having more pain and discomfort, or would you want a plan of care that focuses on relieving pain and discomfort as much as possible, even if that means not living as long?'

This question is used to elicit the perspectives of both patients and staff. Table 3.1 shows results from the post-death family questionnaire, illustrating the caregivers' perspective.

**Table 3.1** Post-death family questionnaire

|  | N | % |
|---|---|---|
| 1. Did the patient prefer treatment that was aimed at extending life as much as possible, or treatment directed towards maximal relief of pain even if meant that his/her death would be hastened? | | |
| Extend life as much as possible | 22 | 27.5 |
| Relieve pain or discomfort as much as possible | 39 | 48.8 |
| Unsure | 19 | 23.8 |
| 2. Were these wishes followed during last weeks of life? | | |
| A great deal | 42 | 51.9 |
| Very much | 14 | 17.3 |
| Moderately | 6 | 7.4 |
| Very little | 1 | 1.2 |
| Not at all | 4 | 4.9 |
| Unsure | 14 | 17.3 |

## 3.6 Family support

In post-death family questionnaires, two-thirds of respondents endorse that the healthcare team spent considerable time during the terminal phase talking to them about the patient and treatment. This is a gratifyingly large proportion, especially since many patients die in the hospital and their final care is assumed by non-dialysis staff.

The RPCI receives tremendous input from its social workers, who emphasize the importance of supporting and attending to the opinions of families. Family members participate in the committees and task forces and their questionnaires are an important source of information about the programme's strengths and weaknesses.

The RPCI team is learning some difficult lessons from the questionnaires, including how to avoid mismanaging family deathbed vigils. For example, it recently became apparent that some loved ones need total access to dying patients. For example, a well-intentioned nurse's aide insisted a family leave the bedside while she cleaned up an incontinent individual. However, the patient died during that brief cleansing process and the family reported in the questionnaire that they remained inconsolable.

## 3.7 Replication advice

The RPCI follows the 'plan, do, study, and act' (PDSA) approach.[23,24] Three fundamental questions are asked:

1. What is our aim?
2. How will we measure whether a change is an improvement?
3. What changes ought we attempt?

The model is based on trial-and-learning, and has been specifically applied to improving end-of-life care.[25] Lynn and associates have concluded that each clinician must examine the shortcomings at their place of practice, and figure out how they can be addressed and improvements accomplished.[26]

The RPCI hypothesizes that dialysis and transplant staff will become more sensitive to end-of-life care issues if they are provided with opportunities to learn about the terminal circumstances of their individual patients. In addition, both the right and left brain of clinicians needs to be stimulated, that is to say, emotional experiences, such as those offered by annual memorial services, need to be supplemented with cognitive experiences, such as those provided by training and education in modern palliative medicine.

The RCPI's experience suggests that:

1. Sincere commitment is necessary on the part of the medical centre and dialysis administration involved.
2. Efforts are best focused on training and using existing staff.
3. Outcomes research ought to be an integral part of the process.

These conclusions mirror the findings of other research on the improvement of performance.[20]

## 3.8 Summary

A demonstration project, the Renal Palliative Care Initiative, has been described. Its primary goal is to integrate palliative medicine into the practice of renal dialysis and transplantation. The programme, now in its fourth year of operation, is developing innovative practice interventions and attempting to catalyse change in the field of nephrology.

Interdisciplinary teams of renal clinicians have undergone intensive training in palliative care, and are encouraged to develop interventions for the RPCI facilities. These now include: treatment protocols to address common symptoms and situations, as well as algorithms for terminal care situations, advance care planning, morbidity and mortality conferences, and bereavement care.

The major barrier to instituting a renal palliative care model is the already impressive staff workload at dialysis facilities. Nephrologists, dialysis, and transplant personnel, all labour together in highly organized, efficient, and demanding environments. At times it seems unimaginable that staff can reasonably add new tasks to their existing clinical responsibilities. However, the RCPI is discovering daily that the satisfaction of learning new ways to manage symptoms and attend to end-of-life issues outweighs all additional burdens.

# References

1. Cohen, L.M., Reiter, G., Poppel, D., Germain, M., (2001). Renal palliative care. In: *Palliative Care for Non-Cancer Patients*, ed. J.M. Addington-Hall, and I.J. Higginson., pp. 103–13. Oxford: Oxford University Press.

2. Cohen, L.M., Germain, M.J. (2003). Palliative and supportive care. In: *Therapy of Nephrology and Hypertension: a Companion to Brenner's the Kidney*, 2nd edn, ed. H. Brady, and C. Wilcox., pp. 753–6 Orlando, FLA: Harcourt.

3. Rabetoy, C.P., Cohen, L.M. (2003). *Integrating Palliative Care into Dialysis Treatment: An American Perspective*. Towards a Closer Understanding: A Psycho/Social Handbook For All Renal Care Workers: Dingwall, R.R., (ed), EDTNA/ERCA Postfach 3052, Luzern, Switzerland, 2003. pp. 87–95.

4. Cohen, L.M., Germain, M. Brennan M., (2003). End-stage renal disease and discontinuation of dialysis. In: *Geriatric Palliative Care*, ed. R.S. Morrison., D.E. Meier., and C.F. Capello., pp. 192–202 Oxford: Oxford University Press. (In press.)

5. Matherlee, K. (2002). Managing advanced illness: a quality and cost challenge to Medicare, Medicaid, and private insurers. In: *NHPF Issue Brief*, No 779. www.nhpf.org/pdfs/8–779

6. National Institutes of Health NIDDK/DKUHD (1999). Excerpts from the United States Renal Data System 1999 annual data report. *Am J Kidney Dis.*, **34**(Suppl. 1).

7. Poppel, D., Cohen, L., Germain, M. (2003). The renal palliative care initiative. *J. Palliative Med.* **6**: 321–6.

8. Poppel, D., Cohen, L.M. (2003). Renal. In: *A Clinician's Guide to Palliative Care*, ed. G.J. Taylor, Malden, M.A., pp. 90–103. Blackwell Publishing. Malden. MA.

9. Cohen, L.M., McCue, J., Germain, M., Kjellstrand, C. (1995). Dialysis discontinuation: a 'good' death? *Arch. Intern. Med.*, **155**: 42–7.

10. Ganzini, L., Cohen, L.M. (2000). Commentary: resolution and ambivalence. *Hastings Center Rep.*, **30**(6): 24–5.

11. Woods, A., Berzoff, J., Cohen, L.M., Cait, C.A., Pekow, P., Germain, M. *et al.* (1999). The family perspective of end-of-life care in end-stage renal disease: the role of the social worker. *J. Nephrol., Social Work* **19**: 9–21.

12. Cohen, L.M. (2002). Renal disease. In: *Textbook of Consultation–Liaison Psychiatry: Psychiatry in the Medically Ill*, 2nd edn, ed. M. Wise, and J.R. Rundell, pp. 557–62. Washington, DC: American Psychiatric Press.

13. Cohen, L.M., Germain, M., Poppel, D.M., Pekow, P.S., Woods, A., Kjellstrand, C.M. (2000). Dying well after discontinuing the life-support treatment of dialysis. *Arch. Intern. Med.*, **160**: 2513–18.

14. Cohen, L.M., Germain, M., Poppel, D.M., Woods, A., Kjellstrand, C.M. (2000). Dialysis discontinuation and palliative care. *Am. J. Kidney Dis.*, **36**(1): 140–4.

15. Germain, M.J., Cohen, L.M. (2001). Commentary: supportive care for patients with renal disease— time for action. *Am. J. Kidney Dis.*, **38**: 884–6.

16. Cohen, L.M., Poppel, D.M., Cohen, G.M., Reiter, G.S. (2001). A very good death: measuring quality of dying in end-state renal disease. *J. Palliative Med.,* **4**: 167–72.

17. Cohen, L.M., McCue, J., Germain, M., Woods, A. (1997). Denying the dying: advance directives and dialysis discontinuation. *Psychosomatics* **38**: 27–34.

18. Ormandy, P. (1998). A memorial service for renal patients. *EDTNA/ERCA J.* **24**(3): 22–4.

19. Cohen, L.M., Steinberg, M.D., Hails, K.C., Dobscha, S.K., Fischel, S.V. (2000). The psychiatric evaluation of death-hastening requests: lessons from dialysis discontinuation. *Psychosomatics* **41**(3): 195–203. [Commentary pp. 193–4.]

20. McHorney, C.A., Ware, J.E., Raczek, A.E. (1993). The MOS 36-item short form health survey (SF-36): II. Psychometric and clinical tests of validity in measuring physical and mental health constructs. *Med., Care* **31**: 247–63.

21. Byock, I.R., Merriman, M.P. (1998). Measuring quality of life for patients with terminal illness: the Missoula-VITAS quality of life index. *Palliative Med.,* **12**: 231–44.

22. Hamel, M.B., Teno, J., Goldman, L., Lynn, J., Davis, R.B., Galanos, A.N., *et al.* (1999). Patient age and decisions to withhold life-sustaining treatments from seriously ill, hospitalized adults. *Ann. Intern. Med.,* **130**: 116–25.

23. Berwick, D.M. (1998). Developing and testing changes in delivery of care. *Ann. Intern. Med.,* **128**: 651–6.

24. Langley, G., Nolan, K., Nolan, T., Norman, C., Provost, L. (1996). *The Improvement Book.* San Francisco: Jossey-Bass.

25. Lynn, J., Schall. M., Milne, C., Kabcenell, A. (2000). Quality improvements in end of life care: insights from two collaboratives. *Jt Comm. J. Qual. Improv.,* **26**: 254–67.

26. Lynn, J., Nolan. K., Kabcenell, A., Weissman, D., Milne, C., Berwick, D.M. (2002). Reforming care for persons near the end of life: the promise of quality improvement. *Ann. Intern. Med.,* **137**: 117–22.

Chapter 4

# Advance directives and advance care planning in patients with end-stage renal disease

Jean L. Holley

## 4.1 Introduction

The traditional focus of advance care planning has been the completion of a written advance directive.[1-3] Most dialysis patients support the concept of advance directives but only 7–35% complete them.[4-6] This chapter addresses the benefits and failures of advance care planning in end-stage renal disease (ESRD) patients by focusing on the purpose, characteristics, and use of advance directives in this population. Current views of advance care planning and advance directives are contrasted with traditional views and discussed within the framework of the Sheffield model[7] of chronic illness applied to chronic kidney disease progressing to ESRD. This model highlights the dynamic nature of advance care planning and defines opportunities for nephrologists and others caring for these patients to stimulate advance care planning. The unique aspects of kidney disease which affect advance care planning are also discussed.

## Case study

Mr J is a 63-year-old White man with Type II diabetes mellitus, coronary artery disease, and peripheral vascular disease. He is seen by a nephrologist for progressive renal failure presumed due to diabetic nephropathy. No reversible cause of his kidney failure is found. His estimated creatinine clearance is 22 ml/min. He has no uraemic signs or symptoms but does have dyspnoea on exertion, three-pillow orthopnoea, and increasing lower-extremity oedema. His past medical history includes myocardial infarctions 3 months and 2 years ago; he underwent percutaneous coronary angioplasty and stent placement with his recent myocardial infarction. His left ventricular ejection fraction last week was 22%. He underwent a right femoral–popliteal bypass procedure 1 year ago. He has a non-healing ulcer on his left great toe. He continues to smoke two packs of cigarettes daily.

Mr J is a retired construction worker and lives with his wife of 43 years. Mr J's overall declining medical condition, including his failing eyesight, peripheral neuropathy, vascular disease, and congestive heart failure, is increasingly preventing him from engaging in activities he enjoys. His wife has always taken care of Mr J's medications and medical appointments; he does not know the names or doses of any of his medications. Mrs J is quite active in church activities but Mr J has never participated in these activities despite his wife's urgings. Mr and Mrs J's daughter, a widowed emergency room nurse, and two of his sons (a copyright law attorney and an automobile salesman) live nearby and see Mr J frequently. He has not completed any form of advance directive.

## 4.2 Defining advance care planning and advance directives and their purpose

Advance care planning is a process of communication among patients, health care providers, families, and other important individuals about appropriate future medical care when the patient cannot make his or her own decisions.[8] Traditionally, the purpose of advance care planning was to prepare for the patient's incapacity by focusing on the completion of a written advance directive (Table 4.1).[1–3] Advance directives are written documents completed by a capable person. An advance directive may stipulate a surrogate decision-maker or medical durable power of attorney (a proxy directive) or outline decisions to be made (an instruction directive). A healthcare proxy is the individual designated as the decision-maker in the event the patient becomes incapable of making his or her own decisions about medical care. Most patients choose a spouse or family member as a healthcare proxy but anyone may be selected for this role. Implicit in the designation of a proxy is the assumption that that individual is the person best able to make decisions the patient would make for him/herself if able.

Living wills and do not resuscitate orders are examples of instruction directives. Instruction directives are developed in accord with the patient's wishes, values, goals, and life experiences, including cultural, religious, and spiritual views. Instruction directives may be intricate attempts to address all foreseeable events or may outline one's wishes in a broad, general way. In both non-dialysis and dialysis populations, instruction directives are more useful if state of health rather than treatment interventions are considered.[3,9,10]

Although completing written advance directives may be goals of advance care planning in ESRD patients,[11] as shown in Table 4.1, the purpose of advance care planning is more complex.[2,3,12–18] Advance care planning prepares for death, strengthens interpersonal and inter-family relationships, relieves burdens on loved ones, and provides a way for patients to achieve and maintain control over present and future healthcare.[2,3,12–18] As illustrated by the Sheffield model, the advance care planning process is a supportive therapy that occurs throughout the course of chronic kidney disease. Other supportive or palliative therapies in chronic kidney

**Table 4.1** Traditional versus modern aspects of advance care planning in ESRD patients (adapted from Singer[3] and Quill[22])

|  | Traditional | Modern |
| --- | --- | --- |
| Purpose | Prepare for incapacity | Prepare for death |
|  |  | Achieve control |
|  |  | Relieve burdens on loved ones |
|  |  | Strengthen interpersonal relationships |
| Desired outcome | Written proxy and instruction directives | Proxy directive Resuscitation status |
| Context | Physician–patient | Patient–family |
| Time of discussion | End of life | Whenever discussing: prognosis, renal replacement therapy options |
|  |  | Following: hospitalizations, acute illnesses |

disease include medical interventions to slow progression of renal disease and planning for renal replacement therapy. Symptom management prior to and during dialysis is another example of palliative care in ESRD.[7] A cornerstone of palliative care within the chronic disease model is advance care planning.[3,7] The chronic, progressive nature of kidney disease provides multiple opportunities for patients to prepare for death, achieve control over their medical care, and strengthen and improve relationships with those close to them (advance care planning). Completion of advance directives may result if the patient, family, and designated surrogate are favourably disposed[2,3] but the advance care planning process may be highly successful in the absence of written advance directives.

## 4.3 Timing of advance care planning in the course of chronic kidney disease

When we meet Mr J, he has progressive renal failure and will soon require dialysis. He has a relatively poor prognosis with an expected survival of approximately 3.5 years or less after starting dialysis.[19] At the initial visit, the nephrologist should encourage Mr J to begin advance care planning with his family. Issues to be raised for discussion with the patient and family include Mr J's prognosis on dialysis, the likelihood of his unacceptability as a kidney transplant recipient, and options for renal replacement, including the 'fourth option' (no dialysis). His clinical condition appears to be declining and questions about Mr J's quality of life, wishes, hopes, and fears are appropriate to assist in defining his state of health. Patients and families deal with bad news in stages.[20] Determining what Mr and Mrs J know about his medical illness and prognosis and how much they are ready to hear will be key aspects to initial discussions about dialysis and prognosis.[20,21] Ambivalence about decisions should be expected as additional medical information is provided.[20,21] Following contemplation of options, an action phase will occur during which Mr J, his family, and healthcare providers develop plans and proceed with advance care planning if Mr J and his family are favourably disposed.[2,3,20,21]

Opportunities to initiate discussions about wishes for the end of life care arise whenever prognosis or new therapies are being discussed.[22] Patients want physicians to be honest and willing to talk about dying.[13,16,21] Discussing the need for dialysis and the poor prognosis of ESRD is an opportune time for a nephrologist to show his or her willingness to address these issues and to introduce concepts of advance care planning like proxy and instruction directives. Talking about ESRD is an example of breaking bad news[21] and a conversation most practising nephrologists will have many times during their careers. The Sheffield model illustrates that dialysis and transplantation are supportive or palliative therapies. Discussing the prognosis of ESRD is therefore integral to the supportive care provided. An inherent aspect of the nephrologist's role is as a conveyor of the information required for informed decision-making.[11] Most nephrologists do not discuss end-of-life care with their dialysis patients[3,23] but adopting palliative care principles into nephrology practice requires that attention be given to this issue. Such discussions should occur early and throughout the course of chronic kidney disease.

Since Mr J will start dialysis within the next few months, it is appropriate for the nephrologist to introduce the concept of voluntary withdrawal from dialysis in the same manner in which he or she discusses management of anaemia, fluid overload, calcium and phosphorus control, dialysis options, and expected survival as all are components of the supportive care to be provided. During this period, the nephrologist will learn more about Mr J's life goals, wishes, values, and will continue to encourage advance care planning within the family. Once Mr J begins dialysis, relationships with dialysis care providers (nurses, social workers, and so on) will develop. As described by Swartz and Perry,[24] Mr J's family may then expand to include his 'medical family'. The medical family remains a step away from the primary participants in advance care planning but accessing the medical family for information and support in medical decision-making may avoid family conflicts and enrich the advance care planning process.[24]

## 4.4 Usefulness of advance care planning and advance directives in patients with chronic kidney disease

Surveys of nephrologists have demonstrated that advance directives facilitate decisions to withhold and withdraw dialysis.[25–27] A major study of hospitalized patients failed to show a benefit of advance care planning[28] but small studies in ESRD patients suggest that advance directives increase the likelihood of reconciled or 'good deaths' and reduce the chances of inappropriate interventions.[29,30] Guidelines for withholding dialysis have been developed based on medical evidence and expert opinion.[11] Withholding and withdrawing from dialysis (see Chapter 13) and dialysis trials for patients in whom the relative benefits of renal replacement therapy are unclear are appropriate topics for nephrologists to address.[11]

Dialysis is withheld from patients in all countries.[31–33] There are some differences in the frequency with which dialysis is withheld but the reasons for withholding dialysis are similar among nephrologists and primary care providers and include the patient's mental status and ability to communicate with his/her environment, surrogate and/or family wishes, and expected survival.[31–33] Since Mr J has been referred for nephrology care, his primary care providers believe he is an appropriate candidate for renal replacement therapy. It is unfortunate that he has been referred late in the course of his chronic kidney disease as opportunities for nephrology care and advance care planning have been lost. Despite his medical problems, Mr J has not completed an advance directive.

Until we ask, we don't know whether Mr J has engaged in advance care planning with his family or physicians. Most dialysis patients welcome discussions of advance directives,[9,34] expect their physicians to initiate such discussions,[3,4,34] centre the process within the patient–family relationship rather than the physician–patient relationship,[35,36] and do not complete written advance directives.[3,34,37] Providing dialysis patients with written information on advance directives increased completion of advance directives only transiently.[38] No other specific intervention has increased completion of advance directives by ESRD patients.[3] Opportunities to address Mr J's wishes for end-of-life care will arise throughout his clinical course. For example, appropriate times to discuss end-of-life care include following hospitalizations, acute illnesses, or change in clinical status.[22] Such ongoing discussions will allow Mr J to reassess his wishes depending on his state of health and experiences. Ongoing patient–family discussions may not completely ready proxies for decision-making[14,15,39] but designation of a proxy will facilitate the provision of appropriate care should Mr J become unable to make his own decisions.

## 4.5 Components of advance care planning: the document and the participants

### 4.5.1 The document

An instruction directive is traditionally based on the treatment preferences of a patient (Table 4.1). The failure of advance care planning is in part due to this focus.[3,10,37] Considering a patient's state of health and specifically focusing on what he or she considers acceptable in terms of the quality of his or her life, the burdens of treatments being considered, and the probability of a successful outcome are integral components of advance care planning that, until recently, have been inappropriately superseded by treatment preferences.[3,10,17,18] The 'checklist' method of discussing treatment preferences (e.g. 'Do you want CPR?', 'Do you want to be put on a ventilator, to receive antibiotics, a feeding tube, to stop dialysis?') overlooks the multifaceted purposes of advance care planning that include relieving suffering, minimizing the burden on families, maintaining control, and strengthening relationships among family members.[2,13,18]

Values-based directives are more appropriate than treatment-based directives and are inherently a more acceptable foundation for developing instruction directives.[3,10,17,18] Questions such as 'Is it more important for you to live as long as possible but with some suffering or to live without suffering but for a shorter period of time?' and 'Under what conditions would living be unacceptable to you?' should replace 'Do you want CPR?' in advance care planning. A patient's values, goals, and beliefs will guide and influence the development of instruction directives (Table 4.1).[2,3] Patients modify their preferences for life-sustaining treatments based on expected functional and cognitive impairments resulting from illness and therapeutic interventions.[9,10,37] The complexity of available medical interventions and conditions precludes the development of a document that addresses wishes for every possible treatment in every possible scenario. Focusing on the goals of care according to patients' values, wishes, and desires, results in more useful instruction directives and advance care planning. Questions like 'What makes life worth living?', 'What are your biggest fears, your most important hopes?', 'Under what conditions would you not want to live?' provide entry to value-based instruction directives.[22] The shift away from treatment-specific and toward value-based instruction directives is compatible with the modern view of advance care planning.[10,22,37,40] The 'Five Wishes' document incorporates these principles and is well received by patients and family (www.agingwithdignity.org).

## 4.5.2 The participants

Just as modern views of the documents and questions to be asked in advance care planning are being clarified, we now realize that centring advance care planning within the patient– physician relationship contributed to the failure of advance care planning in dialysis as well as other patient groups.[14,35,39] A patient-based, family-centred approach to advance care planning is more appropriate.[14,15,35]

Dialysis patients expect their physicians to initiate conversations about end-of-life care[3,4,34] but few nephrologists engage in such discussions.[23] In some dialysis programmes, social workers are more likely to participate in end-of-life discussions with patients.[23,35] Dialysis staff avoid such conversations due to inadequate time, lack of training, and discomfort with these issues.[23] Experiencing a personal loss increases the likelihood that providers will have end-of-life discussions with patients.[23] Providers of dialysis care influence patients' completion of advance directives,[4,5] but most dialysis patients do not believe physicians are integral to the advance care planning process.[35] Although 50% of 400 in-centre haemodialysis patients had spoken with their family members/loved ones about their wishes for end-of-life care, only 6% had discussed these issues with their nephrologists.[35] The designated surrogates in this study were more inclined than the dialysis patients to want physician input (51% of surrogates and 37% of patients want physician input) but the physicians' role envisioned by these patients was as a provider of information necessary for medical decision-making.[35,39] In fact, 62% of surrogates and 48% of patients feared that physicians would not honour patients' wishes.[35,39] Thus, maintaining control and strengthening interpersonal relationships are goals of advance care planning in dialysis patients. Moreover, dialysis patients view physicians as keys to medical information but not as direct participants in advance care planning.[2,35,39]

The strictness with which surrogates follow patients' wishes for end-of-life care varies[14,39,40] and 31% of chronic dialysis patients would give 'complete leeway' to surrogates in decision-making.[41] As previously discussed, emphasizing projected outcomes, quality of life, and state of health rather than treatment interventions will better prepare surrogates for decision-making.[3,10,15,17] The team of dialysis providers may also be helpful in preparing proxies for decision-making.[15,24,39]

## 4.6  Specific issues in advance care planning and advance directives for chronic kidney disease and ESRD patients

The progressive nature of chronic kidney disease (see Sheffield model)[7] provides multiple opportunities for advance care planning. In some instances, renal replacement therapy will be withheld or a trial of therapy will be discussed and offered.[3,11] Withdrawal from dialysis is relatively common[7,11] but dialysis patients rarely include stopping dialysis in end-of-life discussions with their families.[9,40] Nephrologists should encourage dialysis patients and their families to discuss situations in which continuing renal replacement therapy would be burdensome and unacceptable.[11,39,40] Renal palliative care includes the possibility of a comfortable and timely death by discontinuing dialysis.[7,42] Focusing advance care planning discussions on quality of life, goals, and values, will allow consideration of discontinuation of dialysis as part of life assessment and remove it from the 'heroic intervention' category where it has been placed by healthcare providers but not by patients.[9,40]

Completing a general instruction directive is not an appropriate goal of advance care planning[2,3,15,17,18] but some specific instruction directives, such as do not resuscitate orders, should be considered by ESRD patients.[11] Here again, the nephrologist's role is primarily to provide information; he or she should explain the risks and benefits of cardiopulmonary resuscitation (CPR) and encourage the patient and family to consider CPR in advance care planning. In a study of 221 dialysis patients experiencing cardiopulmonary arrest in hospital, 8% of dialysis and 12% of 1201 non-dialysis patient controls survived to hospital discharge.[43] Only 3% of successfully resuscitated chronic dialysis patients were alive 6 months after the arrest.[43] Complications of CPR in dialysis patients are also common with 77% suffering fractured ribs in one study of 56 arrests.[44] When cardiorespiratory arrest occurred in haemodialysis units, 40% of patients reached the hospital alive; long-term survival was not available.[45] Thus, there is some information on survival of dialysis patients after CPR that can be provided to patients and their families. Unfortunately, most patients receive information on CPR from television dramas.[46,47] The unrealistically high survival seen after CPR on television causes most dialysis patients to want CPR in the event of cardiorespiratory arrest.[47] However, despite their personal wishes, most dialysis patients believe a request not to undergo CPR should be honoured.[47] This desire to maintain personal control requires consideration when dialysis units develop policies and procedures for CPR.[11,47]

## 4.7  Strategies to increase advance care planning in ESRD patients

Patients look to healthcare providers for information necessary to enable them to make informed decisions. Patients expect physicians and other healthcare providers to be truthful, sensitive, and timely in introducing such issues for discussion.[13,21,22] Although difficult, breaking bad news is a skill that can be learned.[21,22] Nephrology training programmes should include palliative care in their curricula and emphasize supportive care within the chronic disease model.[11,17,48] Dialysis units are unique in the opportunities they provide for a team approach to advance care planning and education of patients utilizing social workers, nurses, nephrologists, peer counsellors, and others.[3,5,7,23,24,47,49]

As Mr J's renal function declines and he begins dialysis, changes in his healthcare status, e.g. improvement in his anaemia and volume overload, will prompt him to reassess his quality of life and adjust his goals. As additional improvements and/or complications occur, the impact of those changes on his health status and goals should be discussed. If his nephrologist and dialysis care providers regularly address his quality of life and life goals, ongoing medical care should be provided in accord with Mr J's wishes. At this time, asking Mr J to name a healthcare proxy and to consider resuscitation status are appropriate goals of advance care planning. Throughout his chronic disease and ESRD, advance care planning should be an integral part of Mr J's care.

## Ethical analysis

Mr J is a relatively young man with major co-morbidities. He has not assumed responsibility for the treatment of his illness in terms of knowing his medications, and he continues to smoke, the worst thing he could do in terms of maintenance of health. Because of this scenario, one could reasonably predict that Mr J would not be enthusiastic about engaging in advance care planning. To make matters worse, in the absence of advance directives there is an increased likelihood that decision-making with the family may be problematic because of the mix of backgrounds of the children (healthcare, law, and business). Because of Mr J's condition, advance care planning needs to be initiated with the patient. In the discussion, the extent of Mr J's diseases and the consequences of them need to be addressed. Identification of Mr J's values and his attitude toward the use of life-prolonging interventions such as CPR, mechanical ventilation, tube feeding, and dialysis in his present condition and in a worsened condition in which he has lost decision-making capacity need to be explored. His choice for a surrogate decision-maker if he loses decision-making capacity also needs to be determined. With his heart disease and renal failure, it could be argued that CPR should not be offered to him because of its low likelihood of benefit (less than 5% chance of survival to hospital discharge after CPR). The explanation that CPR is not going to be offered should be part of the advance care planning discussion. Starting dialysis would appear to be likely in the next year or so, and because of the patient's co-morbidities that are associated with the worst prognoses for ESRD patients—coronary artery disease, peripheral vascular disease, and diabetes—his survival on dialysis could be anticipated to be quite short. For this reason, it is reasonable to discuss whether Mr J would want to start dialysis, and, if so, under what circumstances (i.e. state of health), if any, he would want to stop. Ideally, Mr J and his family will participate in the advance care planning with his physician. As a result of the process, Mr J's choice for a surrogate decision-maker and his wishes for future care in a variety of states of health will be known by his family and physician and put into writing in a legal document, the advance directive form recognized by law in the state in which he resides. This effort should ensure that Mr J's wishes for future medical care are known and respected.

## References

1. Emanuel, E.J., Emanuel, L.L. (1990). Living wills: past, present, and future. *J. Clin., Ethics* 1: 9–19.
2. Singer, P.A., Martin, D.K., Lavery, J.V., Thiel, E.C., Kelner, M., Mendelssohn, D.C. (1998). Reconceptualizing advance care planning from the patient's perspective. *Arch. Intern. Med.*, 158: 879–84.
3. Singer, P.A. (1999). Advance care planning in dialysis. *Am. J. Kidney Dis.*, 33: 980–91.
4. Perry, E., Buck, C., Newsome, J., Berger, C., Messana, J., Swartz, R. (1995). Dialysis staff influence patients in formulating their advance directives. *Am. J. Kidney Dis.*, 25: 262–8.

5. Holley, J.L., Nespor, S., Rault, R. (1993). Chronic in-center hemodialysis patients' attitudes, knowledge, and behavior towards advance directives. *J. Am. Soc. Nephrol.*, **3**: 1405–8.

6. Cohen, L.M., McCue, J.D., Germain, M., Woods, A. (1997). Denying the dying. Advance directives and dialysis discontinuation. *Psychosomatics* **38**: 27–34.

7. Germain, M.J., Cohen, L. (2001). Supportive care for patients with renal disease: a time for action. *Am. J. Kidney Dis.*, **38**: 884–6.

8. Teno, J.M., Nelson, H.L., Lynn, J. (1994). Advance care planning: priorities for ethical and empirical research. *Hastings Center Rep.*, **24**: S32–S36.

9. Holley, J.L., Finucane, T.E., Moss, A.H. (1989). Dialysis patients' attitudes about cardiopulmonary resuscitation and stopping dialysis. *Am. J. Nephrol.*, **9**: 245–51.

10. Fried, T.R., Bradley, E.H., Towle, V.R., Allore, H. (2002). Understanding the treatment preferences of seriously ill patients. *New Engl. J. Med.*, **346**: 1061–6.

11. Renal Physicians Association and American Society of Nephrology (2000). *Shared Decision-Making in the Appropriate Initiation of and Withdrawal from Dialysis*, pp 41–3. Washington, DC: RPA.

12. Singer, P.A., Martin, D.K., Kelner, M. (1999). Quality end-of-life care: patients' perspectives. *J. Am. Med. Assoc.*, **281**: 163–8.

13. Steinhauser, K.E., Christakis, N.A., Clipp, E.C., *et al.* (2001). Preparing for the end of life: preferences of patients, families, physicians, and other care providers. *J. Pain Symptom Manag.*, **22**: 727–37.

14. Ditto, P.H., Danks, J.H., Smucker, W.D., *et al.* (2001). Advance directives as acts of communication: a randomized controlled trial. *Arch. Intern. Med.*, **161**: 421–30.

15. Hammes, B.J. (2001). What does it take to help adults successfully plan for future medical decisions? *J. Palliative Med.*, **4**: 453–6.

16. Steinhauser, K.E., Christakis, N.A., Clipp, E.C., McNeilly, M., McIntyre, L., Tulsky, J.A. (2000). Factors considered important at the end of life by patients, family, physicians, and other care providers. *J. Am. Med. Assoc.*, **284**: 2476–82.

17. O'Neill, D. (2001). Present, rather than, advance directives. *The Lancet* **358**: 1921–2.

18. Meier, D.E., Morrison, R.S. (2002). Autonomy reconsidered. *New Engl. J. Med.*, **346**: 1087–9.

19. US Renal Data System (2001). Excerpts from the USRDS 2001 Annual Report: atlas of end stage renal diseases I: the United States. *Am. J. Kidney Dis.*, **38**: S1–S248.

20. Levinson, W., Cohen, M.S., Brady, D., Duffy, F.D. (2001). To change or not to change: 'Sounds like you have a dilemma'. *Ann. Intern. Med.*, **135**: 386–91.

21. Buckman, R. (1992). *How to Break Bad News: a Guide for Health Care Professionals*. Baltimore, MD: Johns Hopkins University Press.

22. Quill, T.E. (2001). Perspectives on care at the close of life. Initiating end-of-life discussions with seriously ill patients: addressing the 'elephant in the room'. *J. Am. Med. Assoc.*, **284**: 2502–7.

23. Perry, E., Swartz, R., Smith-Wheelock, Westbrook, J., Buck, C. (1996). Why is it difficult for staff to discuss advance directives with chronic dialysis patients? *J. Am. Soc. Nephrol.*, **4**: 2160–8.

24. Swartz, R.D., Perry, E. (1999). Medical family: a new view of the relationship between chronic dialysis patients and staff arising from discussions about advance directives. *J. Women. Health Gen.-B. Med.*, **8**: 1147–53.

25. Holley, J.L., Foulks, C.J., Moss, A.H. (1991). Nephrologists' reported attitudes about factors influencing recommendations to initiate or withdraw dialysis. *J. Am. Soc. Nephrol.*, **1**: 1284–8.

26. Moss, A.H., Stocking, C.B., Sachs, G.A., Siegler, M. (1993). Variation in the attitudes of dialysis unit medical directors toward decisions to withhold and withdraw dialysis. *J. Am. Soc. Nephrol.*, **4**: 229–34.

27. Singer, P.A., The End-Stage Renal Disease Network of New England (1992). Nephrologists' experience with and attitudes towards decisions to forego dialysis. *J. Am. Soc. Nephrol.*, **2**: 1235–40.

28. The SUPPORT Study (1995). A controlled trial to improve care for seriously ill hospitalized patients. *J. Am. Med. Assoc.*, **274**: 1591–8.

29. Swartz, R.D., Perry, E. (1993). Advance directives are associated with 'good deaths' in chronic dialysis patients. *J. Am. Soc. Nephrol.*, **3**: 1623–30.

30. Cohen, L.M., Germain, M.J., Poppel, D.M., Woods, A.L., Pekow, P.S., Kjellstrand, C.M. (2000). Dying well after discontinuing the life-support treatment of dialysis. *Arch. Intern. Med.*, **160**: 2513–18.

31. Wilson, R., Godwin, M., Seguin, R. *et al.* (2001). End-stage renal disease: factors affecting referral decisions by family physicians in Canada, the United States, and Britain. *Am. J. Kidney Dis.*, **38**: 42–8.

32. Sekkarie, M., Cosma, M., Mendelssohn, D. (2001). Nonreferral and nonacceptance to dialysis by primary care physicians and nephrologists in Canada and the United States. *Am. J. Kidney Dis.*, **38**: 36–41.

33. McKenzie, J.K., Moss, A.H., Feest, T.G., Stocking, C.B., Siegler, M. (1998). Dialysis decision making in Canada, the United Kingdom, and the United States. *Am. J. Kidney Dis.*, **31**: 12–18.

34. Holley, J.L., Stackiewicz, L., Dacko, C., Rault, R. (1997). Factors influencing dialysis patients' completion of advance directives. *Am. J. Kidney Dis.*, **30**: 356–60.

35. Hines, S.C., Glover, J.J., Holley, J.L., Babrow, A.S., Badzek, L.A., Moss, A.H. (1999). Dialysis patients' preferences for family-based advance care planning. *Ann. Intern. Med.*, **130**: 825–8.

36. Swartz, R., Perry, E. (1998). Advance directives in end-stage renal disease inherently involve family and staff. *Adv. Renal Replacement Ther.*, **5**: 109–19.

37. Singer, P.A., Thiel, E.C., Naylor, C.D. *et al.* (1995). Life-sustaining treatment preferences of hemodialysis patients: implications for advance directives. *J. Am. Soc. Nephrol.*, **6**: 1410–17.

38. Holley, J.L., Nespor, S., Rault, R. (1993). The effects of providing chronic hemodialysis patients written material on advance directives. *Am. J. Kidney Dis.*, **22**: 413–18.

39. Hines, S.C., Glover, J.J., Babrow, A.S., Holley, J.L., Badzek, L.A., Moss, A.H. (2001). Improving advance care planning by accommodating family preferences. *J. Palliative Med.*, **4**: 481–9.

40. Holley, J.L., Hines, S.C., Glover, J.J., Babrow, A.S., Badzek, L.A., Moss, A.H. (1999). Failure of advance care planning to elicit patients' preferences for withdrawal from dialysis. *Am. J. Kidney Dis.*, **33**: 688–93.

41. Sehgal, A., Galbraith, A., Chesney, M., Schoenfeld, P., Charles, G., Lo, B. (1992). How strictly do dialysis patients want their advance directives followed? *J. Am. Med. Assoc.*, **267**: 59–63.

42. Cohen, L.M., Germain, M., Poppel, D.M., Woods, A., Kjellstrand, C.M. (2000). Dialysis discontinuation and palliative care. *Am. J. Kidney Dis.*, **36**: 140–4.

43. Moss, A.H., Holley, J.L., Upton, M.B. (1992). Outcomes of cardiopulmonary resuscitation in dialysis patients. *J. Am. Soc. Nephrol.*, **3**: 1238–43.

44. Tzamaloukas, A.H., Murata, G.H., Avasthi, P.S. (1991). Outcome of cardiopulmonary resuscitation in patients on chronic dialysis. *ASAIO Trans.*, **37**: M369–M370.

45. Karnik, J.A., Young, B.S., Lew, N.L., *et al.* (2001). Cardiac arrest and sudden death in dialysis units. *Kidney Int.*, **60**: 350–7.

46. Diem, S.J., Lantos, J.D., Tulsky, J.A. (1996). Cardiopulmonary resuscitation on television: miracles and misinformation. *New Engl. J. Med.*, **334**: 1578–82.

47. Moss, A.H., Hozayen, O., King, K., Holley, J.L., Schmidt, R.J. (2001). Attitudes of patients toward cardiopulmonary resuscitation in the dialysis unit. *Am. J. Kidney Dis.*, **38**: 847–52.

48. Renal Physicians Association and American Society of Nephrology (2002). *Position on Quality Care at the End of Life*. Washington, DC: RPA.

49. Kapron, K., Perry, E., Bowman, T., Swartz, R.D. (1997). Peer resource consulting: redesigning a new future. *Adv. Renal Replacement Ther.*, **4**: 267–74.

Chapter 5

# What determines a good outcome? The selection of patients for renal replacement therapy

Terry Feest

## 5.1 Introduction

### 5.1.1 A 'good' outcome?

Conventionally, a 'good' outcome is usually measured in terms of the longevity of the patient after starting renal replacement therapy. The length of life on renal replacement therapy is easily measured, can be reported by a large national registry, and is amenable to study in more local audits. It is a measure which is easily understood by the general public and, perhaps more importantly, by politicians. Given that renal replacement therapy is very expensive, in the simplistic economical analysis it would appear most reasonable to argue that in a cash-limited health service as is seen in many developed countries such as the United Kingdom, Australia and New Zealand, and to a lesser extent Canada, it would seem appropriate to offer treatment to those who would benefit most. This is often interpreted as those who would live longest. If such an approach were applied vigorously, it would bar most elderly people from starting renal replacement therapy: simply because they are old statistically they have a shorter life expectancy than younger people. People with other significant co-morbid conditions, such as diabetics, or those with malignancy or severe heart disease, which might otherwise shorten their life, would also be excluded.

The following case histories challenge this simplistic concept of a good outcome.

## Case study 1

Mrs AA presented aged 78 with a 3-day history of increasing shortness of breath due to pulmonary oedema. She was found to be in oliguric renal failure, serum creatinine 1500. Renal ultrasound showed normal sized kidneys. Chest X-ray showed a very large right hilar shadow suggestive of carcinoma of the lung. She received haemodialysis pending urgent chest investigations. Investigations showed squamous cell carcinoma of the right lung, and she was referred for radiotherapy.

With dialysis her dyspnoea completely regressed and she felt well. There were no symptoms from the carcinoma. As she was feeling well she requested to continue dialysis so that she could visit her extended family and tidy her affairs. She said she would wish to stop dialysis once she developed symptoms from the carcinoma of the lung. After 7 weeks of dialysis she began to develop dyspnoea and pain related to her carcinoma, and withdrew from treatment with full supportive palliative care.

## Case study 2

Mr BB aged 66 had a history of mitral regurgitation, atrial fibrillation, and left ventricular failure. Investigations revealed stenosis of the left anterior descending coronary artery and the need for mitral valve replacement. He also had an 80% stenosis of his left renal artery and diffuse arterial disease in the right renal artery. It was initially planned that he should receive renal angioplasty and cardiac surgery. However, he shortly became severely unwell with marked deterioration in renal function.

Renal ultrasound showed normal sized kidneys with no obstruction. Left renal angioplasty was not successful in improving renal function. It then became clear that the patient had developed bacterial endocarditis, and widespread thrombocytopaenia due to bone marrow suppression. The unanimous view of the cardiac physicians and surgeons was that he was not suitable for cardiac surgery and had a very poor prognosis. He was hypotensive, could rarely stand, and could rarely tolerate a full dialysis session due to low blood pressure and poor cardiac output. It was the opinion of the attending renal physicians that renal replacement therapy was not appropriate. Despite extensive and detailed counselling with the patient, his wife, and family, the patient was determined to undertake regular haemodialysis, and his wife fully supported this. As a series of problems arose, the patient and his wife were adamant that he wished to continue dialysis, and he refused to discuss the issue. Because of this they would not accept palliative care or counselling. The patient continued on renal replacement therapy for 5 months until he died, during which time he did not leave hospital. The entire prolonged hospital admission caused considerable distress to the patient, and many months later the relatives had still failed to come to terms with the death and the circumstances surrounding it.

The first case, according to many of the guidelines which have been published, should not have been offered dialysis, but this history must be described as a good outcome. Despite the fact that the patient lived for a short period of time, and had malignancy at the start of dialysis, the use of technology to give the patient a few weeks of extra life was of great benefit to both the patient and to the family. This case demonstrates that a 'good outcome' must be defined beyond simple survival.

In the second case, the patient lived considerably longer than the patient in the first history, but was unhappy throughout. There was great distress for the family, and this has continued long after the death of the patient. This must be considered as a poor outcome, not in terms of the length of life, but in terms of the quality of life and distress caused by the inability of the caring team to be able to reconcile the fears and wishes of the patient and his family with his inevitable death. In the first case a good selection for dialysis was made. In the second case it was not possible to apply either good selection or appropriate care.

In assessing a good outcome of renal replacement therapy, it is essential to consider both the quality of life offered and the length of life. Tools for assessing quality of life in renal replacement therapy will be discussed in other chapters. The most difficult task is to predict, when a patient first presents for dialysis, both the likely length of life and the quality of life which might be achieved. Without such predictive tools it is very difficult to offer appropriate advice and treatment to the more frail patients who present to nephrologists.

### 5.1.2 Selection

The very use of the term 'selection' implies that someone—whether it is doctor, manager, or a panel of worthies—is assessing the patient for a potentially life-saving treatment, with the patient as a passive bystander in this critical decision about his or her future. 'Selection' is thus a paternalistic concept which many believe should not be applied to patients, who must be able to choose whether to start or not to start dialysis therapy.[1] The Renal Physicians Association (RPA) (of the USA) states: 'A patient–physician relationship that promotes shared decision making is recommended for all patients. Participants in shared decision making should involve at a minimum the patient and the physician. If a patient lacks decision-making capacity, the decisions should involve the legal agent. With the patient's consent shared decision making may include family members or friends and other members of the renal care team'.[2] Nephrologists are moving towards a general consensus that there should be a process of shared decision-making and informed consent for initiation of renal replacement therapy.[1–4]

In a healthcare system with unlimited resources it is possible to offer patient autonomy, allowing patients to make an informed choice about whether or not they wish to start renal replacement therapy. Not everyone with established renal failure will elect to undertake treatment. Many patients will have such severe co-morbid conditions that renal replacement therapy will simply prolong a difficult and painful life for a few weeks. Patients with impaired mental ability may be unable to comprehend the treatment offered to them, and simply see it as a torture which is inflicted upon them three times a week. Many patients may wish therefore to select themselves not to receive renal replacement therapy. In this situation of unlimited resources patient autonomy is compatible with 'selection'. Such a situation appears to exist in the USA and some European countries.

In many countries, even in the developed world, healthcare resources are limited. Renal replacement therapy is an expensive process which consumes a huge resource for a small number of patients. In the UK over 2% of the National health Service (NHS) budget is spent on renal replacement therapy for less than 0.06% of the population, and the expenditure is rising. There is not enough resource for all patients with established renal failure to receive renal replacement therapy, and in these circumstances selection is part of a 'rationing' process. This rationing is the implicit or explicit denial of beneficial or marginally beneficial medical treatment as a result of insufficient resources to provide treatment to all. If this occurs it is inevitable that a degree of patient autonomy is lost, as treatment may not be available for all those who might elect to receive it. Selection then becomes a rationing process. It is important to understand when selection starts to become rationing.

There is general agreement that rationing should not be according to social worth, age, or ability to pay, but if necessary could be justified according to potential medical benefit.[5] Even in the USA there is evidence that physicians may still be responsible for selected aspects of terminal care independent of patient choice,[6] and with the advent of managed care there is concern that dialysis will be rationed.[5] In a climate in which some form of rationing may be inevitable it is essential that the criteria for judgement are explicit and that transactions are transparent. This leads to a demand for practice guidelines.[5,7,8] One such set of guidelines has been produced by the RPA[2] and will be considered later in this chapter.

## 5.2 Current selection practices

Historically the UK NHS has been notable, amongst others, in limiting resources available for renal replacement therapy, causing the necessity for rationing of renal care. This was highlighted by Berlyne in 1982[9] who observed that few people over the age of 50 could obtain renal replacement therapy in the UK. It was recognized that age was commonly used as a selection criterion for access to therapy.[10] The criteria for allocating the scarce resources were not in the public domain, if indeed they were explicit in the minds of nephrologists. Decisions seemed to

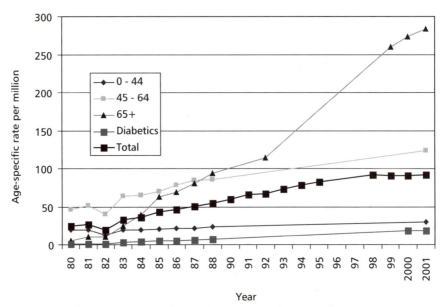

**Fig. 5.1** Age-specific acceptance rates for renal replacement therapy in the UK, 1980–2001.

be dominated by clinicians, but were considered often to be imperfect, and ultimately political.[11] Figure 5.1 shows the changing pattern of acceptance for renal replacement therapy in the UK. Against the background of a steadily increasing acceptance rate, there has been little change for younger people. The most marked change is in the acceptance rate of the elderly, which shows a six-fold increase over some 20 years. This figure illustrates clearly how age was widely used as a criterion for limiting access to care in the early 1980s. It also shows the impact of the recommendation issued by the UK government in 1993 that age was not an acceptable criterion for limiting access to therapy.[12] Acceptance rates for diabetics have also dramatically increased.

Whilst acceptance rates have increased in the last two decades throughout the developed world, there still remain wide differences between different countries (Table 5.1). This wide variation in acceptance from 66 per million population per annum to 333 per million population per annum is unlikely to be explained by differing incidences of renal failure, especially as many of the countries have similar populations. The higher rate in the USA is partly explained by the large Black population which has a high incidence of renal failure, but even in the White population the acceptance rate is 269 per million per annum.[13] There is therefore a strong suggestion that selection practices differ between different countries.

Even within a single country such as the UK, acceptance rates differ widely in different health authorities, from 51 per million per annum to 154 per million per annum.[14] Analysis of possible underlying reasons shows that this is not entirely explained by differing patterns of age or ethnic mix, and therefore differing selection policies must play an important role. These differing practices are covert. Research early in the development of renal replacement therapy showed that the low acceptance rate in the UK was largely due to under-referral of patients to dialysis and transplant units rather than to refusal by consultant renal physicians to treat patients.[15] Attitudes have liberalized significantly since this was published in 1984, but a study in 1996[16] demonstrated that there was still a reluctance of generalists to refer to renal

**Table 5.1** Patients accepted for replacement therapy in different countries (data from USRDS,[13] Ansell *et al.*,[14] Registry of the European Renal Association/European Dialysis and Transplantation Association,[40] Canadian Organ Replacement Register,[41] and Disney and Graeme[42])

| Country | Year | Median age (years) | Rate (pmp) | %DM | DM ESRF rate (pmp) |
|---------|------|--------------------|------------|-----|--------------------|
| Australia | 2000 | 61 | 91 | 22 | 20 |
| Austria | 2000 | 64 | 129 | 33 | 43 |
| Belgium-Dutch | 2000 | 69 | 144 | 20 | 30 |
| Canada | 2000 | | 143 | 32 | 46 |
| Czech Republic | 1998 | | 136 | 37 | 50 |
| Greece | 2000 | 67 | 154 | 26 | 39 |
| Japan | 2000 | | 253 | 37 | 94 |
| Norway | 2000 | 65 | 89 | 15 | 13 |
| Poland | 1998 | | 66 | 18 | 12 |
| Spain, Catalonia | 2000 | 67 | 145 | 20 | 29 |
| Sweden | 2000 | | 125 | 25 | 31 |
| Netherlands | 2000 | 62 | 94 | 16 | 15 |
| New Zealand | 2000 | 58 | 107 | 36 | 39 |
| Basque | 2000 | 65 | 117 | 14 | 17 |
| Germany | 2000 | 66 | 175 | 36 | 63 |
| Croatia | 2000 | 62 | 106 | 28 | 30 |
| USA | 2000 | 64 | 333 | 43 | 142 |
| UK | 2000 | 64 | 95 | 18 | 17 |

DM, primary renal disease diabetes mellitus; ESRF, end-stages renal failure; pmp, annual rate per million population.

physicians, whose attitudes towards acceptance of treatment were much more liberal. That the attitude of referring physicians may still be a dominant feature is illustrated by referrals to the Bristol Renal Unit, which are all sent to the same team of seven physicians. Acceptance rates for renal replacement therapy rates in one health authority served by the unit are 110 per million and in another are consistently low at around 55 per million. Given that the populations served are relatively similar and that all are served by the same nephrologists, the major difference in acceptance rate is likely to be due to under-referral by general practitioners and/or general physicians in some areas. A similar pattern has been observed in the USA and Canada,[17] although the differences between generalists and specialist nephrologists are diminishing.[18]

There have been many studies, usually by means of vignette case history questionnaires, which have assessed the attitude of referring physicians and nephrologists to selection for dialysis.[6–8,15,17–22] In the USA it was clear that nephrologists were more comfortable with-holding dialysis than withdrawing it.[8,22] Overall it was expectation of medical benefit, and not social considerations, which was the main driver in decision-making.[8,22,23] The major factors influencing decisions to recommend non-commencement of dialysis were severe heart disease and severely impaired neurological function. There is, however, strong evidence that resource considerations were influencing these apparently clinical decisions. In the UK,

16 case vignettes were shown to general practitioners, non-nephrologist consultants, and consultant nephrologists. They were asked to consider suitability for dialysis on clinical grounds. The three groups considered respectively an average of 7.4, 6.9, and 4.7 of the patients to be unsuitable for renal replacement therapy.[15] North American nephrologists on average considered only 0.3 of these patients inappropriate for dialysis. It appears highly likely that resource constraints were influencing the apparently clinical opinions of practitioners in the UK. This study also highlighted the importance of non-referral to nephrologists as a limiting factor in acceptance for dialysis. It is interesting that at this time when the age-specific acceptance rate for the over 65s in the UK was very low, the physicians were theoretically willing to accept some of the older patients in this study, suggesting practice differed from principle.

The role of non-referral was confirmed in a Canadian study in 1994,[20] which also demonstrated that age as well as coexisting disease influenced the likelihood of referral. It also concluded that in Canada rationing decisions were being made which prevented access to treatment by patients who might have benefited from it. Whilst acceptance policies in the USA were much more liberal at that time than those of Canada or the UK, 94% of unit directors in the USA reported that they were prepared to make decisions to withhold dialysis. There was marked variation in attitudes and the criteria used for selection,[8] highlighting again the need for explicit guidelines to assist in more open and uniform decision-making.

In a prospective study in one unit in Canada in 1992,[19] one-quarter of patients referred to a dialysis unit were not accepted to the programme. Patients not accepted were predominantly female, with very poor functional capacity as judged by the Karnofsky scale, had a mean age of 74 years, and suffered from a combination of cardiovascular and renovascular disease. Very few of those not accepted survived more than 6 months. Based on their experience the authors suggested the following guidelines for advising against dialysis:

1. Non-uraemic dementia;
2. metastatic or non-resectable solid malignancy or refractory haematological malignancy;
3. end-stage irreversible liver, heart, or lung disease: patient confined to bed or chair needing assistance for activities of daily living;
4. irreversible neurological disease significantly restricting mobility and activities of daily living, e.g. major stroke;
5. multisystem failure making survival extremely unlikely;
6. need to sedate or restrain pain on each dialysis to maintain functioning access.

At this time some believed that doctors with high technology were guilty of having 'tunnel vision in dealings with patients'[24] and that physicians often did things to patients simply because they were able to do them, rather than because they were necessarily correct. It was suggested when counselling patients with impending established renal failure that they should be advised against accepting dialysis if:

1. The patient is physiologically or chronologically old with an estimated life expectancy of less than 2 years.
2. The patient is demented or has impending dementia with no expectations of gaining cognitive function.

3. The patient's life expectancy is under 2 years because of coexisting disease, such as advanced diabetes, vascular disease, heart disease, AIDS, cancer, or other systemic illnesses.

4. The patient has a coexisting illness that will produce intractable pain or suffering should artificial support prolong life long enough to allow this to occur, even though the life expectancy with support may be beyond 2 years.

It was intended to apply these guidelines in a 'sensible' manner. These recommendations were the personal view of one experienced nephrologist, not a consensus statement.

During the 1990s acceptance rates rose throughout the developed world. A study in Virginia in 1998 suggested that only 7% of patients were counselled not to accept treatment.[17] A survey of dialysis decision-making in Canada, the UK, and the USA in 1998[7] showed that American nephrologists were more likely to offer dialysis than Canadian or British nephrologists, and ranked patient/family wishes and fear of lawsuit higher in decision-making than Canadian or British nephrologists. The Americans less frequently used their perceptions of the patient's likely quality of life to make decisions. Two per cent of American nephrologists and 12% of Canadian and British nephrologists had had to refuse dialysis to possibly suitable patients in the last year due to lack of resources. The variation in nephrologists' reported attitudes in the three countries was not great enough to account for the wide variation in acceptance rates between the countries. It was concluded that this variation was partly influenced by financial constraints, and other factors such as differences in rates of referral to the specialist centres.

More recently, in 2000, another study of attitudes in the USA, Canada, and the UK showed that 35% of Canadian and American physicians would operate an age restriction for referral to a specialist, compared with 51% in the UK.[21] Family physicians were still acting as gatekeepers to the system, taking into account the patient's life circumstances, often in concert with the patients and their family. In the USA and Canada, there was still evidence that patients who might benefit from dialysis were not always offered it,[18] and that non-referral by primary care physicians was still an important factor. The reported attitudes of Canadian and American nephrologists were very similar, despite the differing treatment rates in the two countries, again suggesting that attitudes towards acceptance may differ from real practice.

Thus in the development of dialysis programmes in the last 30 years, it is clear that selection for treatment has been significantly influenced by the need for economic rationing. When the first dialysis programme was established in Seattle a citizens committee was set up to allocate places. Analysis showed that perceptions of social worth were influential in decisions.[25] In a fair society access to treatment should be free and not amenable to manipulation by the more able or socially privileged as happened in the UK in the 1980s.[26] As more facilities have been made available, acceptance has become more liberal: concurrently beliefs about who might benefit have also changed, indicating that such apparently clinical decisions are influenced, often subconsciously, by resource and budget constraints.

In the last decade limited resources has become less of an issue in many countries, although it is still present. Nevertheless attitudes to selection have been variable and often not reflected in real practice, which has tended to be more restrictive than the quoted underlying principle. Levinsky[27] reminds us that physicians have not been appointed to resolve economic issues, and that recommendations regarding dialysis must be based on clinical criteria and not on subconscious (or even overt) prejudices or perceptions of social worth.

Thus the situation has now changed. Dialysis is more freely available (even in the UK), and there is a perception that patients who are too sick to benefit may be receiving treatment. By the mid 1990s many nephrologists and renal nurses believed that at least 15% of patients on dialysis had such a poor quality of life they should not be receiving the treatment.[28–30]

The concept of 'selection' is also changing towards patient autonomy, the patient making an informed choice with appropriate counselling from the nephrologist and others. There will be cases where, as in Case 2 above, the patient or family may not be able to accept that advice, but it is hoped this is rare.

On the other hand there are still those who believe that deciding not to offer dialysis is a fundamental responsibility of the nephrologist,[30] and that failure to make these decisions will harm patients, their families, other patients, and staff. Advocates of this approach accept that saying 'no' will demand both careful assessment of the patient and the medical literature on the outcomes of dialysis for someone in the patient's condition. The nephrologist is then obliged to fully explain to the patient why dialysis treatment is not offered. Implementing this advice would be difficult; as it is there is severe doubt about whether the medical literature is adequate to enable nephrologists to predict which patients will experience more harm than benefit on dialysis, and so make such decisions.

Despite these difficulties, paternalism still persists. In a 1-year prospective study in the UK reported in 2000,[31] of 88 patients referred for consideration of dialysis 11 were not started on renal replacement therapy: six of these patients were over 80 and only one had been seen earlier in a renal clinic. Of these 11 not treated, four were considered incapable of making a decision: only one of the other seven was offered a choice.

Even if the nephrologist restricts his or her role to that of informing the autonomous patient, what criteria are to be used to inform a patient, and possibly to advise against accepting treatment? This chapter shows that such criteria have historically been covert and variable, and susceptible to economic and political influences. Even if it is accepted that the major criterion should be an expectation of an acceptable quality of life for a given length of time, is it possible to define and predict this in an individual case?

## 5.3 Is it possible to predict individual outcomes?

Several factors have been shown to have value in predicting outcome for patients starting renal replacement therapy.

### 5.3.1 Age

Whilst age was widely used to exclude people in the early development of dialysis, there is now a majority view amongst nephrologists[7] and governments[12] that age alone is not an acceptable criterion for selection. The concept of fitness rather than chronological age should be applied. Whilst older patients starting dialysis have a shorter prognosis than younger patients (Table 5.2),[13] their relative risk of death compared with the general population of the same age is much less (Fig. 5.2).[14] Additionally some older patients live a long time on treatment. Whilst some older patients are fit, there are many with other significant co-morbidity factors giving them a poor prognosis on the stratification techniques. It is the sum of co-morbidity present which renders many older patients of poor prognosis, rather than age itself.

### 5.3.2 Terminal illness

Many patients present with established renal failure at a time when they have other terminal illness leading to very short life expectancy. Case 1 in this chapter is an example. A few weeks

**Table 5.2** Survival of incident renal replacement therapy (RRT) patients in different age groups, UK (England and Wales only) and USA. Per cent survival is for 1 year after the first 90 days of renal replacement therapy. US data are from the US Renal Data System (USRDS) 2001 annual report.[13] UK data are unpublished data from the UK Renal Registry. Survival in the UK is significantly higher than in the USA in all age bands ($p < 0.05$) with the exception of 20–44-year-old patients where rates were similar. The differences, especially in the elderly, may be due to the fact that in the USA many patients with very high rates of co-morbidity start RRT, whereas in England and Wales, where starting rates are much lower, there is selection bias

| Age range | USA: incident patients 1999 (% survival) | UK: incident patients 2000 (% survival) |
|---|---|---|
| 20–29 | 95.8 | 96.6 |
| 30–39 | 91.6 | 94.1 |
| 40–49 | 90.3 | 94.7 |
| 50–59 | 86.6 | 89.3 |
| 60–69 | 76.3 | 84.6 |
| 70–79 | 69.3 | 75.9 |
| 80+ | 58.3 | 64.9 |

of additional life may be of considerable value to such patients. A study of such patients[32] showed that 62% treated rated their quality of life as good or improved, but only 27% were alive at 5 months. An analysis of cost-effectiveness, however, showed that except for the best prognostic group the cost per quality adjusted life year (QALY) gained was well over the commonly used threshold acceptability of $50 000.

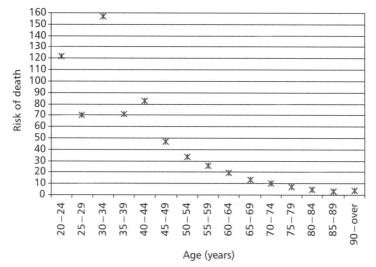

**Fig. 5.2** Relative risk of death in patients with established renal failure compared with the general population in England and Wales.

### 5.3.3 Preparation for dialysis

There have been numerous papers reporting that patients who present late for dialysis have a poorer outcome than those who are referred early. Whilst there has been much debate about the reason for this, an important paper was recently published looking at the influence of the quality of preparation for dialysis on outcome.[33] This shows clearly that frequent visits to the nephrologist in the year of preparation for dialysis is associated with improved survival in the first year of dialysis. In patients with multiple co-morbidities, significant social problems, or of advanced age careful preparation and counselling are likely to be essential for a good outcome.

### 5.3.4 Co-morbidity

Several risk stratification systems have been developed to try to predict survival in different groups of patients, to identify those with good or bad prognosis, and to allow correction for case mix in comparison of survival between centres.[34–36] Whilst they do identify groups of patients at high risk, they were not designed for the purpose of selecting patients suitable for receiving treatment. A recent systematic literature review identified several individual factors as predictors of early death, in particular low serum albumin, poor functional status, and acute myocardial infarct.[2] Patients with an above-knee amputation may have a 73% 1-year mortality. However, interpretation of even an objective measure such as the serum albumin must now be done with caution, given the considerable variation in dialysis patients between the two most commonly used methods of measuring the serum albumin.[14]

A hospital-based cohort study of factors affecting survival and morbidity in patients starting dialysis in a single unit in the UK published in 1999 identified factors significantly affecting survival,[37] which included a poor Karnofsky performance score at presentation, and myeloma. Unplanned presentation for dialysis was also a risk factor. Using several factors, a high-risk group of 26 patients was defined, which had a 19.2% 1-year survival. However, five of these 26 patients did have good long-term survival with apparent good quality of life. Thus excluding this group of 26 patients from dialysis would have excluded a significant number who had a good outcome. It should also be noted that in this study an estimate was made of the cost savings of not treating this group of patients. Savings of some 3% would have been made in the overall dialysis budget. One might observe that those patients who have a short life on dialysis do not consume a huge resource, and that not treating them makes relatively small savings at the risk of excluding a group of patients who would do well.

It would thus appear that whilst groups of patients can be identified who are statistically at high risk, the application of these stratification techniques to the selection of patients for dialysis would exclude significant numbers of patients who would do well.

The difficulties of predicting individual patient outcomes are illustrated by the following two case histories.

## Case study 3

A 60-year-old male with no previous history suffered a severe myocardial infarct. He developed a major ventricular septal defect and profound hypotension, and was transferred to the Regional Cardiothoracic Surgery Unit. Two attempts at closure of the septal defect were not entirely successful and he was left with a small defect and persistent hypotension. He remained in cardiac intensive and high-density care units for 3 months. During his profound hypotension he developed anuria,

**Case study 3** *(continued)*

there was cortical necrosis of his kidneys, and his renal function did not recover. He was considered to have a dreadful cardiac prognosis.

The patient expressed the wish to try dialysis. Multiple central lines had already been used in ICU and he was profoundly hypotensive, so he opted for peritoneal dialysis. This was started and within 3 weeks he had a mild episode of peritonitis which was successfully treated. He was then discharged from hospital, and despite persisting hypotension, remained reasonably well and was not admitted to hospital for a further year. There was then one admission with low-grade peritonitis which recovered rapidly. Eighteen months after starting dialysis he developed myelodysplasia which is now transforming to acute myeloid leukaemia. For those 18 months he has remained ambulant, at home, and independent.

This apparently hopeless case has now been at home on peritoneal dialysis for 15 months, during which time he has not needed hospital admission, and is very grateful to have been given this extension of reasonable life.

## Case study 4

An 86-year-old female presented with established renal failure of unknown cause. She initially started peritoneal dialysis but had several episodes of peritonitis over the subsequent year and was transferred to haemodialysis. Following the death of her husband she moved to live nearer her son and continued therapy at another renal unit. She is now 94 and has been on dialysis for 8 years. She is mobile, independent, and thoroughly enjoys life, particularly participating in the care of her grandchildren. In the course of her 7 years of haemodialysis she has twice needed revision of her vascular access. She has not been admitted to hospital for over 3 years.

This elderly lady may have been refused renal replacement therapy by many centres, especially 8 years ago when her treatment started. Her excellent response to treatment would not have been predicted by any of the systems used for predicting outcomes.

### 5.3.5 Quality of life

Predicting the quality of life which may be attained for patients starting dialysis is notoriously difficult. Furthermore it has been widely shown that physicians' and healthcare professionals' perceptions of a patients quality of life are usually lower than those of the patients themselves. It is regrettable that many renal units do not perform any formal assessment of quality of life or function in their patients, either before or after starting renal replacement therapy, especially as a relatively simple measure such as the Karnofsky score has been shown to be of useful predictive value in terms of outcome.[37] A low level of independence and poor scoring on the Karnofsky index are associated with short survival on treatment. There is growing awareness of the desirability of such measurements, as is indicated by the recommendation for their use in the latest Standards for Renal Replacement Therapy issued by the UK Renal Association.[38]

The patients themselves are the ones who are best placed to determine whether the quality of life they achieve is sufficient to wish to continue therapy. It is important that patients feel no coercion to accept treatment. If a supportive relationship is maintained between the renal team and the patient, which respects the patient's autonomy, then the patient will decide whether or not they wish to continue attending for treatment. In that circumstance it is both presumptuous and unnecessary for the renal team to attempt to make decisions for the patient as to whether their quality of life is worthwhile.

## Case study 5

A 75-year-old female had a long history of thoracic surgery and respiratory problems. She needed to use continuous positive airway pressure (CPAP) ventilatory support at night, but led an active and independent life. She then developed a severe chest infection and was admitted to an intensive care unit. Associated with the infection she developed acute renal failure on the background of moderate chronic renal impairment. A nephrologist had suggested haemofiltration to support this, but the intensive care team was uneasy about starting further interventional therapy. A second nephrologist was asked for a further opinion. He stated that he would give this after reading the notes and talking with the patient. On his way to visit the patient he met the patient's elder sister. She asked, 'What are they going to do to my sister?' The nephrologist responded by saying that he did not know, he was first going to ask the patient what she wanted. At this point the sister burst into tears, saying 'Nobody ever asks us old people what we want'. After discussion with the patient it was agreed that she would undergo haemofiltration or dialysis for a short period to see if she obtained renal recovery. She agreed that if her kidneys did not recover that long-term renal replacement therapy would not be appropriate. The patient received renal replacement therapy for 5 days. Her kidneys recovered, and she is now once more at home and independent.

This case illustrates the widespread anticipation that things will be done to patients by doctors and therapeutic systems, without recognition that the central figure in such decisions who must be consulted is the patient. It was consultation with the patient that resolved the situation and enabled a wise decision to be made.

## 5.4 Guidelines

Guidelines for decision-making on initiation of dialysis may be issued for a variety of reasons. They may be for political purposes, for cost containment and appropriate use of scarce resources, or for good professional practice in the interest of patients.

Governments may issue political statements which are effectively guidelines. For example in 1993 the UK Department of Health stated that age was not an acceptable criterion for judging suitability for dialysis.[12] This was effectively a guideline to those referring patients to nephrologists, and to nephrologists in the UK. It did not, however, come with any funding for the massive increase in acceptance for dialysis which would have occurred had these guidelines been followed at the time, although it did appear to facilitate a progressive increase in treatment of the elderly (Fig. 5.1).

The Wiltshire Health Authority in the UK, faced with considerable cost constraints, issued guidelines for initiation of treatment[39] with the aim 'To prioritise entry onto the programme for those patients who have the most likelihood of health gain from treatment, based on potential life years to be gained from treatment'. The three criteria published were:

1. anticipated survival of at least 12 months;
2. absence of significant co-morbidity;
3. the capability of independent living.

Whilst the document did not define significant co-morbidity it was verbally reported that this was intended to mean significant multiple co-morbidities. Independent living was later defined as not needing nursing home care.

There have been few professional consensus guidelines issued. Two guidelines have already been considered, the personal view of Lowance[24] issued in 1993 and those of Hirsch *et al.*[19] published in 1994 in response to their experience of advising when dialysis was not considered appropriate. More recently, following a detailed literature review and consultation, the RPA and the American Society of Nephrology (ASN) issued a clinical practice guideline on shared decision-making in the appropriate initiation or withdrawal from dialysis.[2] The recommendations are summarized below.

## 5.4.1 Guidelines from the Renal Physicians Association of the USA

1. **Shared decision-making**. A patient–physician relationship that promotes shared decision-making is recommended. Participants in shared decision-making should involve at a minimum the patient and the physician. If a patient lacks decision-making capacity, decisions should involve the legal agent. With the patient's consent, shared decision-making may include family members or friends and other members of the renal care team.

2. **Informed consent or refusal**. Physicians should fully inform patients about their diagnosis, prognosis, and all treatment options, including a time-limited trial of dialysis and stopping dialysis and receiving end-of-life care.

3. **Estimating prognosis**. To facilitate informed decisions about starting dialysis, discussions should occur with the patient or legal agent about life expectancy and quality of life by a doctor who is familiar with prognostic data. Survival for the patient should be estimated, realizing that the ability to predict survival in the individual patient is difficult and imprecise. For patients who experience major complications that may substantially reduce survival or quality of life, it is appropriate to discuss and/or reassess treatment goals, including consideration of withdrawing dialysis.

4. **Conflict resolution**. A systematic approach for conflict resolution is recommended if there is disagreement regarding the benefits of dialysis between the patient or legal agent (and those supporting the patient's position) and the renal care team. If dialysis is indicated urgently, it should be provided while pursuing conflict resolution, provided the patient or legal agent requests it.

5. **Advance directives**. The renal care team should attempt to obtain written advance directives from all dialysis patients. These advance directives should be honored.

6. **Withholding or withdrawing dialysis**. It is appropriate to withhold or withdraw dialysis for patients with either ARF [acute renal failure] or ESRD [end-stage renal disease] in the following situations:

   ◆ Patients with decision-making capacity, who being fully informed and making voluntary choices, refuse dialysis or request dialysis be discontinued.

   ◆ Patients who no longer possess decision-making capacity who have previously indicated refusal of dialysis in an oral or written advance directive.

   ◆ Patients who no longer possess decision-making capacity and whose properly appointed legal agents refuse dialysis or request that it be discontinued.

   ◆ Patients with irreversible, profound neurological impairment such that they lack signs of thought, sensation, purposeful behavior, and awareness of self and environment.

7. **Special patient groups**. It is reasonable to consider not initiating or withdrawing dialysis for those who have a terminal illness from a non-renal cause, or whose medical condition precludes the technical process of dialysis.

8. **Time-limited trials**. For patients requiring dialysis, but who have an uncertain prognosis, or for whom a consensus cannot be reached about providing dialysis, nephrologists should consider offering a time-limited trial of dialysis.

9. **Palliative care**. All patients who decide to forgo dialysis or for whom such a decision is made should be treated with continued palliative care by a team with appropriate expertise.

These recommendations summarize the converging approaches discussed earlier in this chapter. Recommendations 5, 8, and 9 are of particular interest. Advance directives, whilst relatively common in the USA, are infrequently written in the UK.

Similar recommendations are embodied in the standard set by the Renal Association of the UK.[38]

## 5.4.2 Standard from the Renal Association of the UK

The decision to institute active non-dialytic management of the patient with ERF [established renal failure], including nutritional, medical, and psychological support, should be made jointly by the patient and the responsible consultant nephrologist after consultation with relatives, the family practitioner and members of the caring team. Centres should develop guidelines for palliative care of such patients, including liaison with community services.

This standard stresses the concept that the 'no-dialysis' option is not a withdrawal of care but the decision for an active alternative route of care.

The renal team must have adequate resource to appropriately counsel and prepare patients for dialysis, to support them through these difficult decisions, and to enable them to write advanced directives if necessary.

Time-limited trials of dialysis are often decided upon informally in renal units. Many physicians nevertheless find it difficult to stop treatment if a trial is apparently unsuccessful. If such an approach is to be successful it is essential that the patient fully understands the treatment plan, and that some criteria for judging success are decided upon before the trial begins. Again, this proposition can only work if there is a full team available with adequate time and expertise to counsel and support the patient and the family throughout treatment 'trial'.

Finally there is growing interest in palliative care in renal units. The UK Department of Health is giving the topic careful consideration in preparing the British National Service Framework for renal disease, and it is likely to be recommended that all renal units have an appropriately trained and experienced palliative care team to support not only patients who have been on dialysis for a long time and have declining health, but also those patients who elect not to start dialysis.

## 5.5 The 'no-dialysis' option

As has been outlined, if appropriate support and counselling is available for patients, a number of patients will make a well-informed and appropriate decision not to undertake dialysis. It must be stressed that the no-dialysis option is not a no-treatment option. Many patients will live for several weeks or months without dialysis; indeed in elderly patients not undertaking dialysis may not greatly shorten life expectancy. It is important that through this period patients receive full supportive care from the resources of the Renal Service to maximize their physical and mental health, and to optimize their survival and reduce the need for hospitalization. These relatively positive aspects of not undertaking dialysis should be made clear to patients through the counselling process to enable them to make an appropriate decision.

The Renal Association standards document[38] states: 'The most realistic and accurate description of starting or not starting, continuing or not continuing dialysis should be given. If the decision is taken not to initiate, or to stop dialysis, then a management plan of supportive care must be put in place. This must then be carried through in a way that ensures continued support, achieves what seems best *from the patient's point of view* and finally enables the patient to die with dignity, when the time comes. Achieving this will often require co-ordinated work with the palliative care team, which should be involved early in the management plan.'[31]

Continuing medical care should be modified appropriately to the situation. Thus in a patient with a short prognosis it is not sensible to place severe dietary restrictions, or make great efforts to control moderate hyperphosphataemia, in order to prevent long-term complications. However, use of erythropoietin to treat anaemia can dramatically improve a patient's quality of life. The use of appropriate drugs such as ondansetron to relieve pruritus may be of enormous benefit. Continued monitoring of the patient's condition, with appropriate modification of care, and full availability of psychological and palliative support from the renal multiprofessional team and palliative care specialists are essential. In large renal units it is should be possible to have a group within the multiprofessional team who have developed specific palliative care and end-of-life skills.

The majority of patients with end-stage renal failure currently die in hospital. However, renal wards are traditionally designed and equipped for curative and interventional treatments, and not for long-term rehabilitation or care of the dying. In designing renal wards, and the staffing of these wards, the increasing need for appropriate palliative care must be recognized.

## 5.6 Conclusion

Patients, the renal team, politicians, and managers may not entirely agree on what constitutes a 'good' outcome in renal replacement therapy. There are many studies that identify on clinical criteria general groups of patients who may do badly when started on renal replacement therapy, but the uncertainty of the prediction in individuals is such that if these criteria were to be used for selection, 20% of those denied treatment might have done well. It is also clear that assessment of suitability on clinical grounds is not an exact science, and opinions have changed over the years. The evidence suggests that even such apparently objective clinical decisions are influenced by economic factors. Faced with such uncertainty, it is difficult with confidence to simply refuse treatment to an individual.

In addition, it is now no longer acceptable to the general public or to many governments for nephrologists to make unilateral decisions whether or not to offer patients treatment. The nephrologist must respect the patient's autonomy, and be willing to sensitively present carefully considered information concerning likely outcomes, such that the patient and the family, can make a supported and informed decision about whether or not to accept therapy. There is evidence that frequent visits during the preparatory period can improve outcomes. Furthermore, studies on those patients who do not accept dialysis, but who receive good supportive alternative care, show that with good counselling the recommendation of no dialysis therapy is rarely disputed by patients, their families, or referring physicians, and that the no-dialysis option can give a satisfactory outcome to patients and their families.[19] The factor that determines a good outcome is likely to be the existence of an appropriately experienced team, with time to allow frequent contact with the patient and family during the period before dialysis might be recommended. It is important to continue this support during the early phase of dialysis. If dialysis is not undertaken it is equally important to continue both intensive medical and psychological support to maximize the quality of remaining life for the patient and the family.

A 'good' outcome cannot simply be judged on length of life obtained; quality of life, even if short, is equally important. The case histories demonstrate that provision of short periods of dialysis life can be very rewarding for patients, families, and the renal team. A good outcome is one which maximizes the physical, mental, and emotional health available to the patient within the limitations imposed by the illness. Whilst no rigid rules can be applied, careful counselling and preparation, coupled with good support for those not accepting dialysis, should enable a good outcome to be achieved in the large majority of patients, whether or not dialysis is accepted.

## Ethical case analysis

The challenge in trying to establish a framework for selecting patients for renal replacement therapy is that major ethical principles conflict. In some cases such as that of Mr BB (Case 2 in this chapter), the principle of respect for patient autonomy conflicts with non-maleficence, justice, and professional integrity. Despite extensive counselling, Mr BB undertook a course of dialysis therapy that the renal physicians thought likely to cause more harm than good. In the terms of the RPA/ASN guidelines, dialysis was not medically indicated for Mr BB because the expected benefits did not justify the risks. Mr BB experienced considerable distress during his course of dialysis, and he never improved enough to be discharged from the hospital. In terms of quality of life and quantity of life, Mr BB did not benefit from dialysis. The judgment of his nephrologists that dialysis was not appropriate for him was vindicated. Use of the process for conflict resolution in the RPA/ASN guideline (recommendation 5) might have helped in dialysis decision-making with this patient and his family. Unresolved psychosocial and spiritual issues were probably present.

With regard to the case of Mrs AA (Case 1 in this chapter), recommendation 7 of the RPA/ASN guideline is applicable. The RPA/ASN Guideline Working Group resisted using a diagnosis of a terminal illness from a non-renal cause as a reason to preclude dialysis in all cases. The guideline working group anticipated cases just like Mrs AA. She used the 7 weeks of extended life with dialysis to accomplish the tasks of life closure. Dialysis provided her with the opportunity to strengthen her personal relationships and leave a legacy of good memories for her family. Mrs AA clearly benefited from her dialysis. The extension of life that dialysis afforded for Mr BB did not have such a positive effect. In all likelihood intensive counselling based on exploring the issues raised in a 'patient as person' history (see the ethical case analysis in Chapter 14) would have benefited him more than dialysis.

## References

1. Lowance, D.C. (2002). Withholding and withdrawal of dialysis in the elderly. *Semin. Dial.,* **15**(2): 88–90.

2. Renal Physicians Association and American Society of Nephrology (2000). *Clinical Practice Guideline on Shared Decision-Making in the Appropriate Initiation of and Withdrawal from Dialysis.* Washington, DC: RPA/ASN.

3. Kee, F., Patterson, C.C., Wilson, E.A., McConnell, J.M., Wheeler, S.M., Watson, J.D. (2000). Stewardship or clinical freedom? variations in dialysis decision making. *Nephrol. Dial. Transpl.,* **15**(10): 1647–57.

4. Lelie, A. (2000). Decision-making in nephrology: shared decision making? *Patient Educ. Couns.*, **39**(1): 81–9.

5. Glover, J.J., Moss, A.H. (1998). Rationing dialysis in the United States: possible implications of capitated systems. *Adv. Renal Replacement Ther.*, **5**(4): 341–9.

6. Rutecki, G.W., Cugino, A., Jarjoura, D., Kilner, J.F., Whittier, F.C. (1997). Nephrologists' subjective attitudes towards end-of-life issues and the conduct of terminal care. *Clin. Nephrol.*, **48**(3): 173–80.

7. McKenzie, J.K., Moss, A.H., Feest, T.G., Stocking, C.B., Siegler, M. (1998). Dialysis decision making in Canada, the United Kingdom, and the United States. *Am. J. Kidney Dis.*, **31**(1): 12–18.

8. Moss, A.H., Stocking, C.B., Sachs, G.A., Siegler, M. (1993). Variation in the attitudes of dialysis unit medical directors toward decisions to withhold and withdraw dialysis. *J. Am. Soc. Nephrol.*, **4**(2): 229–34.

9. Berlyne, G. (1982). Over 50 and uremic equals death. *Nephron,* **31**: 189–90.

10. Baker, R. (1994). BNHS (British National Health Service) age rationing: a riposte to Bates. *Health Care Anal.*, **2**(1): 39–41.

11. Halper, T. (1985). Life and death in a welfare state: end-stage renal disease in the United Kingdom. *Milbank Mem. Fund Q. Health Soc.*, **63**(1): 52–93.

12. Department of Health (1994). *Report of the Health Care Strategy Unit Review of Renal Services. Part I.* London.

13. US Renal Data System (2001). *USRDS 2001 Annual Data Report.* Bethesda, MD: National Institutes of Health.

14. Ansell, D., Feest, T., Byrne, C. (2002). *The Fifth Annual Report of the UK Renal Registry.* Bristol: UK Renal Registry.

15. Challah, S., Wing, A.J., Bauer, R., Morris, R.W., Schroeder, S.A. (1984). Negative selection of patients for dialysis and transplantation in the United Kingdom. *Br. Med. J.*, **288**(6424): 1119–22.

16. Parry, R.G., Crowe, A., Stevens, J.M., Mason, J.C., Roderick, P. (1996). Referral of elderly patients with severe renal failure: questionnaire survey of physicians. *Br. Med. J.*, **313**(7055): 466.

17. Sekkarie, M.A., Moss, A.H. (1998). Withholding and withdrawing dialysis: the role of physician specialty and education and patient functional status. *Am. J. Kidney Dis.*, **31**(3): 464–72.

18. Sekkarie, M., Cosma, M., Mendelssohn, D. (2001). Nonreferral and nonacceptance to dialysis by primary care physicians and nephrologists in Canada and the United States. *Am. J. Kidney Dis.*, **38**(1): 36–41.

19. Hirsch, D.J., West, M.L., Cohen, A.D., Jindal, K.K. (1994). Experience with not offering dialysis to patients with a poor prognosis. *Am. J. Kidney Dis.*, **23**(3): 463–6.

20. Mendelssohn, D.C., Kua, B.T., Singer, P.A. (1995). Referral for dialysis in Ontario. *Arch. Intern. Med.*, **155**(22): 2473–8.

21. Wilson, R., Godwin, M., Seguin, R., *et al.* (2001). End-stage renal disease: factors affecting referral decisions by family physicians in Canada, the United States, and Britain. *Am. J. Kidney Dis.*, **38**(1): 42–8.

22. Singer, P.A. (1992). Nephrologists' experience with and attitudes towards decisions to forego dialysis. The End-Stage Renal Disease Network of New England. *J. Am. Soc. Nephrol.*, **2**(7): 1235–40.

23. Holley, J.L., Foulks, C.J., Moss, A.H. (1991). Nephrologists' reported attitudes about factors influencing recommendations to initiate or withdraw dialysis. *J. Am. Soc. Nephrol.*, **1**(12): 1284–8.

24. Lowance, D.C. (1993). Factors and guidelines to be considered in offering treatment to patients with end-stage renal disease: a personal opinion. *Am. J. Kidney Dis.*, **21**(6): 679–83.

25. Sanders, D., Dukeminier, J. Jr. (1968). Medical advance and legal lag: hemodialysis and kidney transplantation. *UCLA Law Rev.*, **15**: 357–413.

26. Aaron, H.J., Schwartz, W.B. (1984). *The Painful Prescription: Rationing Hospital Care.* Washington, DC: Brookings Institution.

27. Levinsky, N.G. (2003). Too many patients who are too sick to benefit start chronic dialysis nephrologists need to learn to 'just say no'. *Am. J. Kidney Dis.*, **41**(4): 728–32.

28. Friedman, E.A. (1993). We treat too many dialysis patients but ESRD program is still a success. *Nephrol., News Issues,* **7**: 41–2.

29. Badzek, L.A., Cline, H.S., Moss, A.H., Hines, S.C. (2000). Inappropriate use of dialysis for some elderly patients: nephrology nurses' perceptions and concerns. *Nephrol. Nursing J.,* **27**: 462–70.

30. Moss, A. (2003). Too many patients who are too sick to benefit start chronic dialysis nephrologists need to learn to 'just say no'. *Am. J. Kidney Dis.*, **41**(4): 723–7.

31. Main, J. (2000). Deciding not to start dialysis—a one year prospective study in Teesside. *J. Nephrol.,* **13**(2): 137–41.

32. Hamel, M.B., Phillips, R.S., Davis, R.B., *et al.* (1997). Outcomes and cost-effectiveness of initiating dialysis and continuing aggressive care in seriously ill hospitalized adults. SUPPORT Investigators. Study to Understand Prognoses and Preferences for Outcomes and Risks of Treatments. *Ann. Intern. Med.,* **127**(3): 195–202.

33. Avorn, J., Bohn, R.L., Levy, E., *et al.* (2002). Nephrologist care and mortality in patients with chronic renal insufficiency. *Arch. Intern. Med.,* **162**(17): 2002–6.

34. Khan, I.H., Campbell, M.K., Cantarovich, D., *et al.* (1998). Comparing outcomes in renal replacement therapy: how should we correct for case mix? *Am. J. Kidney Dis.,* **31**(3): 473–8. [Erratum in *Am. J. Kidney Dis.,* **31**(5): 900.]

35. Beddhu, S., Bruns, F.J., Saul, M., Seddon, P., Zeidel, M.L. (2000). A simple comorbidity scale predicts clinical outcomes and costs in dialysis patients. *Am. J. Med.,* **108**(8): 609–13.

36. Fried, L., Bernardini, J., Piraino, B. (2001). Charlson comorbidity index as a predictor of outcomes in incident peritoneal dialysis patients. *Am. J. Kidney Dis.,* **37**(2): 337–42.

37. Chandna, S.M., Schulz, J., Lawrence, C., Greenwood, R.N., Farrington, K. (1999). Is there a rationale for rationing chronic dialysis? A hospital based cohort study of factors affecting survival and morbidity. *Br. Med. J.,* **318**(7178): 217–23.

38. Renal Association (2003). *Treatment of Patients with Renal Failure: Recommended Standards and Audit Measures.* London: Renal Association and Royal College of Physicians.

39. Farmery, E., Milner, P. (1997). *Renal Replacement Therapy: Purchasing Review and Recommendations.* Devizes: Wiltshire Health Authority.

40. Registry of the European Renal Association/European Dialysis and Transplantation Association (2003). www.era-edta-reg.org/

41. Canadian Organ Replacement Register (2002). *2002 Report. Vol 1: Dialysis and Renal Transplantation.* Ottawa: Canadian Institute for Health Information.

42. Disney, A.P.S., Graeme, R. (2001). *Australia and New Zealand Dialysis and Transplant Registry Report 2001.* Adelaide: Australia and New Zealand Dialysis and Transplant Registry.

# Chapter 6

# Health-related quality of life in chronic renal failure

Donna L. Lamping

## 6.1 Introduction

Outcomes in chronic renal failure have traditionally been evaluated using conventional clinical measures such as mortality, morbidity (e.g. access problems, infection), and health service use (e.g. hospitalization, outpatient visits). Although clinical measures provide important information to clinicians and policy-makers, they are often poorly related to patients' reports of health and well-being and do not capture aspects of outcome that are important to patients. This is why there has been increasing interest among patients, clinicians, researchers, policy-makers, and regulators in the evaluation of patient-based outcomes such as quality of life.[1–3]

This chapter provides an overview of quality of life in chronic renal failure from the clinical, research, and policy perspective. We shall begin by defining quality of life and discuss why it has become so important in clinical practice, research, and policy-making. We then discuss measures and methodological challenges in evaluating quality of life and discuss using and choosing measures. Research on health-related quality of life (HRQL) in chronic renal failure is discussed, first by providing an historical overview and then by presenting examples in three areas of research to illustrate the range of studies in this area. Finally, the application of HRQL measures in clinical practice are considered.

## 6.2 What is health-related quality of life?

Patient-based outcomes refer to aspects of subjective well-being that are affected by a condition or its treatment and that can only be assessed by patients themselves: quality of life, health status, symptom distress, disability, patient satisfaction, etc. They are distinct from traditional clinical indicators such as mortality, morbidity, and health service use. Quality of life is one of the most frequently discussed and investigated patient-based outcomes. When talking about quality of life in patients with medical conditions such as chronic renal failure, we generally use the term 'health-related quality of life'. HRQL is different from the broader concept of quality of life in that it includes only those aspects of quality of life that are affected by a health condition. Although there are several similar definitions of the term, there is broad consensus that HRQL refers to a person's subjective perceptions of the impact of a health condition/treatment on different aspects of daily life.[4] This includes the impact of health on well-being in the core areas of physical and mental health, social and role functioning, and general health perceptions. This definition underscores the essential element in any assessment of HRQL—that it is based on a person's own *subjective* evaluation of well-being—and identifies the core or minimum set of concepts that should be included. HRQL may also include other aspects of well-being, such as symptoms, sleep, cognitive functioning, cosmetic appearance, sexual functioning, etc.

HRQL includes both physical and mental components. It is important to differentiate these two components when assessing HRQL so that potential differences in physical and mental HRQL can be evaluated. This is because combining them into a single index may obscure important differences between physical and mental HRQL.

## 6.3 Why the sudden interest in health-related quality of life?

There has been an explosion of interest in HRQL over the last 20 years. In the medical literature, for example, whereas there were only five articles with 'quality of life' as a key reference word in Medline in 1973, this had increased to 1252 articles in 1990–1995.[5] In addition to the growth of research in this area, patient advocacy groups, clinicians, policy-makers, and regulators are demanding that evidence about the impact on HRQL be taken into account when evaluating treatments.[1–3]

There are several reasons why HRQL has become so important in healthcare evaluation in general and in chronic renal failure in particular. First, given the broader definition of health as 'a complete state of physical, mental, and social well-being and not merely the absence of disease or infirmity',[6] any comprehensive evaluation of health outcomes should assess patient-based outcomes in addition to traditional clinical indicators such as mortality and morbidity. Second, because traditional health indicators provide a very limited picture of outcome when evaluating non-curative treatments for chronic diseases, it is important to assess other aspects of outcome that are important to patients. Clinical audit and research in healthcare are now considered inadequate unless the patient's view of treatment outcomes has been assessed, in addition to traditional clinical indicators. Third, there is increased demand for evidence of the cost-effectiveness of new treatments, in which both the costs and benefits—including those to a patient's well-being—must be weighed. Fourth, the evidence-based culture that guides the evaluation of modern healthcare dictates the need for rigorous outcome data based on scientifically robust measuring tools. There is now a plethora of reliable, valid, and responsive measures of HRQL and other patient-based outcomes.[3,7–10]

The clinical relevance of HRQL in chronic renal failure is illustrated in a survey of 533 nephrologists from the UK, Canada, and the USA to examine the criteria for acceptance for dialysis.[11] Nephrologists read five case vignettes and were then asked to indicate whether they would offer dialysis and to rank possible reasons for their choice in order of importance. British and Canadian nephrologists reported their perceptions of patients' HRQL as a reason to provide or not provide dialysis more often than American nephrologists, who offered dialysis more, and ranked patient/family wishes and fear of lawsuit higher, than British or Canadian nephrologists.

HRQL has also been shown to be related to clinically important dialysis outcomes. For example, results from an American study of 1000 haemodialysis patients showed that physical HRQL predicted mortality and hospitalization and, moreover, that HRQL was a better predictor of outcome than diabetes.[12] Similar results were reported in the Netherlands Cooperative Study on Adequacy of Dialysis (NECOSAD) Merkus and colleagues[13] compared 189 patients with good or poor outcome at 12 months (defined on the basis of hospitalizations, serum albumin, physical and mental functioning) and found that HRQL predicted poor outcome. Routine assessment of HRQL in patients with chronic renal failure provides a broader and more comprehensive evaluation of outcome than traditional clinical indicators alone.

# 6.4 Evaluating HRQL

## 6.4.1 Measures of HRQL

There are two main approaches to measuring HRQL:[14] generic and disease-specific measures.

### 6.4.1.1 Generic measures

These include such well-known and widely used measures as the Medical Outcomes Study Short Form-36 (SF-36),[15,16] Nottingham Health Profile (NHP),[17] Sickness Impact Profile (SIP),[18] and the World Health Organization Quality of Life assessment (WHOQOL).[19] Generic measures are applicable across different types of diseases and can therefore be applied to any health condition. The advantage of generic measures is that they allow comparisons across studies of patients with different medical conditions, thereby enabling one to interpret findings about HRQL in a specific patient group in a wider context through comparison with other types of patient. For example, using a generic measure such as the SF-36 allows one to compare HRQL in dialysis patients with patients with other chronic conditions such as cancer, arthritis, cardiovascular disease, etc. This enhances the generalizability of findings about a specific patient group to a wider context.

### 6.4.1.2 Disease-specific measures

These are used to evaluate HRQL in specific conditions such as renal failure, human immuno-deficiency virus/acquired immune deficiency syndrome (HIV/AIDS), hypertension, dementia, etc. The advantage of disease-specific measures is that because they are designed to tap specific areas of the target condition that are not covered in generic measures, they are generally more responsive in detecting clinically important change and/or treatment effects. For example, using a renal-specific measure such as the Kidney Disease Quality of Life Questionnaire (KDQOL)[20] or the Kidney Disease Questionnaire,[21] allows one to assess such renal-specific outcomes as dialysis-related symptoms, staff support and encouragement, etc. This enhances the content validity, relevance, and appropriateness of the HRQL measure for the specific patient group.

## 6.4.2 Challenges in measuring HRQL

### 6.4.2.1 Ensuring scientifically robust measurement

A common misconception is that HRQL is a 'soft' outcome that cannot be rigorously measured. This is an understandable concern, given that HRQL is a much broader and more complex concept than seemingly simple, well-defined clinical outcomes such as death, access problems, and infection. However, rigorous 'gold-standard' scientific methods called psychometrics,[22] borrowed from the social sciences for use in healthcare evaluation,[23] provide well-established methods for measuring subjective judgements using numerical scales and evaluating the quality of measurement scales (i.e. reliability, validity, responsiveness). Rigorous criteria are now available for evaluating the scientific robustness of health outcome measures.[24,25] Measures are only considered scientifically acceptable after they have been put through a comprehensive series of tests to demonstrate that they are reliable, valid, and responsive. These methods allow patient advocacy groups, clinicians, researchers, policy-makers, and regulators to determine whether an instrument is a 'good' measure that provides scientifically credible information.

The use of unvalidated questionnaires to evaluate patient-based outcomes in clinical research can no longer be justified. Tailor-made questionnaires, generally developed using a 'back of the envelope' approach instead of standard psychometric methods, may look appropriate and relevant from a clinical point of view and may even have undergone extensive pilot testing. However, this is no guarantee that the questionnaire is scientifically sound, that is, that patients' responses are unbiased, consistent, and stable and that the questionnaire is measuring what it is intended to measure. There are now a number of gold-standard generic and disease-specific measures available for ensuring scientifically rigorous measurement of HRQL,[3,7–10] including measures developed specifically for use in chronic renal failure.[26,27] The criteria for determining whether a measure is scientifically robust are discussed later.

### 6.4.2.2 Objective versus subjective measures

An unhelpful distinction is sometimes made between 'objective' and 'subjective' measures of HRQL. Referring to a measure as 'objective' has nothing to do with the scientific rigour of an instrument, but erroneously as to whether it is self-completed by the patient (subjective) or observer-rated by a clinician (objective). In the literature on chronic renal failure, many studies that purport to measure HRQL have in fact used the Karnofsky index. The Karnofsky index is a so-called 'objective' measure of physical performance and dependency based on clinician's ratings. The Karnofsky index does not evaluate patients' subjective perceptions or assess psychosocial functioning; it is a measure of functional status not HRQL. Moreover, results from several studies have shown that the Karnofsky index cannot be considered an objective measure, given its poor reproducibility[28] and lack of congruence with several other clinical[29] and patient-based[30] outcomes.

### 6.4.2.3 Weighting scores

It is often assumed that HRQL scores should be weighted in order to reflect differences in how patients rank different domains of HRQL such as physical versus psychological versus social functioning. However, weightings are quite complex and have been shown to be unnecessary. In a study that compared Spitzer QL Index scores with and without ratings of importance in 675 renal patients, weighting scores by personal rating added no benefit to unweighted scores in terms of discrimination, prediction or responsiveness.[31]

## 6.4.3 Choosing and using HRQL measures

The question for potential users of HRQL measures and consumers of HRQL data is how to know whether an instrument is a 'good' measure of HRQL. There are two main criteria to use to judge the appropriateness and scientific rigour of HRQL measures: practical and scientific criteria.

### 6.4.3.1 Practical criteria

From a practical point of view, the measure should be appropriate for use with patients with the specific condition and acceptable to patients and users. That is, the instrument should have been developed and/or validated for use in the specific patient group so that the content is appropriate and relevant to patients with that condition. In addition, the instrument should be feasible for routine use. That is, it should be brief and simple to administer, score and interpret.

## 6.4.3.2 Scientific (psychometric) criteria

In terms of psychometric criteria,[22,23] the measure must be reliable, valid, and responsive or sensitive to change. The availability of population norms helps in interpreting HRQL data by allowing one to compare results from a specific study with results from other patient samples, nationally and internationally. Instruments that have undergone standardized cross-cultural adaptation and translation[32,33] and which are available in validated language versions provide a valuable common metric in international comparisons at the research and/or policy level.

## 6.4.3.3 Which renal-specific HRQL measure to use?

There are several practical and psychometrically sound generic and renal-specific measures for evaluating HRQL. As many of the currently available measures are practically and scientifically equivalent, the question is which one to use. The difficulty of choosing one measure over another is illustrated by findings from two studies. In a study in which 19 different measures were used to assess HRQL in 742 patients, Deniston et al.[34] found that depending on the measure used, there were different conclusions about the relationship between HRQL and demographic characteristics. In a smaller study, Hornberger et al.[35] used six different HRQL measures to assess HRQL in 58 patients and found that the measures were poorly correlated. The Sickness Impact Profile produced scores 20% higher than other methods and, more importantly, differences among measures led to 30% variance in estimated cost-effectiveness ratios. The main requirement is to use a renal-specific measure that is reliable, valid, and responsive. More head-to-head comparisons among measures are needed to evaluate the relative performance of different renal-specific instruments[27] and to determine their relationship to other variables, e.g. medical, treatment-related, and demographic characteristics and other outcome indicators.

# 6.5 HRQL in chronic renal failure

## 6.5.1 Historical overview

The early days of research in this area were generally marked by a doom and gloom view about HRQL in chronic renal failure. The period from 1976 to 1986 has, in fact, been referred to as the 'dark age'.[36] During this time, the potential of renal rehabilitation was seriously questioned. Renal replacement therapy was viewed as merely life-prolonging treatment which was associated with serious complications and poor HRQL. This view was buttressed by findings from two of the earliest and most widely cited studies in this area. In a study of 2481 patients, Gutman et al.[37] found that 40% of patients had not achieved successful rehabilitation and that 40% of non-diabetic patients and 77% of diabetic patients were incapable of a level of physical activity beyond that of caring for themselves. In a subsequent study of 859 patients, Evans et al.[30] found that ESRD patients 'have a poor objective quality of life ... despite the fact that they are enjoying life' compared with the general population. Around the same time, however, there were reports in both the British[38] and the American[39] literature that suggested a more optimistic view.

Research on HRQL in chronic renal failure came to the fore and began to flourish in the 1990s, largely as a result of government quality improvement initiatives in the USA and UK. An influential Institute of Medicine (IOM) report in 1991 led to an IOM sponsored 1993 conference on 'Measuring, Managing and Improving Quality in the ESRD Treatment Setting'.[40] Further developments led to a 1994 IOM workshop 'Assessing Health and Quality of Life

Outcomes in Dialysis'.[27] The task of this 15-member expert panel was to: (i) undertake a critical review of existing HRQL instruments; (ii) consider the use of HRQL assessment to improve care; (iii) develop an agenda for testing and developing measures for routine use; and (iv) develop a database. Based on this extensive review, the expert panel concluded that there are several scientifically validated, clinically useful HRQL instruments that are being used increasingly for routine patient monitoring and management, but no single HRQL instrument can be said to be the best. The panel recommended that more research and experience in clinical settings was needed to determine how to interpret HRQL scores and the relationship between HRQL and other outcomes. The panel also noted a tendency among purchasers of healthcare to overemphasize costs rather than quality in valuing healthcare. There were further developments as a result of a National Institutes of Health 1994 Consensus Conference 'Morbidity and Mortality of Renal Dialysis'[41] about improving the quality of ESRD care. The group highlighted the shift in emphasis from a narrow focus on quality assurance to a more comprehensive assessment of outcomes and processes of care, based on the use of scientifically validated instruments for patient assessment and management in clinical settings. Moreover, the group recommended that the quality of ESRD care should be assessed on the basis of clinical indicators and functional and health status. Other initiatives included the 1997 National Kidney Foundation 'Dialysis Outcomes Quality Initiative Clinical Practice Guidelines', which outlined standards for measuring adequacy of dialysis, management of anaemia, etc.

## 6.5.2 HRQL in dialysis

The availability of scientifically rigorous instruments for assessing HRQL has significantly changed the face of research in this area over the past 15 years. For example, in one of the earliest forays into research on HRQL in dialysis,[42] none of the current gold-standard measures had been developed. As a result, a battery approach was used that included several different, well-established single measures to evaluate specific components of HRQL, such as psychological and social functioning, symptoms, etc. Since then, the development of numerous generic and renal-specific HRQL measures has led to a burgeoning of research on HRQL in chronic renal failure. To illustrate the range of studies in this area, examples in three areas of research on HRQL in chronic renal failure are provided below. Studies have been selected for their policy relevance and methodological rigour.

### 6.5.2.1 HRQL and treatment modality

The majority of studies in this area of research have investigated differences in HRQL among patients undergoing haemodialysis (HD), peritoneal dialysis (PD), including continuous ambulatory peritoneal dialysis (CAPD) and continuous cycling peritoneal dialysis (CCPD), or transplant. A review of studies and UK registry data on survival and HRQL in HD and PD[43] found survival similar in HD and PD patients and better HRQL in home HD and CAPD than centre HD patients. Researchers in The Netherlands[44] used the SF-36 to assess physical and mental HRQL 3 months after the start of dialysis in 120 HD and 106 PD patients in the NECOSAD study. Results showed better mental HRQL in PD than HD patients, but modality explained only 6% of the variance in HRQL scores. One of the largest studies[45] used the SF-36 to assess HRQL in 16 755 HD and 1260 PD (728 CAPD, 532 CCPD) patients. The particular strengths of this study are that it used the current international gold-standard measure to assess physical and mental components of HRQL and included a large sample which allowed adjustment for several case mix variables. Findings showed similar physical and mental HRQL in HD and CAPD patients, similar physical HRQL between HD and PD patients, better mental HRQL in PD than HD patients, and better mental but poorer physical HRQL in CCPD than CAPD or HD patients. Another large study, based on a rigorous meta-analysis of 49 studies, examined differences in HRQL between home and hospital HD, CAPD, and transplant patients.[46] Results showed higher well-being and lower distress in transplant patients than in hospital HD and CAPD patients, higher well-being in CAPD than hospital HD patients, and higher distress in hospital than home HD patients.

Case-mix bias and selection bias are inherent limitations in all observational studies that have investigated differences in outcome by modality, and publication bias may be a problem in meta-analyses. Most studies have, however, examined possible case-mix bias. Publication bias, on the other hand, is difficult to control as negative results are rarely published. Selection bias remains a problem, but because there are no well-controlled, randomized trials of outcomes in HD versus PD, evidence about modality differences in outcome is limited to results from observational studies.

## 6.5.2.2 HRQL in the NECOSAD study

One of the largest programmes of research on HRQL in dialysis has been carried out in a large study in The Netherlands. In the earliest reports from the NECOSAD group, Merkus et al.[44] reported that HRQL in dialysis patients is substantially impaired at 3 months after the start of dialysis compared with the general population. They also found[47] that symptom burden predicted HRQL. Adding symptom burden to clinical and demographic predictors increased the amount of variance explained in physical HRQL from 22% to 39% (HD) and 11% to 39% (PD), and in mental HRQL from 14% to 37% (HD) and 12% to 17% (PD). When the NECOSAD group followed up 230 patients to assess HRQL at 3, 6, 12, and 18 months after the start of dialysis,[48] they found that mental HRQL remained stable but physical HRQL decreased over time (HD advantage). They also found that HRQL in patients who died was lower at baseline and decreased at a faster rate.

## 6.5.2.3 HRQL in elderly people on dialysis

Evidence about patients' HRQL is now a key consideration in developing healthcare policy for renal replacement therapy. Healthcare rationing has become one of the most intensely debated issues in health services worldwide. As one of the more costly health technologies, dialysis features prominently on the rationing agenda. Elderly people with chronic renal failure are particularly vulnerable, as age has been used to ration renal services,[49,50] although not always explicitly. The issue of age rationing in dialysis is a particularly urgent health policy concern in light of the increasing demand for renal replacement therapy for elderly people in the UK and worldwide. This increase is inevitable due to population ageing, the liberalization of acceptance criteria for dialysis, and the age-related increase in the incidence of chronic renal failure.[51]

The arguments for rationing dialysis by age, i.e. that elderly people have poor survival and quality of life, that dialysis is costly, and that older people have a societal obligation to demand less, have been debated extensively.[52,53] However, there is surprisingly little empirical evidence to inform the debate about how elderly people fare on dialysis and to guide decision-making in this area.[54] Although survival is poorer in older than in younger patients, little is known about quality of life and costs to the health service that are associated with reduced life expectancy. To address the need for rigorous evidence to inform decision-making and debate about the effectiveness of dialysis treatment in elderly people, a comprehensive study was carried out of outcomes in 221 elderly people aged 70 years or over on dialysis in the North

Thames Dialysis Study (NTDS).[55] HRQL, hospitalizations, and costs (disease burden) were evaluated in 174 prevalent patients and 1-year survival in 125 incident patients.

Gold-standard generic and renal-specific measures were used to evaluate HRQL in elderly dialysis patients in the NTDS and the findings were compared with elderly people in the general population. Not surprisingly, it was found that physical HRQL in elderly people on dialysis is compromised compared with the general population. Remarkably, however, mental HRQL in elderly people with a chronic life-threatening illness and who are on dialysis was found to be comparable to that of elderly people in the general population. Investigation of modality differences in HRQL showed similar HRQL to that measured by the SF-36 in HD and PD patients at 3, 6, and 12 months.[56] Dialysis-related symptoms/problems, measured by the KDQOL, were lower in PD than HD patients at 3 months but similar at 6 and 12 months.

## 6.6 Applying HRQL in clinical practice

In addition to its numerous applications in research and policy, how is HRQL relevant and useful in clinical practice? One concern of many busy clinicians is that collecting HRQL data is too time-consuming and labour-intensive as time and resources are required to collect, analyse, and report HRQL data. There are several solutions to these practical difficulties. First, the use of less costly postal surveys to collect questionnaire data from patients has proved to be a highly viable option to the more resource-intensive practice of face-to-face administration. In recent studies conducted by postal survey to evaluate patient-based outcomes in prostatectomy[57] and hysterectomy,[58] response rates of 95% and 85% respectively were achieved. Second, there has been a concerted effort among test developers to produce validated short-form versions of standard questionnaires that are often too lengthy for use on a routine basis. Third, many standard questionnaires now include computerized scoring programs that can be easily used in most clinical settings, thus avoiding the time-consuming scoring of questionnaires. Some provide optical scan response sheets to provide a quick option for data entry and computer-generated patient profiles or other graphical summaries of individual and group outcomes. Finally, newer technologies such as the use of touch-screen computerized questionnaires for instantaneous collection, scoring, and analysis of data offer an attractive alternative for routine patient-based outcomes assessment.

Meyer et al.[59] have demonstrated how routine HRQL assessment can be easily incorporated into clinical practice. Nephrologists or nurses/technicians distributed the SF-36 to patients during HD or at routine PD clinic visits. Nurse managers supervised completion of the questionnaires. Based on 496 HRQL assessments, there was only a 5% non-participation rate. The majority of patients (73%) were able to complete the standard self-completion optical-scan version. A further 17% were able to complete the SF-36 using the large-type version, and 10% completed the SF-36 by interview. Most patients (92%) found the SF-36 acceptable (62% excellent, 30% satisfactory). Problems were encountered with a minority of patients (8%); two-thirds of these were due to incomplete questionnaires and one-third to inconsistent responses. Meyer et al. reported that no additional personnel or increase in staffing was required to collect HRQL data. They estimated that 2 h per day for 8 days per year are required for a nurse manager to supervise data collection, 30 min four times per year for a unit administrator to administer the interviewer version, 1-h weekly meetings, and about 20 h four times per year for the audit department to enter data and produce reports.

Meyer et al. discuss some of the potential limitations that need to be considered. First, although language barriers may preclude some patients from participating in HRQL assessments, the increasing availability of validated language versions for measures such as the SF-36[33] makes HRQL measures accessible to more non-English-speaking patients. Second, there is a need for automated methods for scoring data and producing results. The developers of the SF-36 now provide an automated scoring service. Third, more work is needed regarding the clinical interpretation and implications of individual patient results and what HRQL scores mean. Again, there have been major advances in the past few years in this area,[60] with instrument developers putting an increased emphasis on the clinical interpretation of scores.

The main clinical application of HRQL measures is in clinical audit. Routine assessment of HRQL allows clinicians and healthcare managers to evaluate how well patients in their hospital or clinic are doing, based on their own views about their well-being, relative to their performance on other routinely collected indicators of clinical outcome. This provides important additional information about patients' well-being to supplement routine data obtained about mortality, morbidity, and other clinical outcomes. HRQL measures are appropriate for use at the group level, that is, to make inferences and decisions about a group of dialysis patients as a whole based on the average performance for the group. Like most patient-based measures, HRQL measures are not designed for use in decisions about individual patients, as the precision of such instruments is not sufficiently high to make reliable decisions based on the performance of a single individual. However, a great deal of work is currently being done to clarify the interpretation of HRQL scores[60] so that users can be clear, for example, about what a four-point difference on a measures such as the SF-36 means in terms of a patient's actual functional ability.

## 6.7 Summary

HRQL is a key outcome in research, clinical audit, and healthcare policy/decision-making. Rigorous methods, including generic and renal-specific measures that are reliable, valid, responsive, and culturally appropriate, are now available for evaluating HRQL in chronic renal failure. The availability of scientifically rigorous outcome measures, along with the growing emphasis on quality improvement initiatives, has led to the development of a flourishing body of research on HRQL in chronic renal failure, particularly in dialysis. Routine assessment of HRQL in clinical practice allows healthcare professionals to evaluate how well patients are doing, based on their own views about well-being, relative to performance on other routinely collected indicators of clinical outcome, thus allowing the patient's perspective to be included as an integral part of the evaluation of outcomes in chronic renal failure.

## References

1. Fitzpatrick, R., Fletcher, A., Gore, S., Jones, D., Spiegelhalter, D., Cox, D. (1992). Quality of life measures in health care. I: Applications and uses in assessment. *Br. Med. J.*, **305**: 1074–7.

2. Editorial (1995). Quality of life and clinical trials. *The Lancet*, **346**: 1–2.

3. Bowling, A. (2001). *Measuring Disease*, 2nd edn., Buckingham: Open University Press.

4. Bullinger, M., Anderson, R., Cella, D., Aaronson, N. (1993). Developing and evaluating cross-cultural instruments: from minimum requirements to optimal models. *Qual. Life Res.*, **2**: 451–9.

5. Testa, M.A., Simonson, D.C. (1996). Assessment of quality-of-life outcomes. *New Engl. J. Med.*, **334**: 835–40.

6. World Health Organization (1947). The constitution of the World Health Organization. *WHO Chronicles*, **1**: 29.

7. Bowling, A. (1997). *Measuring Health: a Review of Quality of Life Measurement Scales*, 2nd edn. Milton Keynes: Open University Press.

8. Fayers, P.M., Machin, D. (2000). *Quality of Life: Assessment, Analysis and Interpretation.* Chichester: Wiley.

9. McDowell, I., Newell, C. (1996). *Measuring Health: a Guide to Rating Scales and Questionnaires,* 2nd edn. Oxford: Oxford University Press.

10. Wilkin, D., Hallam, L., Doggett, M.A. (1991). *Measures of Need and Outcome for Primary Health Care.* Oxford: Oxford University Press.

11. McKenzie, J.K., Moss, A.H., Feest, T.G., Stocking, C.B., Siegler, M. (1998). Dialysis decision making in Canada, the United Kingdom, and the United States. *Am. J. Kidney Dis.,* **31**: 12–18.

12. DeOreo, P.B. (1997). Hemodialysis patient-assessed functional health status predicts continued survival, hospitalization, and dialysis-attendance compliance. *Am. J. Kidney Dis.,* **30**: 204–12.

13. Merkus, M.P., Jager, K.J., Dekker, F.W., de Haan, R.J., Boeschoten, E.W., Krediet, R.T., for the NECOSAD Study Group (2000). Predictors of poor outcome in chronic dialysis patients: The Netherlands Cooperative Study on the Adequacy of Dialysis. *Am. J. Kidney Dis.,* **35**: 69–79.

14. Patrick, D.L., Deyo, R.A. (1989). Generic and disease-specific measures in assessing health status and quality of life. *Med. Care,* **27**(3): S217–S232.

15. Ware, J.E., Snow, K.K., Kosinski, M., Gandek, B. (1993). *SF-36 Health Survey Manual and Interpretation Guide.* Boston, MA: New England Medical Centre, The Health Institute.

16. Ware, J.E., Kosinski, M., Keller, S.D. (1994). *SF-36 Physical and Mental Health Summary Scales: a User's Manual.* Boston, MA: The Health Institute.

17. Hunt, S.M., McKenna, S.P., McEwan, J., Williams, J., Papp, E. (1981). The Nottingham Health Profile: subjective health status and medical consultations. *Soc. Sci. Med.,* **15A**: 221–9.

18. Bergner, M., Bobbitt, R.A., Carter, W.B., Gibson, B.S. (1981). The Sickness Impact Profile: development and final revision of a health status measure. *Med. Care,* **19**: 787–805.

19. The WHOQOL Group (1998). The World Health Organization Quality of Life assessment (WHOQOL): development and general psychometric properties. *Soc. Sci. Med.,* **46**: 1569–85.

20. Hays, R.D., Kallich, J.D., Mapes, D.L., Coons, S.J., Carter, W.B. (1994). Development of the kidney disease quality of life (KDQOL) instrument. *Qual. Life Res.,* **3**: 329–38.

21. Laupacis, A., Muirhead, N., Keown, P., Wong, C. (1992). A disease-specific questionnaire for assessing quality of life in patients on hemodialysis. *Nephron,* **60**: 302–6.

22. Nunnally, J.C., Bernstein, I.H. (1994). *Psychometric Theory,* 3rd edn. New York: McGraw Hill.

23. Streiner, D.L., Norman, G.R. (1995). *Health Measurement Scales: a Practical Guide to their Development and Use,* 2nd edn. Oxford: Oxford University Press.

24. McDowell, I., Jenkinson, C. (1996). Development standards for health measures. *J. Health Services Res. Policy,* **1**(4): 238–46.

25. Scientific Advisory Committee of the Medical Outcomes Trust (2002). Assessing health status and quality-of-life instruments: attributes and review criteria. *Qual. Life Res.,* **11**: 193–205.

26. Edgell, E.T., Coons, S.J., Carter, W.B., Kallich, J.D., Mapes, D., Damush, T.M., *et al.* (1996). A review of health-related quality-of-life measures used in end-stage renal disease. *Clin. Therapeutics,* **18**: 887–938.

27. Rettig, R.A., Sadler, J.H., Meyer, K.B., Wasson, J.H., Parkerson, G.R., Jr., Kantz, B., *et al.* (1997). Assessing health and quality of life outcomes in dialysis: a report on an Institute of Medicine workshop. *Am. J. Kidney Dis.,* **30**: 140–55.

28. Hutchinson, T.A., Boyd, N.F., Feinstein, A.R. (1979). Scientific problems in clinical scales, as demonstrated in the Karnofsky index of performance status. *J. Chron. Dis.,* **32**: 661–6.

29. Kimmel, P.L., Peterson, R.A., Weihs, K.L., Simmens, S.J., Boyle, D.H., Verme, D., *et al.* (1995). Behavioral compliance with dialysis prescription in hemodialysis patients. *J. Am. Soc. Nephrol.,* **5**: 1826–34.

30. Evans, R.W., Manninen, D.L., Garrison, L.P., Hart, L.G., Blagg, C.R., Gutman, R.A., *et al.* (1985). The quality of life of patients with end-stage renal disease. *New Engl. J. Med.,* **312**: 553–9.

31. Mozes, B., Shabtai, E. (1996). The contribution of personal rating to the clinimetric functioning of a generic quality of life instrument. *J. Clin. Epidemiol.,* **49**: 1419–22.

32. Guillemin, F., Bombardier, C., Beaton, D. (1993). Cross-cultural adaptation of health-related quality of life measures: literature review and proposed guidelines. *J. Clin. Epidemiol.,* **46**: 1417–32.

33. Ware, J.E., Keller, S.D., Gandek, B., Brazier, J.E., Sullivan, M., and the IQOLA Project Group (1995). Evaluating translations of health status questionnaires: methods from the IQOLA Project. *Int. J. Technol. Assessment Health Care,* **11**: 525–51.

34. Deniston, O.L., Carpenter-Alting, P., Kneisley, J., Hawthorne, V.M., Port, F.K. (1989). Assessment of quality of life in end-stage renal disease. *Health Services Res.,* **24**: 555–78.

35. Hornberger, J.C., Redelmeier, D.A., Petersen, J. (1992). Variability among methods to assess patients' well-being and consequent effect on a cost-effectiveness analysis. *J. Clin. Epidemiol.,* **45**: 505–12.

36. Oberley, E.T., Sadler, J.H., Alt, P.S. (2000). Renal rehabilitation: obstacles, progress, and prospects for the future. *Am. J. Kidney Dis.,* **35**(Suppl. 1): S141–S147.

37. Gutman, R.A., Stead, W.W., Robinson, R.R. (1981). Physical activity and employment status of patients on maintenance dialysis. *New Engl. J. Med.,* **304**: 309–13.

38. Editorial (1980). Quality of life in renal failure. *Br. Med. J.,* **281**: 97–8.

39. Johnson, J.P., McCauley, C.R., Copley, J.B. (1982). The quality of life of hemodialysis and transplant patients. *Kidney Int.,* **22**: 286–91.

40. Rettig, R.A., Lohr, K.N. (1994). Measuring, managing, and improving quality in the end-stage renal disease treatment setting: conference overview. *Am. J. Kidney Dis.,* **24**: 228–34.

41. Consensus Development Conference Panel (1994). Morbidity and mortality of renal dialysis: an NIH Consensus Conference statement. *Ann. Intern. Med.,* **121**: 62–70.

42. Maher, B.A., Lamping, D.L., Dickinson, C.A., Murawski, B.J., Olivier, D.C., Santiago, G.C. (1983). Psychosocial aspects of chronic hemodialysis: the National Cooperative Dialysis Study. *Kidney Int.,* **23**(Suppl. 13): S50–S57.

43. Gokal, R., Figueras, M., Olle, A., Rovira, J., Badia, X. (1999). Outcomes in peritoneal dialysis and haemodialysis–a comparative assessment of survival and quality of life. *Nephrol. Dial. Transpl.,* **14**(Suppl. 6): 24–30.

44. Merkus, M.P., Jager, K.J., Dekker, F.W., Boeschoten, E.W., Stevens, P., Krediet. R.T., and the NECOSAD Study Group (1997). Quality of life in patients on chronic dialysis: self-assessment 3 months after the start of treatment. *Am. J. Kidney Dis.,* **29**: 584–92.

45. Diaz-Buxo, J.A., Lowrie, E.G., Lew, N.L., Zhang, H., Lazarus, J.M. (2000). Quality-of-life evaluation using Short Form 36: comparison in hemodialysis and peritoneal dialysis patients. *Am. J. Kidney Dis.,* **35**: 293–300.

46. Cameron, J.I., Whiteside, C., Katz, J., Devins, G.M. (2000). Differences in quality of life across renal replacement therapies: a meta-analytic comparison. *Am. J. Kidney Dis.,* **35**: 629–37.

47. Merkus, M.P., Jager, K.J., Dekker, F.W., de Haan, R.J., Boeschoten, E.W., Krediet, R.T., for the NECOSAD Study Group (1999). Physical symptoms and quality of life in patients on chronic dialysis: results of The Netherlands Cooperative Study on Adequacy of Dialysis (NECOSAD). *Nephrol. Dial. Transpl.,* **14**: 1163–70.

48. Merkus, M.P., Jager, K.J., Dekker, F.W., de Haan, R.J., Boeschoten, E.W., Krediet, R.T., for the NECOSAD Study Group (1999). Quality of life over time in dialysis: The Netherlands Cooperative Study on the Adequacy of Dialysis. *Kidney Int.,* **56**: 720–8.

49. Varekamp, I., Krol, L.J., Danse, J.A.C. (1998). Age rationing for renal transplantation? The role of age in decisions regarding scarce life extending medical resources. *Soc. Sci. Med.,* **47**: 113–20.

50. Mallick, N., El Marasi, A. (1999). Dialysis in the elderly, to treat or not to treat? *Nephrol. Dial. Transpl.,* **14**: 37–9.

51. Roderick, P.J., Ferris, G., Feest, T.G. (1998). The provision of renal replacement therapy for adults in England and Wales: recent trends and future directions. *Q. J. Med.*, **91**: 581–7.

52. Grimley Evans, J. (1997). Rationing health care by age: the case against. *Br. Med. J.*, **314**: 822–5.

53. Williams, A. (1997). Rationing health care by age: the case for. *Br. Med. J.*, **314**: 820–2.

54. Lamping, D.L. (2000). Health-related quality of life in elderly people on dialysis. *Br. J. Renal Med.*, Spring: 21–4.

55. Lamping, D.L., Constantinovici, N., Roderick, P., Normand, C., Henderson, L., Harris, S., et al. (2000). Clinical outcomes, quality of life and costs from the North Thames Dialysis Study of elderly people on dialysis: a prospective cohort study. *The Lancet*, **356**: 1543–50.

56. Harris, S.A.C., Lamping, D.L., Constantinovici, N., Brown, E.A., for the NTDS Group (2002). Clinical outcomes and quality of life in elderly patients on peritoneal dialysis versus haemodialysis. *Periton. Dialysis Int.*, **22**: 463–70.

57. Lamping, D.L., Rowe, P., Black, N., Lessof, L. (1998). Development and validation of an audit instrument: the Prostate Outcomes Questionnaire. *Br. J. Urol.*, **82**: 49–62.

58. Lamping, D.L., Rowe, P., Clarke, A., Black, N., Lessof, L. (1998). Development and validation of the Menorrhagia Outcomes Questionnaire. *Br. J. Obstet. Gynaecol.*, **105**: 766–79.

59. Meyer, K.B., Espindle, D.M., DeGiacomo, J.M., Jenuleson, C.S., Kurtin, P.S., Davies, A.R. (1994). Monitoring dialysis patients' health status. *Am. J. Kidney Dis.*, **24**: 267–79.

60. Ware, J.E., Kosinski, M., Dewey, J.E. (2000). *How to Score Version 2 of the SF-36® Health Survey.* Lincoln, RI: QualityMetric.

# Symptoms of renal disease: dialysis-related symptoms

## Michael Germain and Sharon McCarthy

## 7.1 Introduction

Patients with chronic kidney disease (CKD) are amongst the most symptomatic of any chronic disease group. Prior to dialysis uraemia can affect all organ systems. Pruritus, fatigue, gastrointestinal symptoms, sexual dysfunction, neuropathy, and arthropathy are all common symptoms. Erythropoietin prior to dialysis can improve the fatigue and weakness of early renal failure and on initiation of dialysis it can improve some uraemic symptoms, though distressing ones remain. Experience with daily or nocturnal dialysis has demonstrated a significant reduction in symptoms, and peritoneal dialysis eliminates those that are directly related to haemodialysis such as intradialytic hypotension, vomiting, cramps, and post-dialysis 'washout'. Since 90% of American dialysis patient are on haemodialysis three times a week, these symptoms remain prevalent. Forty per cent of dialysis treatments are complicated by intradialytic symptoms.[1] As CKD patients are often elderly, they also have a high incidence of co-morbid conditions. Over 40% are diabetic and 80% are hypertensive. Cardiomyopathy, severe peripheral vascular disease (PVD), bone disease, skin diseases, arthropathies, and psychiatric conditions are all common co-morbidities that contribute significantly to the symptoms of these patients. In this part of the chapter we discuss treatment of common dialysis-related symptoms.

In a survey involving 80 patients receiving haemodialysis, the majority complained of being fatigued, while more than a third reported insomnia, cramping, and pruritus.[2] Neuropathic symptoms were reported by 29%, while 24% admitted to being of 'poor spirits'. We are unaware of any ongoing, systematically tested symptom-treatment protocols, but we have utilized the protocols listed in Table 7.1 at six dialysis units caring for 650 patients. The protocols are kept in the order book that is used on physician and nurse practitioner rounds. We have also utilized a symptom assessment tool that patients fill out on a weekly basis. The patients rate their symptoms on a scale of 1–10 and note those that are most distressing. It has been difficult to get patients to complete these on a regular basis and to get the physicians to review them.

## 7.2 Intradialytic symptoms

Intradialytic symptoms are those relating directly to the dialysis procedure rather than to the co-morbid conditions suffered by CKD patients; however, those with high co-morbidity have an increase in these symptoms. Approximately 40% of haemodialysis sessions are associated with symptomatic hypotension, cramps, nausea and vomiting, and pruritus. In addition post-dialysis hypotension and a 'washed out' feeling lasting up to 24 h is also common. Those symptoms occurring early in the dialysis are commonly related to a lack of appropriate vasoconstriction, while those occurring later may be related to or caused by the target dry weight being too low. Many of these symptoms are reduced or eliminated by peritoneal dialysis or frequent, slow haemodialysis, such as nocturnal or daily. Shorter dialysis treatments, high-flux dialysis, elderly patients, and high co-morbid burden correlate with increased symptoms on dialysis. The majority of symptomatic treatments occur in a minority of patients who are recurrently symptomatic. Fig 7.1 is an algorithm for the treatment of intradialytic symptoms. The most benign and inexpensive treatments are listed first. Recent studies have supported the value of changes in the dialysis prescription in decreasing intradialytic symptoms. Monitoring blood volume, decreasing the dialysis temperature, and modelling of dialysate sodium and ultrafiltration rates are effective and inexpensive.

## 7.3 Specific symptoms

### 7.3.1 Symptomatic hypotension

Symptomatic hypotension can occur early in dialysis and a trial of low dialysate temperature (36 °C) or isothermic control of the dialysis machine has been shown in a controlled trial to decrease its incidence.[3] If this is ineffective or not tolerated, raising the dialysate sodium with profiling, ultrafiltration profiling, or 'mirroring' the sodium and ultrafiltration profiles can be effective.[4,5,6] Continuous monitoring of the blood volume has also been shown to be effective in preventing symptoms by preventing too rapid or large intravascular volume changes. The addition of biofeedback control of ultrafiltration with volume monitoring has also been used.[1,7] For sudden hypotension thought to be due to loss of autonomic nervous system control, Sertraline 50–100 mg four times a day (q.i.d.) has been preventative.[8,9] Midodrine, an oral alpha adrenergic agonist, 2.5–10 mg pre and mid treatment is also quite effective at preventing hypotension.[10,11] For patients resistant to the above treatments, intravenous carnitine during dialysis has been successful.[12,13]

For patients with symptoms late in the treatment, the problem is usually related to the target dry weight being too low. The dry weight should be raised by 0.5 kg each treatment until the symptoms resolve. Continuous monitoring of blood volume can be quite helpful in determining the correct dry weight.

### 7.3.2 Pruritus

Uraemic pruritus[14–23] is one of the most common and frustrating symptoms experienced by patients with end-stage renal disease (ESRD). Approximately 60% of dialysis patients suffer from it, and it is sometimes worse during the dialysis session. A specific aetiology has not been identified but a number of factors have been shown to contribute to the condition. Secondary hyperparathyroidism,[15] hyperphosphataemia,[18] increased calcium phosphate deposition in the skin, dry skin,[16] inadequate dialysis,[20] anaemia,[21] iron deficiency, and low grade hypersensitivity[22] to products used in the dialysis procedure have all been identified as possible contributory factors to the pruritus seen in the dialysis patient.

#### 7.3.2.1 Management

Patients should be well dialysed with a $Kt/V > 1.2$.[20,24] Compliance with dietary restriction and phosphate-binding therapy should be encouraged and the parathyroid hormone should be kept within the target range of 2–4 times normal[25] with active forms of vitamin D.[17–19] Erythropoietin therapy should be given and optimized according to haematocrit values.[21]

If the patient has xerosis, an emollient such as oatmeal moisturizer, oil, or ammonium lactate cream should be tried. If there is only a partial response, then an emollient with an antipruritic such as doxepin cream could be used.[16] If pruritus occurs only during dialysis, the formulation of heparin could be changed to the beef type, Some patient are allergic to the type of membrane and other types can be substituted.[22] Thus, if an ethylene oxide sterilized dialysis membrane is used, it could be changed to a gamma-irradiated membrane.

If pruritus continues sequential 2-week trials of the following can be tried:

- Oral antihistamine therapy is inexpensive and safe so should be tried first, though there is not much evidence to support its efficacy.[23]
- Phototherapy with UVB ultraviolet light three times weekly is quite effective but is inconvenient.[19]
- A trial of naltrexone has been shown to be effective in small controlled trials.[26]
- If the naltrexone interferes with opioids for pain or is not tolerated by patient, capsaicin cream 2–4 times a day can be tried.[27]
- Ketotifen, a mast cell stabilizer, 2 mg twice a day (b.d.)[28] or ondansetron, a 5-hydroxytryptamine 3 (5-HT$_3$) antagonist, 4 mg b.d.[29] have been found to be effective in limited trials.
- Colestyramine 5 mg b.d.[30] or activated charcoal 6 g per day in 4–6 divided doses for 8 weeks,[31] is effective but can interfere with absorption of other medications
- Intravenous lidocaine (100 mg) during dialysis is reserved for severe and refractory cases[32] as it can be associated with seizures.
- Thalidomide 100 mg at bedtime has been shown to be effective in a randomized trial with refractory pruritus in dialysis patients, though care must be taken in handling pills and avoiding exposure to pregnant women.[33]

## 7.3.3 Anorexia

Nutrition is a major problem in dialysis patients and anorexia is common. It is a non-specific symptom that may be an indication of inadequate dialysis and uraemia. There are many other causes, however, including anaemia, depression, and taste disorders, embracing a dry mouth and mechanical causes. Many gastrointestinal problems can contribute to anorexia such as nausea, constipation, diarrhoea, and diabetic gastroparesis. Anorexia and resulting poor nutrition are also common in patients with other co-morbidities and in the elderly.

### 7.3.3.1 Management

The first step is to make sure that the patient is well dialysed (a $Kt/V$ of at least 1.2) and that any anaemia has been treated adequately with erythropoietin; Antidepressants should be considered if appropriate. If nausea is present, then an antiemetic should be offered. Other disorders should be treated appropriately.

Taste disorders are common in patients on dialysis and can lead to anorexia; assuming the patient does not have sinusitis, zinc deficiency should be considered and a trial of oral zinc (220 mg daily) should be given.[34] A dry mouth is also very common in dialysis patients. The first step is to review medication and reduce, if possible, any drug contributing to it, such as clonidine (an antihypertensive central adrenergic blocker), compazine, (a phenothiazine), or tricyclic antidepressants such as amitriptyline, and discontinue any that are no longer necessary.

A saliva substitute, every 1–2 h, or a saliva stimulant such as pilocarpine 5–10 mg three times per day (t.i.d.) can be helpful.[35] Finally a trial of appetite stimulants such as megestrol 40–400 mg,[36–38] dronabinol 2.5–5 mg 2–3 times a day,[39] or prednisone 10–20 mg 1–2 times a day have been used.

## 7.3.4 Constipation

Constipation is a common complaint in the dialysis patient and is multifactorial in origin. The dietary restriction of high potassium fruits and vegetables decreases the fibre content of food ingested. Fluid restriction, physical inactivity, and medications such as aluminium and calcium phosphate binders, iron supplements, and opioids can all contribute to constipation.[40]

### 7.3.4.1 Management

Important steps include an attempt to increase dietary fibre and encourage regular exercise. Often a combination of A stool softener such as docusate or lactulose, or polyethylene glycolate needs to be combined with a stimulant laxative like bisacodyl or casanthranol to be effective. These are all safe in dialysis patients, but those containing magnesium, citrate, or phosphate should be avoided in ESRD patients.

## 7.3.5 Cramps

Cramps are a common complaint amongst patients on haemodialysis and are especially frequent during dialysis, particularly if large amounts of fluid have to be removed.

### 7.3.5.1 Management

Prevention may be easier than treatment. The use of dialysate with appropriate sodium and potassium levels will help as can sodium modelling. This can be accomplished without post-dialysis thirst[6] by starting with a high dialysate sodium (150–155 milliequivalents/litre (meq/l)), then using a programmed linear or step decrease to 135–140 meq/l at the end of treatment. To prevent cramps with quinine use 260–325 mg PO prior to symptoms, i.e. before dialysis or sleep; the dose should not exceed three doses per day.[41]

If quinine is ineffective vitamin E, 400 IU by mouth (PO) per day, or oxazepam, 5–10 mg 2 h before dialysis, could be tried. If cramping continues then consider adding carnitine 1000–2000 mg intravenously (IV) during dialysis for a 3-month trial.[42]

It is important to assess dry weight frequently to prevent patients going below that estimated for them. Also they should be encouraged to adhere to fluid restrictions to prevent large intra-dialytic fluid gains.[43,44] In order to abort a cramp during dialysis administer hypertonic (23.4%) saline 5–20 ml over 3–5 min; hypertonic (50%) glucose (50 ml) may be preferred in non-diabetics since it will not cause post-dialysis thirst.[45] Practical measures that can be helpful in the prevention of cramps include stretching of the affected muscle, for example through dorsiflexion of the foot, either manually or by standing, and the application of heat to the muscle group.[45]

## 7.3.6 Insomnia

Problems of sleep disturbance have been reported by 50% to 90% of dialysis patients surveyed.[46–50] Research has also shown that these patients have a high incidence of specific primary sleep disorders such as sleep apnoea syndrome,[49,50] periodic leg movement disorder, and restless legs syndrome.

### 7.3.6.1 Management

A complete history and physical examination should be performed to assess for signs of sleep apnoea or restless legs syndrome. If these conditions are suspected the patient should be referred for diagnostic sleep studies. In addition it may be necessary for the patient to first make the following lifestyle changes to achieve improved sleep. The avoidance of caffeinated beverages after noon and the limitation of these to no more than two cups per day, not to smoke just before bedtime or during the night, the avoidance of alcoholic beverages in the evening, and not to nap during the day. If sleep apnoea has been excluded a hypnotic can be prescribed. As this may be a long-term measure, drugs with a short duration of action and reduced potential for addiction should be considered first with attention to sleep hygiene concomitantly: zolpidem 5–10 mg at bedtime (q.h.s.), temazepam 7.5–30 mg q.h.s., flurazepam 15–30 mg q.h.s., and triazolam 0.125–0.25 mg q.h.s. are generally safe in dialysis patients.

## 7.3.7 Lethargy

Persistent fatigue as well as post-dialysis fatigue have been attributed to a number of causes including the rapid osmotic changes of the extracellular fluid space during haemodialysis, depletion of specific substances such as carnitine, ultrafiltration and its effect on blood pressure, blood membrane interactions, depression, insomnia, poor nutrition, anaemia, and medication.[51–55]

### 7.3.7.1 Management

Lethargy is one of the most difficult symptoms to help; it is important to exclude and treat any potentially treatable condition that may be contributing to it, while seeking realistic goals with the patient. Thus it will be important to manage insomnia effectively if possible. The patient should be well dialysed ($Kt/V$ of at least 1.2) and the haemoglobin (Hb) kept between 11 and 12 g/dl, while considering a trial of a higher level to see if that improves the situation. At the same time, any depression or hypotension should be treated. Lack of activity can lead to further lethargy, so it is important to encourage activity and regular exercise during the day.[56] If the patient is deconditioned they may be helped by inpatient or home physical therapy.[56] Poor nutrition[57] may contribute to a feeling of lethargy, so it is important to encourage adequate nutritional intake. A course of megestrol acetate with protein supplements[58] may be helpful in patients who are clinically malnourished. A review of medication should be undertaken with the aim of reducing, stopping, or substituting any that may be contributing to the tiredness.[46] If the lethargy is severe and having a large impact on quality of life the use of a psychostimulant such as ritalin10 mg in the morning and at noon could be considered.[59] Carnitine 10 mg/kg IV after each dialysis treatment has been used, but convincing evidence of its efficacy is lacking.[13]

## 7.3.8 Neuropathy

Uraemic neuropathy is a mixed motor and sensory polyneuropathy that is distal and symmetrical.[60] It was common years ago due to thiamine deficiency, as the vitamin is well dialysed. Since the routine of replacing water-soluble vitamins in dialysis patients this is now rarely a cause of neuropathy.[61] Currently the condition is attributed to one or more toxins retained in uraemia and not adequately removed by dialysis.[62]

### 7.3.8.1 Management

Strategies aimed at prevention include ensuring that the patient is adequately dialysed with a $Kt/V$ of at least 1.2 with a high-flux membrane to ensure good middle-molecule clearance.[63]

It is of course important to ensure that the patient is not thiamine deficient. Symptom management is as for neuropathic pain and may include the use of tricyclic antidepressants such as amitriptyline 25–100 mg/day,[64] though side-effects may limit its use, or gabapentin, an anticonvulsant, licensed for this use in the UK. If gabapentin is used it should be started at a low dose (100 mg every other day (q.o.d.)) in renal patients since it is excreted unchanged by the kidney and accumulates in renal failure with the result that sedation is common. It is necessary to titrate to maximum dose of 100–300 mg three times a day (t.i.d).[65] Carbamazepine may also be tried starting at a dose of 100 mg twice a day (b.d)., gradually increasing in increments of 100 mg b.d. to a maximum of 400–800 mg daily; alternatively blood levels can be monitored.[66]

## 7.3.9 Restless legs syndrome

The prevalence of uraemia-associated restless legs syndrome (RLS) is estimated to be between 20% and 40% and it is unclear to what extent this condition is related to uraemic neuropathy.[67,68] Anaemia, low serum ferritin levels, low serum levels of parathyroid hormone, and inadequate dialysis are also associated with the presence of RLS in dialysis patients.[69]

### 7.3.9.1 Management

Preventive treatment is aimed at ensuring adequate dialysis,[69,70] avoiding medication that may be aggravating the condition, such as tricyclic antidepressants, lithium, neuroleptics, and caffeine,[71] and treating any contributing conditions. Thus one should treat anaemia with erythropoietin,[72,73] and low ferritin levels with iron replacement.[69–71,74] If the above treatments are inadequate then a trial of benzodiazepines such as clonazepam 0.5–2.0 mg q.h.s., temazepam 7.5–3.0 mg q.h.s., or triazolam 0.125–0.5 mg q.h.s., as needed,[75] is usually well tolerated in dialysis patients and may be effective. If not one can consider trying a dopaminergic agent such as Carbidopa/Levodopa[76,77] either as a regular formulation of 12.5/50–75/300 mg in divided doses through the day and at bedtime or a sustained release 25/100 to 100/400 mg as a next step. Newer agents such as pergolide 0.10–1.00 mg q.h.s.[78] may also be effective. Other drugs that can be used include bromocriptine 2.5 to 20.0 mg, gabapentin,[79] and clonidine 0.1 to 1.0 mg daily.[80] In resistant and severe cases an opioid has been shown to be quite effective.[81] Patients commonly become resistant to any of these agents, due to tachyphylaxis, and require an escalation of dose. After 3 to 4 months the patient should be rotated to a different agent; they will typically then respond to the first agent again at the initial lower dose. Furthermore RLS is associated with anxiety and stress;[82] perhaps because it is multifactorial it can be very difficult to treat effectively.

## 7.3.10 Nausea and vomiting

There are numerous possible causes of nausea and vomiting in the dialysis patient; it may be a manifestation of uraemia, fluid and electrolyte changes, or hypotension during the dialysis procedure.[40] Alternatively co-morbid conditions or side-effects from other medication may contribute significantly to the symptoms.

### 7.3.10.1 Management

Initial management is to and ensure adequate dialysis (equilibrated $Kt/V$ ($eKt/V$) > 1.2) and to treat any associated hypotensive episode. It then helps to try to postulate the cause and choose an antiemetic from the appropriate group. Thus if the nausea and vomiting is due to gastroparesis, metoclopramide in a small starting dose (5 mg b.d.) with similar increments until results are seen should be tried. Uraemia and some drugs, such as the opioids may stimulate the area postrema (chemoreceptor trigger zone), in which case dopamine receptor antagonists such as haloperidol are likely to be effective. More broad-spectrum antiemetics include: prochloperazine 5–10 mg PO, IM, IV t.i.d. prn, 25 mg PR t.i.d. prn, trimethobenzamide 250 mg PO, 3–4 times daily, PR, IM 200 mg 3–4 times daily, or promethazine 25 mg PO, PR q.i.d. prn. In resistant cases chlorpromazine 10–25 mg PO t.i.d prn, 25 mg PR t.i.d. prn, 25–50 mg IM t.i.d. prn can be used with caution, though this may be very sedating. There is evidence for the use of 5-HT$_3$ antagonists such as ondansetron in anaesthetic-induced vomiting and that induced by radiation and chemotherapy; however, their use empirically in other situations may be effective and is safe in this population (see also Chapter 8)

## 7.4 Conclusion

It can be seen that unpleasant symptoms are common and can be very troublesome for patients, having a significant impact on their quality of life. The myriad of treatments demonstrates the lack of non-toxic, effective, evidence-based treatments for many situations. Here, as in all areas of medicine, it is essential to make a full assessment of the symptom and its effect on the patient's functioning and quality of life as this will guide the physician in determining how aggressive the treatment should be. All new drug regimens should be vigorously monitored for efficacy and toxicity; those which are ineffective or have unacceptable side-effects should be discontinued before considering an alternative. It remains important not to replace one symptom with another, e.g. treating neuropathic pain with amitriptyline and then precipitating RLS. This necessitates a frequent review of medication. Listening to a patient and acknowledging their distress are also important parts of the prescription, which if attended to by the physician will affirm the patient's worth and contribute to the therapeutic environment.

## Case study 1

Mr P is an 92-year-old Italian–American male. He is a retired businessman who presented 5 years ago with a glomerular filtration rate (GFR) of 14 ml/min. He had known ischaemic cardiomyopathy with a left ventricular ejection fraction (LVEF) of 25%. The complaint that caused him most distress was pruritus. It was resistant to antihistamines and moisturizing creams. UVB light treatments ultimately provided relief. At the time of presentation erythropoietin was prescribed for fatigue and a Hb of 9 gm/dl. Four years ago, haemodialysis was begun when the GFR dropped below 10 ml/min.

Throughout the last 4 years on dialysis the patient suffered from restless legs syndrome, post-dialysis hypotension, and fatigue particularly for the 24 h post-dialysis. Recently severe back pain secondary to osteoarthritis has plagued him. His symptoms were controlled with supportive treatments. He has remained at home with his wife with no hospitalizations during this period until this last time, when he fell at home requiring a brief hospitalization and rehabilitation stay. The patient, his wife, and daughters were aware of the option of withdrawal of dialysis from the first meeting with the nephrologists 5 years ago. This was rediscussed at the time of the last hospitalization. Initially he chose to remain on dialysis; he did not qualify for hospice coverage while remaining on dialysis because his LVEF was >20%. One week later the patient decided to stop dialysis: in his word 'I have had enough'. He went home with hospice care and 4 days later died in no discomfort with his wife, daughters, and nephrologist present. Minutes prior to his death he was reminiscing about his life and looking at old photographs, this was his 92nd birthday. He had missed only two dialysis treatments.

## Ethical analysis of Case 1

Mr P is an elderly hemodialysis patient with at least one major comorbidity, congestive heart failure. His long-term prognosis is poor. The USRDS 2002 Annual Report lists 1.6 years as the average mean survival for a male patient starting dialysis who is over the age of 85 years. Following recommendation 3 in the Renal Physicians Association/American Society of Nephrology (RPA/ASN) guidelines, the nephrologist estimated prognosis and informed the patient and family of the option of stopping dialysis when the patient deemed his quality of life unsatisfactory. Having established that the patient wants to start dialysis, the ethical question for the nephrologist is 'What should I do?' Ethically speaking, there are two general things the nephrologist should do: manage the patient's pain and symptoms well and engage the patient in advance care planning. In the latter regard, exploring spiritual issues— those that concern life's ultimate meaning and value—would be very helpful. In a patient with a limited prognosis, the nephrologist provides an important service to the patient and family by assisting them to determine how to best make use of their remaining time together. To do so, the nephrologist should ask questions such as 'What do you still want to accomplish during your life?', 'What might be left undone if you were to die today?', 'Given that your time is limited, what legacy do you want to leave to your family?', 'Is faith important to you in this illness?', 'Do you have someone to talk to about spiritual matters?'. These are spiritual questions that are appropriate for the end of life. The nephrologist can prepare Mr P and his family for the final stage of his life and help them to receive the comfort and support they need.

The nephrologist caring for Mr P communicated well with him and his family, because at the end of life after a rehospitalization, the patient was able to say he had 'had enough'. He received hospice care at home, and in his final minutes, he was working on life closure by reviewing old photographs and reminiscing. This case demonstrates the best aspects of recommendation 9 in the RPA/ASN guidelines; the patient was helped to have a comfortable, peaceful, and reconciled death at home.

## References

1. Santoro, A., Mancini, E., Basile, C., Amoroso, L., Di Giulio, S., Usberti, M., *et al.* (2002). Blood volume controlled hemodialysis in hypotension-prone patients: a randomized, multicenter controlled trial. *Kidney Int.,* **62**(3): 1034–45.

2. Cohen, L.M., Germain, M.J. (2003). Palliative and supportive care. In: *Therapy of Nephrology and Hypertension: a Companion to Brenner's The Kidney*, 2nd edn, ed. H.R. Brady, and C.S. Wilcox, pp. 753–6. Philadelphia, PA: Elsevier Science.

3. http://www.kidney.org/professionals/doqi/guidelines/doqiuphd_vi.html#16

4. Maggiore, Q., Pizzarelli, F., Santoro, A., *et al.* (2002). The effects of control of thermal balance on vascular stability in hemodialysis patients: results of the European randomized clinical trial. *Am. J. Kidney Dis.,* **40**(2): 280–90.

5. Staver, B., De Vries, P.M., Donker, A.J., Ter Wee, P.M., (2002). The effect of profiled haemodialysis on intradialytic hemodynamics when a proper sodium balance is applied. *Blood Purif.,* **20**(4): 364–9.

6. Song, J.H., Lee, S.W., Suh, C.K., Kim, M.J. (2002). Time-averaged concentration of dialysate sodium relates with sodium load and interdialytic weight gain during sodium-profiling hemodialysis. *American Journal of Kidney Diseases.,* **40**(2): 291–301.

7. Sherman, R.A. (2002). Intradialytic hypotension: an overview of recent, unresolved and overlooked issues [review]. *Semin. Dial.,* **15**(3): 141–3.

8. Dheenan, S., Venkatesan, J., Grubb, B.P., Henrich, W.L. (1998). Effect of sertraline hydrochloride on dialysis hypotension. *Am. J. Kidney Dis.,* **31**(4): 624–30.

9. Perazella, M.A. (2001). Pharmacologic options available to treat symptomatic intradialytic hypotension [review]. *Am. J. Kidney Dis.*, **38**(4)(Suppl. 4): S26–S36.

10. Cruz, D.N., Mahnensmith, R.L., Perazella, M.A. (1997). Intradialytic hypotension: is midodrine beneficial in symptomatic hemodialysis patients? *Am. J. Kidney Dis.*, **30**: 772.

11. Flynn, J.J., Mitchell, M.C., Caruso, F.S., McElligott, M.A. (1996). Midodrine treatment for patients with hemodialysis hypotension. *Clin. Nephrol.*, **45**: 261.

12. Riley, S., Rutherford, S., Rutherford, P.A. (1997). Low carnitine levels in hemodialysis patients: relationship with functional activity status and intra-dialytic hypotension. *Clin. Nephrol.*, **48**: 3.

13. Garabed, E., Latos, D., Linberg, J. (2003). Practice recommendations for the use of L-carnitine in dialysis related carnitine disorders. National Kidney Foundation Carnitnine Consensus Conference. *Am. J. Kidney Dis.*, **41**(4): 868–76.

14. Mettang, T., Fritz, P., Weber, J., *et al.* (1990). Uraemic prutitius in patients on hemodialysis or continuous ambulatory peritoneal dialysis: the role of plasma histamine and skin mast cells. *Clin. Nephrol.*, **34**: 136.

15. Hampers, C.L., Katz, A.I., Wilson, R.E., Merrill, J.P. (1968). Disappearance of uraemic itching after subtotal parathyroidectomy. *New Engl. J. Med.*, **279**: 695.

16. Cawley, I.P., Hoch-Ligeti, C., Bond, G.M. (1961). The eccrine sweat glands of patients in uremia. *Arch. Dermatol.*, **84**: 51.

17. Massry, S.G., Popovtzer, M.M., Coburn, J.W., *et al.* (1968). Intractable pruritus as a manifestation of secondary hyperparathyroidism in uremia. *New Engl. J. Med.*, **279**: 697.

18. Parfitt, A.M., Massry, S.G., Winfield, A.C., *et al.* (1971). Disordered calcium and phosphorus metabolism during maintenance hemodialysis. *Am. J. Med.*, **51**: 319.

19. Blachley, J.D., Blankenship, M., Menter, A., *et al.* (1985). Uremic pruritus: skin divalent ion content and response to ultraviolet therapy. *Am. J. Kidney Dis.*, **5**: 237.

20. Hiroshige, K., Kabashima, N., Takasugi, M., Kuroiwa, A. (1995). Optimal dialysis improves uremic pruritus. *Am. J. Kidney Dis.*, **25**: 413–19.

21. De Marchi, S., Ceddhin, E., Villaltgra, D. *et al.* (1992). Relief of pruritus and decreases in plasma histamine concentrations during erythropoietin therapy in patients with uremia. *New Engl. J. Med.*, **326**: 969.

22. Kessler, M., Moneret-Vautrin, D.A., Cao-Huu, T., *et al.* (1992). Dialysis pruritus and sensitization. *Nephron*, **12**: 330.

23. Robertson, K., Mueller, B. (1996). Uremic pruritus. *Am. J. Health-Syst. Pharm.*, **53**: 2159.

24. http://www.kidney.org/professionals/doqi/guidelines/doqiuphd_ii.html#4

25. http://www.kidney.org/professionals/doqi/bonemeta.cfm

26. Peer, G., Kivity, S., Agami, O., *et al.* (1996). Randomised crossover trial of naltrexone in uraemic pruritus. *The Lancet.*, **348**: 1552.

27. Tarng, D.C., Cho, Y.L., Liu, N.H., Huang, T.P. (1996). Hemodialysis-related pruritus: a double-blind, placebo-controlled, crossover study of capsaicin 0.025% cream. *Nephron* **72**: 617.

28. Francos, G., Kauh, V., Grittlen, S. (1991). Elevated plasma histamine in chronic uremia: effects of ketotifen on pruritus. *Int. J. Dermatol.*, **30**: 884.

29. Balaskas, E., Bamihas, G., Karamouzis, M., *et al.* (1998). Histamine and serotonin in uremic pruritis: effect of ondansetron in CAPD-pruritic patients. *Nephron*, **78**: 395.

30. Silverberg, D., Ianina, A., Reisin, E. (1997). Cholestryramine in uraemic pruritus. *Br. Med. J.*, **1**: 752.

31. Giovanetti, S., Barsotti, G., Cupisti, A. (1995). Oral activated charcoal in patients with uremic pruritus. *Nephron*, **70**: 193.

32. Tapia, L., Cheigh, H., David, D. (1977). Pruritis in dialysis patients treated with parenteral lidocaine. *New Engl. J. Med.*, **296**: 261.

33. Silva, S.R.B., Vianna, P.C.F., Lagon, N.V., *et al.* (1994). Thalidomide for the treatment of uremic pruritis: a crossover randomized double-blind trial. *Nephron*, **67**: 270–4.

34. Vreman, H.J., Venter, C., Leegwater, J., Oliver, C., Weiner, M.W. (1980). Taste, smell and zinc metabolism in patients with chronic renal failure. *Nephron*, **26**: 163.

35. Miller, L.J. (1993). Oral pilocarpine for radiation-induced xerostomia. *Cancer Bull.*, **45**: 549.

36. Lien, Y.H., Ruffenach, S.J. (1996). Low dose megestrol increases serum albumin in malnourished dialysis patients. *Int. J. Artificial Organs*, **19**: 147.

37 Boccanfuso, J.A., Hutton, M., McAllister, B. (2000). The effects of megestrol acetate on nutritional parameters in a dialysis population. *J. Renal Nutrition*, **10**: 36.

38. Bruera, E., Macmillan, K., Kuehn, N., Hanson, J., *et al.* (1990). A controlled trial of megestrol acetate on appetite, caloric intake, nutritional status, and other symptoms in patients with advanced cancer. *Cancer*, **66**: 1279.

39. Beal, J.E., Olson, R., Laubenstgein, L., *et al.* (1995). Dronabinol as a treatment for anorexia associated with weight loss in patients with AIDS. *J. Pain Symptom Manag.*, **10**: 89.

40. Lew, S.Q., Albertini, B., Bosch, J.P. (2000). The digestive tract. In: *Handbook of Dialysis*, ed. J.T. Daugirdas, P.G. Blake, T.S. Ing, p. 601. Philadelphia, P.A., Lippincott, Williams & Wilkins.

41. Kaju, D.M., Ackad, A., Nottage, W.L., Stein, K.M., *et al.* (1976). Prevention of muscle cramps in haemodialysis patients by quinine sulphate. *The Lancet*, **2**: 66–7.

42. Ahmad, S., Robertson, H.T., Golper, T.A., *et al.* (1990). Multicenter trial of L-carnitine in maintenance hemodialysis patients. Clinical and biochemical effects. *Kidney Int.*, **38**: 912–18.

43. Daugirdas, J.T. (2000). Acute hemodialysis prescription. In: *Handbook of Dialysis*, 3rd edn, ed. J.T. Daugirdas, and T.S. Ing, pp. 192–220. Philadelphia, P.A., Lippincott, Williams & Wilkins.

44. Canzanello, B.J., Burkart, J.M. (1992). Hemodialysis associated muscle cramps. *Semin. Dialysis*, **5**: 299.

45. Sherman, R.A., Goodling, K.A., Eisinger, R.P., *et al.* (1982). Acute therapy of hemodialysis related muscle cramps. *Am. J. Kidney Dis.*, **8**: 287.

46. Holley, J.L., Nespor, S., Rault, R. (1992). A comparison of reported sleep disorders in patients on chronic hemodialysis and continuous peritoneal dialysis. *Am. J. Kidney Dis.*, **14**: 156.

47. Walker, S., Fine, A., Kryger, M.H. (1995). Sleep complaints are common in a dialysis unit. *Am. J. Kidney Dis.*, **28**: 372.

48. Kimmel, P.L., Miller, G., Mendelson, W.B. (1989). Sleep apnea in chronic renal disease. *Am. J. Med.*, **86**: 308.

49. Mendelson, W.B., Wadhwa, N.K., Greenberg, H.E., Gujavarty, K., Bergofsky, E. (1990). Effects of hemodialysis on sleep apnea syndrome in end-stage renal disease. *Clin. Nephrol.*, **33**: 247.

50. Pressman, M.R., Benz, R.L., Peterson, D.D. (1995). High incidence of sleep disorders in end-stage renal disease patients. *Sleep Res.*, **25**: 321.

51. Sklar, A., Riesenberg, L.A., Silber, A.K., Ahmed, W., *et al.* (1996). Postdialysis fatigue. *Am. J. Kidney Dis.*, **28**: 732.

52. Sklar, A., Newman, N., Scott, R., Semenyuk, L., *et al.* (1999). Identification of factors responsible for postdialysis fatigue. *Am. J. Kidney Dis.*, **34**: 464.

53. Robertson, H., Kaky, N., Gurthrie, M., Cardenas, D., *et al.* (1990). Recombinant erythropoietin improves exercise capacity in anemic hemodialysis patients. *Am. J. Kidney Dis.*, **4**: 325.

54. Brass, E., Adler, M., Sietsema, M., Hiatt,W. (2001). Intravenous L-carnitine increases plasma carnitine, reduces fatigue, and may preserve exercise capacity in hemodialysis patients. *Am. J. Kidney Dis.*, **37**: 1018.

55. Wuerth, D., Finkelstein, S., Ciarcia, M., Peterson, R., *et al.* (2001). Identification and treatment of depression in a cohort of patients maintained on chronic peritoneal dialysis. *Am. J. Kidney Dis.*, **37**: 1011.

56. Kouidi, E.J. (2001). Central and peripheral adaptations to physical training in patients with end-stage renal disease. *Sports Med.,* **31**: 651.

57. Sobh, M., Hussein, S., Tantawy, A., Ghoneim, M. (1998). Study of effect of optimization of dialysis and protein intake on neuromuscular function in patients under maintenance hemodialysis treatment. *Am. J. Nephrol.,* **18**: 399.

58. Johansen, K., Mulligan, K., Schambelan, M. (1999). Anabolic effects of nandrolone decanoate in patients receiving dialysis. *J. Am. Med. Assoc.,* **281**: 1275.

59. Breitbart, W., Rosenfeld, B., Kaim, M., Funesti-Esch, J. (2001). A randomized, double-blind, placebo-controlled trial of psychostimulants for the treatment of fatigue in ambulatory patients with human immunodeficiency virus disease. *Arch. Intern. Med.,* **161**: 411.

60. Fraser, C.L., Arieff, A.I. (1988). Nervous system complications in uraemia. *Ann. Intern. Med.,* **109**: 143.

61. Hung, S.C., Hung, S.H., Tarng, D.C., *et al.* (2001). Chorea induced by thiamine deficiency in hemodialysis patients. *Am. J. Kidney Dis.,* **37**: 4127.

62. Lindsay, R.M., Bolton, C.F., Clark, W.F., *et al.* (1983). The effect of alterations of uraemic retention products upon platelet and peripheral nerve function. *Clin. Nephrol.,* **19**: 110.

63 Tattersall, J.E., Cramp, M., Shannon, M., Farrington, K., Greenwood, R.N. (1992). Rapid high-flux dialysis can cure uraemic peripheral neuropathy. *Nephrol. Dial. Transpl.,* **7**: 539.

64. Portenoy, R.K. (1993). Adjuvant analgesics in pain management. In: *Oxford Textbook of Palliative Medicine,* ed. D. Doyle, G.W. Hanks, and N. MacDonald, pp. 187–203. New York: Oxford University Press.

65. Rose, M.A., Kam, P.C. (2002). Gabapentin: pharmacology and its use in pain management. *Anaesthesia,* **158**: 451.

66. Covington, E.C. (1998). Anticonvulsants for neuropathic pain and detoxification. *Cleve. Clin. J. Med.,* **65**: 121.

67. Callaghan, N. (1966). Restless legs syndrome in uraemic neuropathy. *Neurology,* **16**: 359.

68. Walker, S., Fine, A., Kryger, M.H. (1995). Sleep complaints are common in a dialysis unit. *Am. J. Kidney Dis.,* **26**: 751.

69. Collado-Seidel, V., Kohnen, R., Samtleben, W., *et al.* (1998). Clinical and biochemical findings in uremic patients with and without restless legs syndrome. *Am. J. Kidney Dis.,* **31**: 132.

70. Winkelman, J.W., Cherow, G.M., Lazarus, J.M. (1996). Restless legs syndrome in end-stage renal disease. *Am. J. Kidney Dis.,* **28**: 372.

71. Hening, W.A. (1997). Therapeutic approaches to restless legs syndrome and periodic limb movement disorder. *Hospital Med.,* **33**: 135.

72. Harris, D.C., Chapman, J.R., Stewart, K.H. *et al.* (1991). Low dose erythropoietin in maintenance haemodialysis: improvement in quality of life and reduction in true cost of haemodialysis. *Aust. NZ J. Med.,* **21**: 693.

73. Roger, S.D., Harris, D.C.H., Stewart, J.H. (1991). Possible relation between restless legs and anaemia in renal dialysis patients. *The Lancet* **337**: 1551.

74. O'Keefe, S.T., Gavin, K., Lavan, J.N. (1994). Iron status and restless leg syndrome in the elderly. *Age Ageing* **23**: 200.

75. Schenck, C.H., Mahowald, M.W. (1996). Long-term, nightly benzodiazepine treatment of injurious parasomnias and other disorders of disrupted nocturnal sleep in 170 adults. *Am. J. Med.,* **100**: 333.

76. Allen, R.P., Earley, C.J. (1996). Augmentation of the restless leg syndrome with carbidopa/levodopa. *Sleep* **19**: 205.

77. Von Scheele, C., Kempe, V. (1990). Long-term effect of dopaminergic drugs in restless legs: a 2-year follow-up. *Arch. Neurol.,* **47**: 1223.

78. Silber, M.H., Shepart, J.W. Jr, Wisbey, J.A. (1997). Pergolide in the management of restless legs syndrome: an extended study. *Sleep* **20**: 878.

79. Thorp, M.L., Morris, C.D., Bagby, S.P. (2001). A crossover study of gabapentin in treatment of restless legs syndrome among hemodialysis patients. *Am. J. Kidney Dis.,* **38**: 104.

80. Wagner, M.L., Walters, A.S., Coleman, R.G. *et al.* (1996). Randomized, double-blind, placebo-controlled study of clonidine in restless legs syndrome. *Sleep* **19**: 52.

81. Walters, A.S., Wagner, M.L., Hening, W.A., *et al.* (1993). Successful treatment of the idiopathic restless legs syndrome in a randomized double-blind trial of oxycodone versus placebo. *Sleep* **16**: 32.

82. Takaki, J., Nishi, T., Nangaku, M., *et al.* (2003). Clinical and psychological aspects of restless legs syndrome in uremic patients on hemodialysis. *Am. J. Kidney Dis.,* **41**(4): 833–9.

83. Altamura, A.C., Moro, A.R., Percudani, M. (1994). Clinical pharmacokinetics of fluoxetine. *Clin. Pharmacokin.,* **26**: 201–14.

84. Anderson, R.J., Gambertogolio, J.G., Schrier, R.W. (1976). *Clinical Use of Drugs in Renal Failure.* Springfield, IL: Charles, C. Thomas.

85. Aronoff, G.R., Berns, J.S., Brier, M.E., *et al.* (1999). *Drug Prescribing in Renal Failure Dosing Guidelines for Adults,* 4th edn. American College of Physicians/American Society of Internal Medicine. Philadelphia.

86. Borison, R.L. (1979). Amantadine-induced psychosis in a geriatric patient with renal disease. *Am. J. Psychiatry* **136**: 111–12.

87. Brater, D.C. (2003). *Drug Dosing in Renal Failure in Therapy in Nephrology and Hypertension, A companion to Brenner and Rector's The Kidney,* pp. 641–53. Sanders, New York.

88. Davies, G., Kingswood, C., Street, M. (1996). Pharmacokinetics of opioids in renal dysfunction. *Clin Pharmacokinet.,* **31**: 410–22.

89. Dheenan, S., Venketesan, J., Grubb, B.P., Henrich, W.L. (1998). Effect of sertraline hydrochloride on dialysis hypotension. *Am. J. Kidney Dis.,* **31**: 624–30.

90. Facca, A., Sanchez-Ramos, J. (1996). High-dose pergolide monotherapy in the treatment of severe levodopa-induced dyskenisias [letter]. *Move. Disord.,* **11**: 327–9.

91. Garzone, P.D., Kroboth, P.D. (1994). Pharmacokinetics of the newer benzodiazepines. *Clin. Pharmacokin.,* **16**: 337–64.

92. Hoppmann, R.A., Peden, J.G., Ober, S.K. (1991). Central nervous system side effects of non-steroidal anti-inflammatory drugs. *Arch. Intern. Med.,* **151**: 1309–13.

93. Inturrisi, C.E. (1977). Disposition of narcotics in patients with renal disease. *Am. J. Med.,* **62**: 528–9.

94. Lam, Y.W.F., Banerji, S., Hatfield, C., Talbert, R.L. (1997). Principles of drug administration in renal insufficiency. *Clin. Pharmacokin.,* **32**: 30–57.

95. Laurijssens, B.E., Greenblatt, D.J. (1996). Pharmacokinetic–pharmacodynamic relationships for benzodiazepines. *Clin. Pharmacokinet.,* **30**: 52–76.

96. Levy, N.B. (1990). Psychiopharmacology in patients with renal failure. *Int. J. Psychiatry, Med.,* **20**: 325–34.

97. Ochs, H.R., Greenblatt, D.J., Labedzki, L., Smith, R.B. (1986). Alprazolam kinetics in patients with renal insufficiency. *J. Clin. Psychopharmacol.,* **6**: 292–4.

98. Olyaei, A.J., deMattos, A.M., Bennet, W.M. (2000). Prescribing drugs in Renal Disease. In: *The Kidney,* ed. B. Brenner, pp. 2606–53. W.B. Sanders.

99. Preskorn, S.H. (1997). Clinically relevant pharmacology of selective serotonin reuptake inhibitors. *Clin. Pharmacokinet.,* **32**(Suppl. 1): 1–21.

100. Product information (1999). Ambien®, zolpidem. Skokie, IL: G.D. Searle and Company.

101. Product information (1994). Halcion®, triazolam. Kalamazoo, MI: UpJohn Laboratories.

102. Product information (August 2000). Poxicodone™, oxycodone. Columbus, OH: Roxane Laboratories, Inc.

103. Product information (1999). Sonata®, zaleplon. Philadelphia, PA: Wyeth Laboratories.

104. Product information (1995). Stelazine®, trifluoperazine. Philadelphia, PA: SmithKline & French.

105. Product information (1999). Talacen®, pentazocine and acetaminophen. New York: Sanofi-Synthelabo Inc.

106. Product information (April 1999). Thorazine®, chlorpromazine. Philadelphia, PA: SmithKline Beecham Pharmaceuticals.

107. Product information (October 2000). Zyprexa®, olanzapine. Indianapolis, IN: Eli Lilly and Company.

108. Rubin, A., Lemberger, L., Dhahir, P. (1981). Physiologic disposition of pergolide. *Clin. Pharmacol. Ther.*, **30**: 258–65.

109. Sandoz, M., Vandel, S., Vandel, B., Bonin, B., Hory, B., *et al.* (1984). Metabolism of amitriptyline in patients with chronic renal failure. *Eur. J. Clin. Pharmacol.*, **26**: 227–32.

110. Schmith, V.D., Piraino, B., Smith, R.B., Kroboth, P.D. (1991). Alprazolam in end stage renal disease. *J. Clin. Pharmacol.*, **31**: 571–9.

111. Schwenk, M.H., Verga, M.A., Wagner, J.D. (1995). Hemodialyzability of sertraline. *Clin. Nephrol.*, **44**: 121–4.

112. Wad, N., Guenat, C., Kramer, G. (1997). Carbamazepine: detection of another metabolite in serum, 9-hydroxymethyl-10-carbamoyl acridan. *Ther. Drug Monit.*, **19**: 314–17.

113. Wagner, B.K.J., O'Hara, D.A. (1997). Pharmacokinetics and pharmacodynamics of sedatives and analgesics in the treatment of agitated critically ill patients. *Clin. Pharmacokinet.*, **33**: 426–53.

114. Wong, M.O., Eldon, M.A., Keane, W.F., Turck, D. Bockbrader, H.N. *et al.* (1995). Disposition of gapapentin in anuric subjects on hemodialysis. *J. Clin. Pharmacol.*, **35**: 622–6.

115. Wood, K.A., Harris, M.J., Morreale, A., Rizos, A.L. (1988). Drug-induced psychosis and depression in the elderly. *Psych. Clin. N. Am.*, **11**: 167–93.

116. Bateman, D.N. (1983). Clinical pharmacokinetics of metoclopramide. *Clin. Pharmacokinet.*, **8**: 523–9.

117. Bauer, T.M., Ritz, R., Huberthur, C., *et al.* (1995). Prolonged sedation due to accumulation of conjugated metabolites of midazolam. *The Lancet* **346**: 145–7.

**Table 7.1** Symptom guidelines

| Symptom | Treatment | Dosage | Comments |
|---|---|---|---|
| Cramps | Quinine | 260–325 mg PO | Limit to three doses daily |
| | Vitamin E | 400 IU PO | |
| | Carnitine | 1000–2000 mg IV during dialysis | Also used for cardiomyopathy and refractory anaemia |
| Restless legs | Clonazepam | 0.5–2 mg q.h.s. prn | |
| | Carbidopa/levodopa | 25–100 mg q.h.s. prn | |
| | Pergolide | 0.05–0.2 mg q.i.d. | |
| | Bromocriptine | 2.5–20 mg q.h.s. | |
| | Gabapentin | 100 mg q.o.d., 100–300 mg t.i.d. | |
| | Clonidine | 0.1–1.0 mg q.h.s. | |
| Pruritus | H1 antagonists | | Try any H1 antagonist |
| | Skin moisturizer | | |
| | Hydrourea cream | | |
| | Activated charcoal | 6 g q.i.d. for 8 weeks | |
| | UVB light | | |
| | Lidocaine IV | 100 mg IV during dialysis | Potential seizures |
| | Ketotifen | | Mast cell stabilizer |
| | Ondanstron | 4 mg b.d. | High cost |
| | Plasmapheresis | | 3–4 exchanges |
| Hypotension (intradialytic or persistent) | Alterations to the dialysis bath, temperature, sodium, ultrafltration | | |
| | Midadrine | 1–10 mg t.i.d. prn or predialysis | Oral $\alpha$-adrenergic agonist |
| | Sertraline | 25–50 mg predialysis | |
| Anorexia | Megestrol | 40–400 mg has been used in ESRD | |
| | Dronabinol | 2.5–5 mg b.d./ t.i.d. | |
| Lethargy and fatigue | Methylphenidate | 5–10 mg a.m. and noon | Psychostimulant |

Abbreviations: PO, by mouth; IV, intravenous; q.h.s., at bedtime; q.i.d., four times a day; b.d., twice a day; t.i.d., three times a day; q.o.d., every other day; ESRD, end-stage renal disease; prn, as needed.

**Table 7.2** Commonly used drugs for symptoms in patients with chronic kidney disease

| Drug | Active metabolite | Reaction | Typical adult dose | $t_{1/2}$ | Adult dose in ESRD | $t_{1/2}$ in ESRD | Removed by dialysis? | Comment | Reference |
|---|---|---|---|---|---|---|---|---|---|
| Sertraline | No active metabolites | Anxiety, agitation | 50–200 mg | 24 h | 50–200 mg | 42–96 h | HD: minimal | Minimal changes in kinetics in ESRD. Useful in sudden H hypotension | 87, 89, 98, 99, 111, 115 |
| Alprazolam | α-hydroxy-alprazolam (αHA) (<15% of alprazolam) | Hallucinations | 0.25–5 mg t.i.d. | 9–19 h | 0.25–5 mg t.i.d. | 9–19 h | HD: minimal | Increased free fraction in ESRD. Minimal differences in dialysis-dependent patients | 85, 90, 91, 95–98 |
| Lorazepam | No active metabolites | | 1–2 mg b.d.–t.i.d. | 9–16 h | 0.5–2 mg b.d | 32–70 h | HD: no | Manufacturer does not recommend in ESRD | 85, 96, 98, 113 |
| Midazolam | α-hydroxymi-dazolam conjugate (AHM-C) | Prolonged sedation | 1.25 mg IV, titrate to response | 1.2–12.3 h | 1.25 mg IV, titrate to response | 1.2–12.3 h. AMH-C. 50 4–76.8 h | | Increased effect due to reduced protein binding | 85, 98, 113, 116 |
| Oxazepam | No active metabolites | | 30–120 mg/day | 6–25 h | 30–120 mg/day | 25–90 h | HD: no | | 85, 96, 98 |
| Temazepam | No active metabolites | | 15–30 mg q.h.s. | 4–10 h | 15–30 mg q.h.s. | | HD: no, CAPD: no | | 85, 96, 98 |
| Triazolam | α-hydroxytri azolam | Hallucinations, paranoia | 0.125–0.5 mg | 2–4 h | 0.125–0.5 mg | 2.3 h | HD: no. CAPD: no | | 85, 98, 111 |

**Table 7.2** (continued) Commonly used drugs for symptoms in patients with chronic kidney disease

| Drug | Active metabolite | Reaction | Typical adult dose | $t_{1/2}$ | Adult dose in ESRD | $t_{1/2}$ in ESRD | Removed by dialysis? | Comment | Reference |
|---|---|---|---|---|---|---|---|---|---|
| Zaleplon | No active metabolites | | 5–20 mg q.h.s. | 1 h | 5–10 mg | | | No dose adjustment necessary per manufacturer for mild to moderate renal impairment. Not studied in ESRD | 85 |
| Zolpidem | No active metabolites | | 10 mg | 2–3 h | Reduce dose by 50% | 4–6 h | | Increased free fraction | 83, 100 |
| Carbamazepine | Carbamazepine 10-11-epoxide. Also: 9-hydroxymethyl-10-carbamoyl acridan | | 100 mg b.d. to 400 mg q.i.d. | 12–17 h (with chronic dosing) | 100 mg b.d. to 400 mg q.i.d. | Similar to normal renal function | HD: no. CAPD: no | Used for neuropathy pain | 85, 112 |
| Gabapentin | | | 300–600 mg t.i.d. | 5–7 h | 300 mg q.o.d or 200–300 mg after each 4 h haemodialysis | 132 h | HD: yes. CAPD: partial | Used for neuropathy pain. And restless leg syndrome | 85, 114 |
| Pergolide | Multiple activity | | 0.025 mg/day up to 3 mg t.i.d. | | | | | 55% renal clearance. Not studied in renal insufficiency. Used for restless legs syndrome | 90, 108 |
| Pentazocine | Inactive glucuronide metabolite | Confusion, hallucinations | 50–100 mg PO every 3–4 h | 1.5–10 h | 25–50 mg PO every 3–4 h | | HD: no | Partial antagonist should not be used for individuals receiving chronic opioids. 60–70% renal excretion with 5–8% excreted as unchanged drug | 85, 87, 115 |

| Drug | Active metabolite | Toxicity | Dose (normal) | Half-life (normal) | Dose (renal) | Half-life (renal) | Dialysis | Comments | References |
|---|---|---|---|---|---|---|---|---|---|
| Propoxyphene | Nor-propoxyphene (NP) | CNS + respiratory depression | 65 mg PO t.i.d.–q.i.d. | 12–15 h. NP 23–36 h | Avoid | 12–20 h accumulation of NP | HD: negligible. CAPD: negligible | Avoid in ESRD | 85, 87, 88 |
| Sulindac | Active sulfide metabolite (SS) | Psychosis, aseptic meningitis with delirium, stupor | 200 mg b.d. | 7.8 h. SS 16.4 h | 200 mg b.d. | | HD: negligible | Prostaglandin inhibition may result in renal dysfunction, uraemic bleeding, and GI bleeding. Nephorotic syndrome, interstitial nephritis, hyperkalaemia. More renal sparing | 87, 92, 98, 115 |
| Ibuprofen | Metabolites—? activity | Aseptic meningitis with lethargy, coma | 200–800 mg t.i.d. | 2–3.2 h | 200–800 mg t.i.d. | 2–3.2 h | HD: no. CAPD: no | Prostaglandin inhibition may result in renal dysfunction, uraemic bleeding, and GI bleeding. Nephorotic syndrome, interstitial nephritis, hyperkalaemia | 85, 92, 98 |
| Indomethacin | Inactive metabolites | Visual hallucinations, paranoid delusions | 25–50 mg t.i.d. | 4–12 h | 25–50 mg t.i.d. | 4–12 h | HD: no. CAPD: no | Prostaglandin inhibition may result in renal dysfunction, uraemic bleeding, and GI bleeding. Nephorotic syndrome, interstitial nephritis, hyperkalaemia | 85, 98, 115 |
| Methadone | N-dimethyl-methadone (NDM) | | 2.5–10 mg every 6–8 h | 13–58 h | 1.25–5 mg every 6–8 h | | HD: negligible. CAPD: negligible | Not significantly different in ESRD; titrate to effect | 85, 87, 93, 98 |

**Table 7.2** (continued) Commonly used drugs for symptoms in patients with chronic kidney disease

| Drug | Active metabolite | Reaction | Typical adult dose | $t_{1/2}$ | Adult dose in ESRD | $t_{1/2}$ in ESRD | Removed by dialysis? | Comment | Reference |
|---|---|---|---|---|---|---|---|---|---|
| Meperidine | Nor-meperidine (NM) | Hallucinations, seizures, stupor | 50–100 mg IM every 3–4 h | 2–7 h. NM: 14–20 h | Avoid | 7–32 h. NM: 34 h | HD: negligible. CAPD: negligible | NM accumulation in renal failure significant and increases risk of seizures | 85, 87, 88, 93, 98, 115 |
| Morphine | Morphine 3- and 6-glucuronides (M3 + M6) | | 20–25 mg PO every 4 h. 2–10 mg IV | 1.7 2.5 h | 10–12 mg PO every 4 h. 1–5 mg IV | 1.2–4.5 h | HD: no | Accumulation of metabolites in ESRD; accumulation of M3 associated with some antagonist properties | 85, 88, 98, 113 |
| Oxycodone | Metabolites—activity | Hallucinations | 10–30 mg PO every 4 h | 3.2 h | | | | Manufacturer recommends caution | 112, 115 |
| Codeine | Codeine 6-glucoronide, morphine | Hypotension, sedation, CNS | 30–60 mg every 4–6 h | 2.5–4 h | 15–30mg every 4–6 h | 18 h | | Hypotension, sedation in ESRD has been reported depression | 85, 88, 98 |
| Naltrexonee | | | 50 mg/day PO | 1–1.5 h | | No data | No change | Used in pruritus | 26 |
| Carbidopa (C)/ levodopa (L) | Active metabolites | Hallucinations, agitation | 25/100 t.i.d. | C:2 h. L:0.8–1.6 h | 50% dose reduction | Active metabolites | No change | Used for restless legs syndrome | 85, 115 |
| Amantadine | | Hallucinations, agitation | 100 mg every 8–12h | 12 h | 100 mg every 7 days | 500 h | HD: variable reports | Accumulation in renal failure | 85–87, 94, 115 |
| Cimetidine | Inactive metabolites | Depression, confusion, auditory + visual hallucinations | 400 mg b.d. or 400–800 mg q.h.s. | 1.5–2 h | 100–200 mg b.d. or 200–400 mg q.h.s. | 5 h | HD: 10–20%. CAPD: negligible | Accumulation in renal failure | 85, 87, 94, 98, 115 |

| Drug | Metabolite | Side effect | Dose | Half-life | Renal dose | Renal half-life | Dialysis | Comment | Ref |
|---|---|---|---|---|---|---|---|---|---|
| Diphenhy-dramine | Inactive metabolites | Confusion | 25 mg t.i.d.–q.i.d. | 3.4–9.3 h | 25 mg t.i.d.–q.i.d. | | HD: no. CAPD: no | Anticholinergic effects including urinary retention | 85 |
| Ranitidine | Inactive metabolites | Depression | 150–300 mg q.h.s. | 1.5–3 h | 75 mg q.h.s. | 6–9 h | HD: 50–60%. CAPD: negligible | Accumulation in renal failure | 85, 87, 98, 115 |
| Methylphenidate | Active metabolite | Hallucinations | | | | | | | 115 |
| Metoclopramide | Active metabolite | Anxiety, agitation, tardive dyskinesia | 05–10 mg q.i.d. | 2.5–4 h | 5 mg q.i.d. | 14–15 h | HD: none. CAPD: no data | Increased extrapyramidal side-effects in ESRD | 116 |
| Midodrine | | | 5–10 mg every 8 h | 0.5 h | 5–10 mg every 8 h | No data | HD: none | Used for dialysis hypotension | 10, 11 |
| Ondansetron | | | 4–32 mg IV or PO | 2.5–5.5 h | No change | 2.5–5.5 h | No data | Used with nausea and pruritus | 110 |

Abbreviations: HD, haemodialysis; CAPD, continuous ambulatory peritoneal dialysis; GI, gastrointestinal; CNS, central nervous system; IV, intravenous; IM, intramuscular; PO, by mouth; ESRD, end-stage renal disease; b.d., twice a day; t.i.d., three times a day; q.h.s., at bedtime; q.i.d., four times a day.

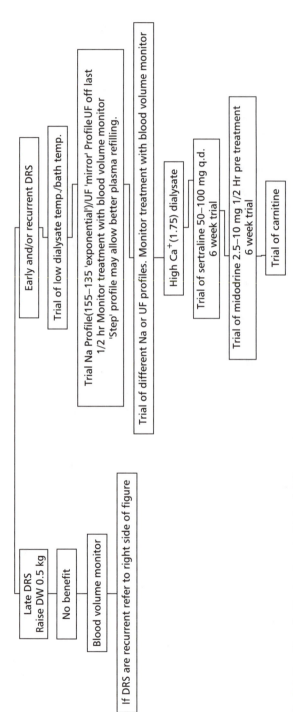

**Fig. 7.1** Algorithm for the treatment of intradialytic symptoms.

# Symptoms of renal disease: the treatment and palliation of symptoms due to co-morbidity in end-stage renal disease

Mohamed Abed Sekkarie and Richard Swartz

## 7.5 Introduction

Dialysis itself is 'palliative' therapy—we cannot cure progressive chronic kidney disease (CKD) and we can only offer enough dialysis to control uraemic symptoms. In addition, the disease processes that lead to end-stage renal disease (ESRD) do not necessarily disappear when chronic dialysis is initiated. As characterized in the case study at the end of the chapter, patients with ESRD are subject to a myriad of complications that are either consequences of chronic dialysis itself or ongoing manifestations of the patient's underlying medical condition. In addition, the older age of ESRD patients, the high prevalence of diabetes, and the accelerated atherosclerotic process in this population predispose to co-morbid conditions.

It would be impractical in a single chapter to review a comprehensive list of co-morbid conditions. Therefore, we are using the case study in order to focus on a subset of common complications that are representative of the symptoms arising in ESRD patients which are not the direct result of the dialysis. In the final analysis, accumulating co-morbidity increases the degree of suffering for the patient and the need for assistance from caregivers. Ultimately, it is the burden of co-morbid conditions, not ESRD or dialysis, that leads to death or to withdrawal from dialysis.[1]

## 7.6 Diabetic gastroenteropathy

Diabetic patients with ESRD have generally had diabetes for more than a decade and are likely to have developed signs and symptoms of visceral autonomic neuropathy, which involves many systems including the gastrointestinal tract. Diabetic gastroparesis and diabetic enteropathy are the most important forms of this involvement.

### 7.6.1 Diabetic gastroparesis

Diabetic gastroparesis is characterized by symptoms that include anorexia, nausea, vomiting, and a feeling of fullness with early satiety. These symptoms are non-specific and do not necessarily denote the diagnosis. Other diagnoses such as inadequate dialysis, peptic ulcer disease, and gastro-oesophageal reflux should be considered, since the treatment of these other disorders may prove easier than that of diabetic gastroparesis itself. Chronic kidney disease, at least in its advanced stages, leads to delayed gastric emptying that can cause dyspeptic symptoms.[2] The diagnosis of diabetic gastroparesis can be confirmed by scintigraphic gastric emptying studies or breath tests.

Treatment to minimize acute hyperglycaemia may help to alleviate symptoms, as hyperglycaemia has been shown to delay gastric emptying. A low-fat diet, frequent small meals, and liquid diets should be considered. In young patients with insulin-dependent diabetes mellitus (IDDM) combined kidney–pancreas transplantation improves gastric emptying and symptoms of gastroparesis, suggesting a pathogenic role for diabetic control in the development of gastrointestinal complications.

There are several pharmacological agents available for treating gastroparesis.[3,4] The most widely used agents are the dopamine receptor antagonists metoclopramide and domperidone. In adults with normal renal function metoclopramide is used at doses of 5–20 mg orally, intramuscularly (IM) or intravenously (IV) before meals and at bedtime. Dose adjustment in patients with severe renal failure is required, and only 25% of the normal dose is recommended. Side-effects of metoclopramide are largely neurological and include anxiety, alteration of mental status, and acute dystonic reactions with extrapyramidal movements due to central blocking of dopamine. Diarrhoea is a further common side-effect. In addition some patients develop tachyphylaxis following prolonged use, which limits its usefulness. Domperidone is another benzamide-class dopamine receptor inhibitor. Its advantage over metoclopramide is that it does not cross the blood–brain barrier and thus does not have the neurological side-effects of metoclopramide. The usual dose is 20 mg four times a day (q.i.d.) and no dose adjustment in renal failure is required. This drug is not available in the United States.

Cisapride is reputed to be more effective than metoclopramide and is administered at doses of 5 to 20 mg before meals and at bedtime. It has fewer neurological side-effects, but the drug can be arrythmogenic. Metabolism of cisapride via the P-450–3A4 cytochrome pathway is inhibited by a number of other drugs, leading to higher cisapride levels and thus a high risk of torsades de pointes in some settings. Because of the high prevalence of cardiac disease and polypharmacy in ESRD patients, the risk of developing arrhythmias while on cisapride is relatively high.[5] In the UK its licence has been suspended for this reason. Using lower dosages, avoiding recognized drug interactions, and limiting use in patients known to have severe heart disease should lower the risk.

Erythromycin, given orally or intravenously in modest doses, promotes gastric emptying. Lack of experience with prolonged use and concerns about toxicity, such as the development of pseudomembranous colitis, limit the use of this drug. It too is a potent inhibitor of the cytochrome P-450–3A4 pathway and is itself arrythmogenic. Its use in conjunction with cisapride is contraindicated.

More drastic measures to treat diabetic gastroparesis include bypassing the stomach by jejunostomy feeding, often in conjunction with a gastrostomy tube; thus feeding can be accomplished through the jejunal tube while gastric emptying can be achieved through the gastric tube to avoid vomiting. Parenteral nutrition and high-frequency gastric electric pacing are also used in some patients with severe diabetic gastroparesis. This latter methodology is still under investigation.

## 7.6.2 Diabetic enteropathy

Diabetic enteropathy, characterized by diarrhoea that alternates with constipation, is another manifestation of diabetic autonomic neuropathy of the gastrointestinal tract. The diarrhoea is watery, painless, occurs at night, and might be associated with faecal incontinence. As with diabetic gastroparesis, other more easily treated causes (iatrogenic, infection, etc.) for the diarrhoea should be considered first.[6]

Specific pathogenic mechanisms for diabetic enteropathy include abnormalities of motility, bacterial overgrowth, and/or anorectal dysfunction. It may not be easy to distinguish between causes, but empirical treatment which addresses these mechanisms is sometimes successful. For example, bacterial overgrowth can be treated with a single course of antibiotics and may remit for several months at a time. Other patients will respond to a rotating regimen of two or three different antibiotics, each given for up to 1 week out of each month. Aerobic and anaerobic coverage should be included. For a single course doxycycline 100 mg twice a day (b.d.) or a combination of cephalexin 250 mg three times a day (t.i.d.) with metronidazole 250 mg t.i.d. could be tried. A suggested rotating regimen includes ciprofloxacin 250 mg b.d., doxycycline 100 mg b.d., and metronidazole 250 mg t.i.d. A lactose-free, low-carbohydrate diet may also be of some help.

Symptomatic treatment of diarrhoea due to accelerated gastric transit can be accomplished using loperamide 2–4 mg q.i.d. or diphenoxilate 5 mg q.i.d. The use of the alpha-2 sympathetic-agonist clonidine has also been shown to be beneficial, although relatively large doses are sometimes needed. Dry mouth and hypotension at dialysis are common side-effects. In refractory cases that do not respond to common symptomatic therapy or clonidine, it is suggested by some case histories that octreotide, a somatostatin analogue, can provide relief. It is given subcutaneously at a dose of 50 μg b.d.[7] A long-acting formulation that is administered IM at doses of 30–90 mg monthly could be used instead. The drug may raise blood pressure with improvement of diabetic autonomic neuropathy-associated hypotension but severe hypertensive responses have been reported with its use.[8]

Loperamide, by reducing stool volume and increasing the tone of the anal sphincter, should be tried in incontinent patients. Biofeedback training, aimed at lowering the threshold for rectal sensation, has been suggested to cure incontinence in some diabetic patients.

## 7.7 Non-autonomic diabetic neuropathies

Diabetic neuropathy may appear in different forms, including symmetric distal polyneuropathy, diabetic polyradiculopathy, and several forms of mononeuropathies. Symmetric distal polyneuropathy is the most common type. Symptoms include paraesthesias, sensory loss, pain, and at later stages motor weakness. These problems can lead to complications including the development of skin ulcers, with an increased risk from burns and trauma, and foot deformities caused by Charcot joint. Early detection of diabetic neuropathy by periodic examination of diabetic patients facilitates the institution of preventive measures and early therapy of complications. Patients or their caregivers should be encouraged to make inspection of the feet at home a daily routine.

Several medications can be used to alleviate the pain of diabetic peripheral neuropathy.[9] Tricyclic antidepressants have been shown to be effective in symptom relief. Improvement is not immediate but appears within 2 weeks of initiating therapy and increases throughout the first 6 weeks. Sedative and antidepressant effects might be additional benefits. Other common side-effects include constipation, dry mouth, orthostatic hypotension, and occasional cardiac ectopy. Concern over these latter side-effects when using high doses in patients with renal failure has discouraged use of these agents and limits their effectiveness. Recommended doses for amitriptyline and nortriptyline are 10 to 50 mg at bedtime, with relief sometimes achieved at higher doses. Doxepin is another agent of this class that has the advantage of being less cardiotoxic, and the recommended dose is 10 to 75 mg daily.

If treatment with tricyclic agents fails, patients may obtain relief with the addition of topical capsaicin. When it is started it can cause local burning and skin irritation; side-effects that improve with continued use. Symptoms will persist in some patients despite this combination. In these patients, carbamazepine, starting at low doses, can be added. The dose can be gradually increased, using drug levels to monitor therapy and minimize its side-effects which include dizziness, rash, nausea, and leucopaenia.

Many physicians now begin therapy for peripheral neuropathy with gabapentin,[10] but this drug requires significant dosage reduction in patients with impaired renal function. In ESRD patients, 150 mg daily or 300 mg after each haemodialysis is the usual recommended dose. Somnolence, dizziness, ataxia, and tremor are side-effects that respond to dose reduction. The drug is expensive but its pharmacokinetic characteristics in patients with renal failure make the drug more affordable. Other pharmacological agents for peripheral neuropathy include opioids and mexilitine, a drug with pro-arrhythmic properties.

In patients with ESRD, where nephrotoxicity is not a concern, non-steroidal anti-inflammatory agents (NSAIDs) can also be used. The newer COX-2 inhibitors have the possible advantage of less gastrointestinal (GI) toxicity but are more expensive. Transcutaneous electric nerve stimulation (TENS) is a non-pharmacological approach that can be applied in difficult cases.

## 7.8 Coronary artery disease

Heart disease is the leading cause of death in patients with renal dysfunction. Coronary atherosclerosis, left ventricular hypertrophy, and valvular diseases are also more common in this population. Symptoms include exertional angina and dyspnoea, haemodialysis-induced chest pain and hypotension, diastolic dysfunction and 'flash' pulmonary oedema due to ischaemia in the absence of volume overload, and palpitations and arrhythmias. It would be foolhardy to attempt to review the entire gamut of coronary disease, modification of risk factors, or anatomical correction in this chapter; therefore we will concentrate simply on non-specific symptom relief.

Beta-blockers, calcium channel blockers, and nitrates can all be used to treat angina in ESRD patients. Special attention should be paid to pharmacokinetic considerations and to the risk of precipitating hypotension during haemodialysis. Thus, the combination of beta-blockade with angiotensin-converting enzyme (ACE) inhibition is particularly useful in treating angina associated with hypertension and with 'flash' pulmonary oedema. In the meantime, strict control of interdialysis volume accumulation and keeping total body fluid weight near the 'dry weight' target is pivotal in controlling these symptoms. Treatment of dialysis-induced hypotension itself has many facets and is discussed in Part 1 of this chapter.

Increasing red blood cell (RBC) mass acutely with transfusion or more durably with increased doses of erythropoietin can sometimes ameliorate the symptoms of angina in dialysis patients. Although the optimal haemoglobin goal is not well established, in a population of haemodialysis patients with asymptomatic ischaemic cardiomyopathy a goal haemoglobin level of 13.5 g/dl, compared with a goal of 10 g/dl, led to better quality of life indices but no evidence of regression of left ventricular hypertrophy or dilatation.[11] In another study of haemodialysis patients with coronary artery disease or congestive heart failure, a target haematocrit of 42% was compared with that of 30%. There was no survival benefit to the higher-haematocrit group; in fact the trend was toward higher mortality.[12] Considering our current knowledge haemoglobin levels between 11 and 12 g/dl are desirable.

If volume overload is present, then diligent volume removal by ultrafiltration during haemodialysis or by increased osmotic fluid removal at peritoneal dialysis should be carried out. Afterload-reducing therapy can sometimes be of substantial benefit. In patients with severe cardiomyopathy and severely impaired left ventricular function who suffer refractory hypotension at haemodialysis, peritoneal dialysis can be very effective. In patients with biventricular failure and severe right-sided signs of ascites and oedema, volume management by removing excess volume during peritoneal drainage can be very effective for some as an adjunct to diffusive removal of uraemic metabolites during peritoneal equilibration. We have seen surprising success using peritoneal dialysis in the setting of severe cardiomyopathy when haemodialysis proved impractical.[13]

Interventional therapy for treatable coronary disease should be offered in appropriate ESRD patients. The experience with conservative treatment and with re-stenosis in angiographic treatment in the ESRD setting is discouraging. However, selected ESRD patients do very will with coronary bypass grafting and should be considered for this treatment whenever reasonable.[14]

## 7.9 Peripheral vascular disease

Peripheral vascular disease (PVD) is common in patients with chronic kidney disease due to the high prevalence of both general risk factors such as diabetes and smoking, factors unique to renal disease such as hyperhomocysteinaemia, and metastatic vascular calcification related to hyperphosphataemia and high calcium–phosphate product. In a recent cross-sectional study of a haemodialysis population, duration of dialysis, malnutrition, and low parathyroid hormone (PTH) were found to be associated with higher prevalence of PVD.[15] This condition contributes substantially to the co-morbidity in ESRD patients and is often progressive and poorly responsive to revascularization.[16,17]

PVD is frequently quite advanced before ESRD patients are symptomatic. Symptoms, when they begin, range from intermittent claudication to rest pain, ischaemic ulceration, and gangrene. The diagnosis of PVD relies on the history and physical examination, the ankle brachial index, and some more accurate tests such as the toe brachial index, transcutaneous partial pressure of oxygen measurement, and toe pulse volume recordings.

Management includes invasive and non-invasive measures. Smoking, a significant risk factor for kidney disease, is common among ESRD patients and accelerates PVD. Smoking cessation and regular exercise have been shown to improve symptoms of intermittent claudication and are very important in affected ESRD patients. Preventive foot care has a valuable role too and is discussed in Section 7.10 on care of the diabetic foot.

Several pharmacological agents for the treatment of symptoms of PVD have been studied.[18] Pentoxifylline and vitamin E have not proven useful in ESRD patients. Antiplatelet agents may improve exercise tolerance and prevent complications. The best results have been reported with ticlopidine, but this drug can have serious haematological side-effects. The new agent, cilastazol, improves symptoms in non-ESRD patients, but the drug has not been studied nor has its safety been established in ESRD patients. Antiplatelet agents or warfarin are recommended following peripheral reconstructive procedures, but the risk of atheroembolism, both spontaneously and after intervention, is increased by the use of systemic anticoagulation.[19]

Angioplasty and surgical revascularization are invasive methods that may be indicated in the management of intermittent claudication and the more severe manifestations of PVD. Revascularization is often used in conjunction with limited amputations. The incidence of amputation is several-fold higher in ESRD patients than the normal population, even after adjusting for diabetes. Compared with the general population, patients with kidney disease are also at increased risk of peri-operative complications including mortality, technical problems, atheroembolism, and limb loss.[17,20] In addition, PVD is now recognized as a major comorbidity influencing the decision for some patients ultimately to withdraw from dialysis.

## 7.10 The diabetic foot

Lower extremity amputations are common in diabetic patients, especially those with kidney failure, with an amputation rate of 14/100 person-years. Appropriate care may prevent or delay many of these. Diabetic foot lesions result from ischaemic and neuropathic complications in varying proportions. Prophylaxis of diabetic foot problems is crucial. Avoidance of trauma and thermal injuries, exercise, daily foot inspection by someone with good vision, and local skin care should be emphasized for all diabetics. Appropriate educational programmes are thought to reduce amputation rates by 50%.[21]

Patients with gangrene or ulcers require aggressive care. Measures include infection control by local debridement and systemic antibiotics, assessing the need for revascularization, orthotic devices and/or special shoes to unload the lesions, glycaemic control, and nutritional support. When these treatment measures fail, then pain control generally requires amputation. To facilitate healing, the need for revascularization should be assessed before local debridement or amputation. Other approaches that have been suggested to expedite ulcer healing include the use of hyperbaric oxygen, topical phenytoin, and granulocyte-colony stimulating factor.

## 7.11 Calciphylaxis

Calciphylaxis is a condition that is seen mainly in ESRD patients during the course of dialysis or immediately after transplantation. It is characterized by occlusive vascular calcifications in small arteries and causes ischaemic necrosis of the dermis, subcutaneous tissues, and distal extremities. Skin changes include livedo reticularis and painful subcutaneous nodules with necrosis, occurring largely in the lower trunk and lower extremities. The condition was originally thought to be rare and to develop only after considerable time on chronic dialysis with uncontrolled high calcium–phosphate product. However, the syndrome is now recognized much more frequently, particularly in diabetic patients simultaneous with, or even shortly before, chronic dialysis begins. The pathogenesis of calciphylaxis is not well understood, and a host of factors have been proposed as possible contributors, including hyperparathyroidism, hyperphosphataemia, hypercalcaemia, elevated alkaline phosphatase, White race, obesity, protein malnutrition, and hypercoagulable states. More aggressive use of calcium-containing phosphate binders and of vitamin D analogues in treating the osteodystrophy of ESRD may actually facilitate more frequent development of calciphylaxis. Other drugs such as prednisone and warfarin are also possible risk factors but have not been shown conclusively to contribute to the syndrome in ESRD patients.[22,23]

The management of this problem is very difficult and often is not successful. Anecdotally, patients with severe secondary hyperparathyroidism can have a dramatic response to parathyroidectomy.[24] Avoidance of calcium-containing phosphate binders and discontinuation of vitamin D analogues, together with aggressive lowering of serum phosphorus by dietary measures and non-calcium, non-aluminium binders are recommended. Wound care and treatment of secondary infections are essential.[25] A role for hyperbaric oxygen has been suggested but not conclusively demonstrated.[26,27] Except in cases that respond to parathyroidectomy, the prognosis is generally poor. Pain management is the most important therapeutic measure in refractory cases, and relatively high short-term mortality can be expected. Calciphylaxis results in voluntary withdrawal from dialysis in many cases due to intractable pain.

## 7.12 Falls

Patients with chronic kidney disease, because of their age, co-morbidities, medications, and dialysis-related hypotension are at high risk for falling. Bone disease and bleeding tendencies may make these falls more dangerous. Hip fractures, for example are 4.4 times more likely in ESRD patients than in non-ESRD patients matched for age and gender.[28] Postural hypotension, already a significant problem for patients with diabetes, is accentuated after volume removal at haemodialysis. Thus, extra precautions immediately after haemodialysis are important for vulnerable ESRD patients.

Measures to prevent falls should be emphasized in this population. Some of these measures include avoidance of postural hypotension by optimizing dry weight, paying attention to medications and teaching patients certain manoeuvres such as ankle pumps and gradual rather than abrupt assumption of upright posture. Attention to the patient's environment should be considered. Shower chairs, raised toilet seats, grab bars, and hazard removal are some of these measures. Gait training including proper use of assist devices such as walkers is also essential.

## 7.13 Decubitus ulcers

Immobility, incontinence, malnutrition, and physical injuries during transportation predispose many patients with chronic kidney disease, especially those on dialysis, to decubitus ulcers. The most important step in the management of decubitus ulcers is their prevention.[29] Identification of patients at risk, regular evaluation of patients, and correction of risk factors are essential. Guidelines are published by the Agency for Healthcare Research and Quality.[30] Patient positioning, pressure-reducing devices, management of incontinence, proper transportation techniques, nutritional support, and avoiding unnecessary sedation or immobilization are approaches that should be used to prevent bed sores. These steps are also important in the management of patients who already have decubiti. In these patients the treatment depends on the stage of the ulcer. Patients with partial-thickness skin loss (stage II) are treated by occlusive or semipermeable dressings. Deeper ulcers require tissue debridement which can be achieved by wet to dry dressings, hydrotherapy, sharp debridement, or other methods. Infections are treated by topical and/or systemic antibiotics. Diverting colostomies in the management of sacral decubiti are sometimes needed and can lead to good outcome. Adequate pain relief is essential.

## 7.14 Conclusion

Patients with renal disease often suffer from other chronic conditions that may not necessarily be related to their kidney disease. These conditions complicate the lives of these patients and make their management more challenging. Medical literature which addresses these topics and that is specific to the ESRD patient is sparse, so care offered is often extrapolated from knowledge related to the non-renal setting and utilizes personal experience. Additional considerations necessarily include the number and severity of co-morbid conditions, the patient's prognosis and personal wishes, the drug kinetics and side-effects profile in that patient, and the balance of benefit versus further complications from any proposed intervention. When quality of life, as judged by the patients or their proxies, is felt to be unacceptable, then withdrawal of renal replacement therapy should be considered as the most humane option.

## Case study 2

At age 65, after some 20 years of non-insulin dependent diabetes, Mrs AB reached ESRD. She had already suffered a unilateral below-knee amputation, and she was ambulating with a prosthesis. She was hypertensive and moderately obese but had never smoked. She was not a transplant candidate because of diffuse atherosclerosis.

After 2 years of haemodialysis, she began having hypotension at the end of her treatments. Discontinuation of her antihypertensives and adjustment of her dry weight led to transient improvement, but she developed increasing dyspnoea with evidence of reduced left ventricular contractility and ischaemia. Heart catheterization showed three-vessel disease, she underwent coronary artery bypass grafting, and her haemodialysis was more stable thereafter.

Within the next year, she developed frequent diarrhoea for which no aetiology other than autonomic neuropathy could be found. She responded somewhat to anti-diarrhoea drugs, treatment for bacterial overgrowth, and clonidine, but weight loss, fatigue, and hypoalbuminaemia progressed. Within a few months she suffered progressive muscle wasting, became bed-ridden, and had to be cared for in a nursing home. A decubitus ulcer developed requiring aggressive local treatment and parenteral nutrition. She showed some signs of improvement but remained bed ridden. Over the next 6 months she developed necrotic areas in the lower abdomen and upper thighs, typical of 'calciphylaxis' with infectious complications. These lesions became increasingly painful, and she became septic and confused. Based on her advance directives she received palliative care at the nursing home, she was not hospitalized, and her dialysis was discontinued. She died peacefully a few days later.

## Ethical Analysis of Case 2

This case demonstrates the benefit of the application of six of the nine recommendations in the Renal Physicians Association/ American Society of Nephrology (RPA/ASN) guidelines to a fairly frequent case of a dialysis patient with a common set of co-morbidities and a typical course. Because of her age, diabetes, and peripheral vascular disease, she could be predicted to have an expected remaining lifetime based on Table 29 (survival in diabetic ESRD patients after amputation) in the RPA/ASN guidelines and US Renal Data System (USRDS) data of 2 to 3 years. In the light of this limited life expectancy, it was especially important for her renal care team to involve her in shared decision-making, obtain informed consent for dialysis, and estimate prognosis (RPA/ASN Recommendations 1–3). Advance care planning needed to be conducted with the patient to determine under what health states she would not want to continue dialysis and other life-sustaining treatments as well as to identify whom she would prefer to make decisions for her if she lost decision-making capacity (RPA/ASN Recommendation 5). Because the patient had completed advance directives, at the time the patient's condition deteriorated and she lost decision-making capacity, her renal team knew how to care for her according to her wishes. This care included withdrawing dialysis (RPA/ASN Recommendation 6) and providing her with palliative care (RPA/ASN Recommendation 9) in the nursing home where she resided, sparing her one last hospitalization. The final outcome, a peaceful death, was the result of applying the RPA/ASN guideline recommendations throughout her care, not just at the end when she became very sick and confused. In this case the application of the guideline recommendations achieved the stated purpose for clinical practice guidelines, to assist practitioner and patient decisions about appropriate healthcare for specific clinical circumstances, and demonstrated their benefit for ESRD patients.

# References

1. Collins, A., Hanson, G., Umen, A., Kjellstrand, C., Keshaviah, P. (1990). Changing risk factor demographics in ESRD patients entering haemodialysis and the impact on long-term mortality. *Am. J. Kidney Dis.*, **15**: 422–32.

2. Van Vlem, B., Schoonjans, R., Vanholder, R., *et al.* (2000). Delayed gastric emptying in dyspeptic chronic haemodialysis patients. *Am. J. Kidney Dis.*, **36**: 962–8.

3. Koch, K.L. (1999). Diabetic gastropathy: gastric neuromuscular dysfunction in diabetes mellitus: a review of symptoms, pathophysiology, and treatment. *Digest. Dis. Sci.*, **44**: 1061–75.

4. Rabine, J.C., Barnett, J.L. (2001). Management of the patient with gastroparesis. *J. Clin. Gastroenterol.*, **32**: 11–18.

5. Sekkarie, M.A. (1997). Torsades de pointes in two chronic renal failure patients treated with cisapride and clarithromycin. *Am. J. Kidney Dis.*, **30**: 437–9.

6. Valdovinos, M.A., Camilleri, M., Zimmermann, B.R. (1993). Chronic diarrhoea in diabetes mellitus: mechanisms and an approach to diagnosis and treatment. *Mayo Clin. Proc.*, **68**: 691–702.

7. Dudl, R.J., Anderson, D.S., Forsythe, A.B., Ziegler, M.G., O'Dorisio, T.M. (1987). Treatment of diabetic diarrhoea and orthostatic hypotension with somatostatin analogue SMS 201–995. *Am. J. Med.*, **83**: 584–8.

8. Pop-Busui, R., Chey, W., Stevens, M.J. (2000). Severe hypertension induced by the long-acting somatostatin analogue sandostatin LAR in a patient with diabetic autonomic neuropathy. *J. Clin. Endocrinol. Metab.*, **85**: 943–6.

9. Waldman, S.D. (2000). Diabetic neuropathy: diagnosis and treatment for the pain management specialist. *Curr. Rev. Pain,* **4**: 383–7.

10. Morello, C.M., Leckband, S.G., Stoner, C.P., *et al.* (1999). Randomized double-blind study comparing the efficacy of gabapentin with amitriptyline on diabetic peripheral neuropathy pain. *Arch. Intern. Med.,* **159**: 1931–7.

11. Foley, R.N., Parfrey, P.S., Morgan, J., *et al.* (2000). Effect of haemoglobin levels in haemodialysis patients with asymptomatic cardiomyopathy. *Kidney Int.,* **58**: 1325–35.

12. Besarab, A., Bolton, W.K., Browne, J.K., *et al.* (1998). The effects of normal as compared with low hematocrit values in patients with cardiac disease who are receiving hemodialysis and epoetin. *New Engl. J. Med.,* **339**: 584–90.

13. Swartz, R. (1999). The use of peritoneal dialysis in special situations. *Adv. Perit. Dial.,* **15**: 160–6.

14. Szczech, L.A., Reddan, D.N., Owen, W.F., *et al.* (2001). Differential survival after coronary revascularization procedures among patients with renal insufficiency. *Kidney Int.,* **60**: 292–9.

15. O'Hare, A.M., Hsu, C.Y., Bacchetti, P., Johansen, K.L. (2002). Peripheral vascular disease risk factors among patients undergoing haemodialysis. *J. Am. Soc. Nephrol.,* **13**: 497–503.

16. O'Hare, A., Johansen, K. (2001). Lower-extremity peripheral arterial disease among patients with end stage renal disease. *J. Am. Soc. Nephrol.,* **12**: 2838–47.

17. Eggers, P.W., Gohdes, D., Pugh, J. (1999). Nontraumatic lower extremity amputations in the Medicare ESRD population. *Kidney Int.,* **56**: 1523–33.

18. Girolami, B., Bernardi, E., Prins, M.H., *et al.* (1999). Antithrombotic drugs in the primary medical management of intermittent claudication: a meta-analysis. *Thromb. Haemost.,* **81**: 715–22.

19. Mayo, R.R., Swartz, R.D. (1996). Redefining the incidence of clinically detectable atheroembolism. *Am. J. Med.,* **100**: 524–9.

20. Edwards, J.M., Taylor, L.M., Porter, J.M. (1998). Limb salvage in ESRD: comparison of modern results in patients with and without ESRD. *Arch. Surg.,* **123**: 1164–8.

21. Schomig, M., Ritz, E., Standl, E., Allenberg, J. (2000). The diabetic foot in the dialysed patient. *J. Am. Soc. Nephrol.,* **11**: 1153–9.

22. Block, G.A., Hulbert-Shearon, T.E., Levin, N.W., Port, F.K. (1998). Association of serum phosphorus and calcium phosphate product with mortality risk in chronic haemodialysis patients: a national study. *Am. J. Kidney Dis.*, **31**: 607–17.

23. Mazhar, A.R., Johnson, R.J., Gillen, D., *et al.* (2001). Risk factors and mortality associated with calciphylaxis in ESRD. *Kidney Int.*, **60**: 324–32.

24. Girotto, J.A., Harmon, J.W., Ratner, L.E., Nicol, T.L., Wong, L., Chen, H. (2001). Parathyroidectomy promotes wound healing and prolongs survival in patients with calciphylaxis from secondary hyperparathyroidism. *Surgery* **130**: 645–50.

25. Hess, C.T. (2002). Calciphylaxis: identification and wound management. *Adv. Skin Wound Care.*, **15**: 64.

26. Podymow, T., Wherrett, C., Burns, K.D. (2001). Hyperbaric oxygen in the treatment of calciphylaxis: a case series. *Nephrol. Dial. Transpl.*, **16**: 2176–80.

27. Wilmer, W.A., Voroshilova, O., Singh, I., Middendorf, D.F., Coslo, F.G. (2001). Transcutaneous oxygen tension in patients with calciphylaxis. *Am. J. Kidney Dis.*, **37**: 797–806.

28. Alem, A.M., Sherrard, D.J., Gillen, D.L., *et al.* (2000). Increased risk of hip fracture among patients with end stage renal disease. *Kidney Int.*, **58**: 396–9.

29. Pressure ulcers in adults: prediction and prevention. *Clinical Practice Guideline Number 3*, AHCPR Publication No. 92–0047. May 1992. Retrieved from *www.ahcpr.gov*

30. Treatment of pressure ulcers. *Clinical Practice Guideline Number 15*. AHCPR Publication No. 95–0652. December 1994. Retrieved from *www.ahcpr.gov*

Chapter 8

# Management of pain in renal failure

Charles J. Ferro, Joanna Chambers,
and Sara N. Davison

Even thinking of pain is like tapping at a high voltage wire with the back of your finger to see if it's live

## 8.1 Introduction

Pain has been defined by the International Association for the Study of Pain as 'an unpleasant sensory and emotional experience associated with actual or potential tissue damage, or described in terms of such damage'.[1] This definition reminds us of the emotional associations of pain including fear and depression. There are numerous potential causes for pain in the patient with end-stage renal disease (ESRD); the experience of pain will, however, be unique to each individual as pain is a subjective experience and can only be described and measured by that individual. The term 'total pain', first used by Cicely Saunders[2] to describe cancer pain, emphasizes the contribution of psychological, spiritual, and social factors to the experience of pain. This concept is equally applicable to pain in ESRD. A unidimensional approach to pain management is likely to be unsuccessful, until the whole person, in the context of their disease and personal life, is taken into account.[3]

> It seems to me that pain in itself, though a pretty nasty piece of work, wouldn't have half the street cred if it wasn't like all bullies joined at the hip with that cringing lickspittle, fear.

## 8.2 Incidence and types of pain

Pain is a very common problem for ESRD patients and may be due to their primary disease (e.g. polycystic kidney disease), concurrent co-morbidity (e.g. diabetic neuropathy or peripheral vascular disease), or disease consequent upon renal failure (e.g. calciphylaxis, bone pain from renal osteodystrophy, and dialysis-related amyloid arthropathy). Pain may also result from the treatment of ESRD. Painful chronic infections such as osteomyelitis and discitis are complications seen from central lines. Arteriovenous fistulae can lead to painful ischaemic neuropathies, including the 'steal syndrome' in which blood that would normally flow to the palmar arch is diverted by the creation of an arteriovenous fistula. Patients on peritoneal dialysis often contend with recurrent pain due to abdominal distension, recurrent peritonitis, and lower back strain.

Pain in patients with ESRD includes most of the same types of pain experienced by cancer patients, namely nociceptive, somatic and visceral, neuropathic, and possibly complex regional pain syndromes. Patients with ESRD frequently experience more than one type of pain,[4] a not unexpected finding in view of the diverse causes of pain in this population. However, the full extent of the problem is not known, as there is little research into the prevalence, nature, aetiology, and impact of pain in these patients. The literature has focused on either pain in the context of a quality of life study,[4,5] non-specific symptoms including pain, or the pathophysiology of particular painful syndromes, e.g. joint pain,[6] rather than the study of pain itself. Despite improvements in dialysis technology and the care of the renal patient, the incidence of chronic pain appears to be increasing and probably reflects an ageing dialysis population with greater co-morbidity so that pain due to peripheral vascular disease, peripheral polyneuropathy, and osteoarthritis is becoming more common.

Although the incidence of pain in ESRD is not clear, preliminary results from ongoing studies in Bristol, UK (verbal communication, C. Cornish) and Edmonton, Canada[7] suggest that approximately 50% of haemodialysis patients report a problem with pain and over 30% rate their current pain as severe. This is consistent with a study citing a 37% prevalence of chronic pain in a population of Italian haemodialysis patients[8] and a more recent study indicating that 20% of in-centre haemodialysis patients experience pain severe enough to require consultation with palliative care for pain management.[9] In North America approximately 20% of dialysis patients die following withdrawal of dialysis, the second most common cause of death for this group of patients.[10] In this subset of patients, almost 50% are known to have significant pain as well as other distressing symptoms as they die.[11–13] However, it is not dialysis withdrawal itself that results in pain. Pain is a part of living with ESRD as opposed to dying following withdrawal of dialysis. While dialysis sustains life, underlying systemic diseases and painful syndromes such as ischaemic limbs and painful neuropathies continue their inexorable course. Non-specific pain is also a concern for the majority of dialysis patients. Another study[4] reported cramps and headaches in 81% and 62% respectively of patients for around one-third of each dialysis session, while 62% and 43% respectively of patients report these symptoms for a significant duration of time off dialysis as well. For post-transplant patients the most common pains were headaches (59%) and bone pain (30%).[4] In a separate study[5] cramps, headache, and joint pain featured as three of the top six symptoms rated by ESRD patients; with a prevalence of 56%, 41%, and 43% respectively. Of those with severe cramps, 68% recorded that it had an adverse effect on daily living. These painful conditions present significant challenges to the patient and the nephrology team throughout the patient's life on dialysis.

## 8.2.1 Quality of life

Pain carries only two messages to the sufferer 'You are broken. Mend or die.'

Pain is one of the most distressing and feared symptoms experienced by patients with advanced terminal illnesses. It can have a significant impact on perceptions of health-related quality of life[14–19] and is the most common reason to seek medical consultation. In an ongoing study of pain in haemodialysis patients, 62% of patients with pain reported extreme interference in their ability to participate in and enjoy recreational activities, and 51% reported extreme suffering due to their pain. Forty-one per cent of patients with pain had considered stopping dialysis due to the pain.[9] A study of pain[4] which included a subset of dialysis patients who completed the Beck Depression Inventory showed a positive correlation between pain and depression. Pain may increase anxiety and impair function affecting both social activities and work. A reduction in both of these can further contribute to low mood or depression. Although not well studied, it appears that chronic pain may be a factor in decisions to withdraw from dialysis.[12,20] If this is confirmed it would be contrary to extensive studies in other populations of terminally ill patients where decisions to hasten death are more commonly related to depression, hopelessness, loss of control, and fear of being a burden.[21–25] This underlines the need to address pain and symptom management in this population.

## 8.2.2 Categories of pain

### 8.2.2.1 Nociceptive pain

Tissue damage in the skin, muscle, and other tissues causes stimulation of sensory receptors with electrical discharge to the spinal cord along mainly Aδ and C fibres. Pain is characteristically felt at the site of damage and may be described using terms such as sharp or like a knife. This is the mechanism of joint pain in dialysis-related amyloid arthropathy. Visceral nociceptors may be stimulated in a similar way by chemical or mechanical irritation, experienced as a sharp pain from liver capsule distension in polycystic kidney and liver disease or a dull, poorly localized pain from gut ischaemia.

### 8.2.2.2 Neuropathic pain

Neuropathic pain results from damage to and changes in the nervous system resulting in either dysfunction or pathological change in the nerve, either at the site of damage or at the level of the dorsal horn. A complex series of changes can occur leading to an increase in excitation. This is contributed to by a reduction in descending (noradrenergic and serotonergic) inhibitory pathways and an increased local activation of excitatory neurotransmitters and N-methyl-D-aspartate (NMDA) receptors. Common descriptors of neuropathic pain include burning, shooting, and stabbing. It characteristically occurs in an area of abnormal sensation, and may be felt at a site distant from its cause, in the distribution of a nerve for example. It may be associated with episodes of 'spontaneous pain', hyperalgesia, and allodynia. The presence of the latter is pathognomonic. The pain of peripheral neuropathy belongs in this category. Many cancer pains have both nociceptive and neuropathic elements. It is likely that the situation is similar for the pains of ESRD; for example the severe pain seen in limb ischaemia and the soft tissue pain of calciphylaxis.

## 8.2.3 Types of pain

### 8.2.3.1 Acute pain

Acute pain occurs following tissue damage and activation of nociceptors at the site of injury and is normally seen as serving an important protective physiological function. The dialysis patient may experience repeated episodes of acute pain during dialysis, such as headaches and muscle cramps, as well as short-lived but severe pain in other sites such as the abdomen. These may occur over long periods of time, though the patient will also be free from them for long periods. These recurring pains need distinguishing from chronic pain, as the management is different. The term recurrent pain has been used to describe this;[26] drawing attention to the fact that it increases the amount the illness intrudes on everyday life. In addition anticipation of pain before each dialysis has an impact on quality of life and may increase the distress from the pain (see Case study 1).

## Case study 1: to illustrate management of temporary but excruciating pain during dialysis

Y is a 31-year-old female with a 13-year history of insulin-dependent diabetes. Both parents had diabetic nephropathy; her mother had died with renal failure and her father had a renal transplant. Renal insufficiency was first diagnosed 4 years previously at routine screening during her first pregnancy, with further deterioration following the birth of her second child. Recently, admission was precipitated by extensive infected oedema of her anterior abdominal wall with full thickness necrosis in the lateral margins of her abdominal apron. Daily haemodialysis, alternating with ultrafiltration, was started to reduce the fluid overload, together with antibiotic treatment.

**Case study 1: to illustrate management of temporary but excruciating pain during dialysis** (continued)

Y had two pains. The first was across her anterior abdomen and was present at all times though eased at rest by tramadol 50 mg 8-hourly. Within minutes of starting dialysis, a second excruciating pain, described as such a strong burning pain she expected to smell burning, would occur across her abdomen, particularly in the 'apron', starting laterally and working medially. The pain lasted throughout dialysis and for approximately 30 min after completion. Anxiety about this pain dominated her feelings.

She had been taking hydromorphone, first 1.3 mg, then 2.6 mg and finally 3.9 mg during dialysis without benefit despite the dose being repeated.

## Actions

Day 1. Fentanyl 25 μg given subcutaneously (SC) prior to dialysis and available hourly as needed plus clonazepam 0.5 mg at night. This led to a better night's sleep but no real improvement in dialysis pain.

Day 2. Fentanyl 50 μg SC before dialysis and as needed (prn). There was some improvement, but by the time she got subsequent doses of fentanyl, she had already started to lose control over the pain. Clonazepam was increased to 1 mg at night and amitriptyline added, working up to a dose of 40 mg at night.

Day 6. Changed to short SC fentanyl infusion of 50 μg/h, starting 30 min before dialysis and running for 30 min after dialysis stopped. This was extremely effective and she was able to tolerate dialysis comfortably on this regimen.

Since this episode it has been possible to stop the SC fentanyl regimen during dialysis as the infected, loculated fluid on her abdominal wall has been managed with plastic surgery. Her background pain control 3 months after this episode is with transdermal fentanyl. Similar excruciating dialysis pain in another patient has been treated successfully in the same way.

### 8.2.3.2 Chronic pain

Chronic pain is usually initiated by tissue injury but is perpetuated by neurophysiological changes which take place within the peripheral and central nervous system leading to continuation of pain in the absence of the pain stimulus. The intensity of the pain may be out of proportion to the original injury or tissue damage. As pain persists, other factors, such as the psychosocial and spiritual distress relating to the disease or unrelated situations can influence the experience of pain. Chronic pain is not defined by duration but rather in the context of someone who continues to experience pain in the absence of persistent nociceptor damage. This pain has no useful biological function. The many causes of recurrent pain in ESRD can be perpetuated by continued physical damage from disease processes, such as dialysis-related amyloid arthropathy, in addition to neurophysiological changes in the nervous system. They are therefore better described as repetitive acute pain or recurrent pain,[26] though they are chronic in the sense of occurring over many years. Patients may in addition experience chronic pain as defined above and thus the total picture is complex with mixed categories.

### 8.2.3.3 Episodic, incident, or breakthrough pain

These are terms used to describe pain that breaks through or occurs despite regular analgesic medication. They fall into three main categories: incident pain where movement precipitates the pain; breakthrough pain where the background medication is inadequate for continuous pain control so pain occurs towards the end of a dosing period; and paroxysmal pain arising without obvious precipitators and which is often neuropathic in nature. All three kinds of episodic pain occur in patients with ESRD.

Categorizing pain helps the physician choose an appropriate management strategy which may include both drug and non-drug therapies. Generally nociceptive pain responds well to opioids whereas neuropathic pain may be poorly responsive or require doses for response that are associated with unacceptable toxicity. The handling of opioids by patients with ESRD increases the likelihood of this toxicity occurring before useful pain relief. Diagnosing neuropathic pain reminds the physician to consider the use of adjuvant analgesics such as antidepressants and anticonvulsants where there is evidence for their efficacy.[27,28] Good descriptive studies of the types of pain seen in cancer have helped its management, the same is likely to be true for ESRD.

## 8.2.4 Barriers to adequate pain relief

The high prevalence of unrelieved pain is not unique to ESRD. Despite the availability of effective pain management interventions[28] and published guidelines for its management,[29] many patients with cancer have considerable pain and receive inadequate analgesia.[30] Inadequate pain assessment, reluctance of the patient to report pain, and lack of staff time and training in the basic principles of pain management have been identified as barriers to adequate pain management in cancer patients.[31] Many of these apply to ESRD; however, the management of pain in ESRD is more complex for several reasons:

◆ **Lack of recognition of the problem**: patients may under-report pain, assuming that pain is an integral part of their condition. Others may have cognitive dysfunction preventing effective communication. If pain is reported, it may not be acknowledged and managed effectively by the nephrology team as pain management may not have sufficient priority in dialysis units.

◆ **Lack of research/knowledge**: there is a lack of a discrete medical literature that synthesizes pain management and nephrology. Studies of the pattern and types of pain seen in ESRD are needed in addition to those evaluating the efficacy of analgesia with particular reference in this group of patients to the toxicity and pharmacokinetic and pharmacodynamic data.

◆ **Altered pharmacokinetics and pharmacodynamics of analgesics in ESRD**: the absorption and clearance of drugs are more complex in renal failure. ESRD patients are much more likely to run into problems of opioid toxicity, such as confusion, myoclonus, and sedation (see later section on opioids).

◆ **Adverse effects** of analgesics are common and may be mimicked by uraemic symptoms resulting in the inappropriate withdrawal of analgesics. Unfortunately even after appropriate withdrawal or reduction they are often not restarted when the acute crisis resolves. In our experience, the most common presentation of opioid toxicity necessitating opioid switch in the ESRD population is confusion and cognitive impairment.

◆ **Co-morbid disease and an increase in susceptibility to some adverse drug effects** often limit the use of analgesics. Patients with ESRD are frequently on multiple drugs, with the consequent increase in risk of adverse interactions between these drugs. For example warfarin increases the risk of gastrointestinal bleeding associated with NSAIDS, some of which potentiate the action of warfarin itself, by inhibiting its metabolism. In addition there is known to be an increase in the non-nephrotoxic adverse effects of NSAIDS in patients with ESRD, particularly relating to the gastrointestinal tract.

◆ **Lack of training in pain management**: pain management has not been a focus of training in renal medicine, resulting in the lack of a systematic approach to the problem of pain.

Patients and their families may be denied the right to effective pain management through lack of understanding of effective pain evaluation and management.

◆ **Many patients will have more than one cause for their pain**: this makes the diagnosis and management of pain challenging. However, it is of clinical importance to try and distinguish the types or components of a patient's pain in order to treat them effectively.

◆ **Limb preservation**: ESRD patients may experience severe pain from ischaemic limbs for a considerable time in an effort to preserve a limb or defer high-risk surgery.

Adequate pain management in ESRD will require:

◆ Recognition of the need to work collaboratively with other teams, including palliative care and pain management teams.

◆ Better education in pain management of the nephrology team.

◆ Recognition of the spiritual and psychosocial aspects of pain.

◆ Increased study and understanding of the pharmacology of analgesics in patients with ESRD.

## 8.2.5 Evaluation of pain and its management

The study of pain management in ESRD is limited; however, the principles of its management are similar to those of managing acute and chronic pain in other conditions. The aim of pain relief is to provide effective analgesia without undue or unacceptable toxicity. This requires regular assessment and recording of the intensity of pain, its effect on functioning and quality of life, and the impact of analgesic medications on these factors.

Evaluation starts at the bedside with a good pain history, documentation of sites, severity, and postulated causes of the pain (Table 8.1). It will include previous measures of pain relief, their effectiveness, and toxicity. It should also embrace the effects of the pain on social functioning and psychosocial and spiritual issues that may impact on the perception of the pain. Pain can be recorded either as pain intensity or pain relief using verbal or numerical scales. Despite there being no objective measure of pain relief it has proved reliable to work on the principle that pain is what the patient says it is and he or she is the only person who can measure it. This can then safely be used as a measure of severity and gauge of effectiveness. It is also important to listen to the patient to validate the significance of their pain and suffering. This expression of understanding of their situation is an important part of the therapeutic intervention.

Studies where pain has been measured have used the McGill Pain Questionnaire (MPQ),[32] or the Brief Pain Inventory (BPI)[7,9,3] which incorporates quality-of-life questions such as effect on sleep, daily activities, relationships, and enjoyment of life.

Pain measurement tools (PMTs) have been used extensively in cancer patients both as research tools and for bedside evaluation of therapy. They range from simple unidimensional bedside tools that can be used by all physicians and nurses; such as visual analogue scales and verbal and numerical rating scales, to more sophisticated multidimensional tools (e.g. BPI or MPQ) which include diagrammatic representation of pain and information on the other dimensions of the pain. Both of these multidimensional PMTs have been validated in cancer care across a wide variety of cultural and linguistic backgrounds. The BPI uses numerical scales to score worst, least, average, and current pain. It covers medications, percentage pain relief, and interference with mood, physical activity, and other functional areas. It is self-administered

**Table 8.1** Suggested contents of a pain history

| Pain dimension | Relevant questions |
| --- | --- |
| Site of pain | Where do you feel this pain?<br>Does it go anywhere else?<br>Is there numbness or other strange sensation at the site of the pain? |
| Character of pain | Describe your pain. Is it dull, burning, or shooting? |
| History of pain | How long have you had it?<br>How did it start?<br>Did something appear to cause it or did it appear out of the blue? |
| Relieving factors | Does anything make it better, such as position, medication? |
| Accentuating factors | Does anything make it worse? |
| Pattern | Is there any pattern to the pain?<br>Is it worse at any particular time of day? |
| Sleep disturbance | Does the pain prevent you getting to sleep?<br>Does it wake you in the night? |
| Activities | Does the pain stop you doing things you would otherwise do? |
| Previous treatments | What have you used in the past for you pain?<br>What was helpful/What was not helpful and why? |

Adapted from: *Relief of chronic malignant pain?* Henry McQuay at http:www.jr2.ox.ac.uk/bandolier/booth/painpag/-wisdom/493HJM.html

and easy to use. The MPQ is also self administered. It asks the patient to specify subjective pain experience using classes of word descriptor; sensory, affective, and evaluative. In a review of PMTs in clinical research in palliative care both the BPI and the MPQ were felt to be appropriate tools for measuring pain outcomes.[34] Many of the recommendations in this review could be transferred for use in ESRD.

## 8.3  Treatment strategy

Following assessment of the pain, a straightforward explanation of the postulated cause(s) and a proposed management plan should be given to the patient. Where treatment is likely to be complex it is important to give the patient achievable goals, and an explanation of the steps to be taken. These may need to be staged, initially aiming for freedom from pain at rest and at night, progressing to relief of more difficult pain such as that which is movement related. It is important to the patient that the clinician is honest and does not raise unrealistic expectations. The patient should also be reassured that the clinician will continue to address the patient's pain management needs if unsuccessful initially. Since relief of all pain is not always possible, an important treatment target can be that pain will be reduced sufficiently for it to cause less interference with the individual's desired lifestyle. Attention to psychosocial and spiritual issues must not be forgotten as part of the pain management strategy (see Case study 2). The incidence of depression in dialysis patients is known to be high, possibly up to 50% of those who dialyse.[35,36] Pain is also known to be associated with depression[37] and appropriate pharmacological management should be instituted where indicated clinically.

## Case study 2: Psychosocial issues matter

A 62-year-old West Indian had phantom limb pain following amputation for peripheral vascular disease. Pain relief had been successfully achieved using a fentanyl 75 μg/h transdermal patch. Severe infection, without a change in the level of pain or other parameters, led to an episode of opioid toxicity, necessitating reversal of narcosis. Fentanyl was stopped but his pain returned. He described his pain as starting in his absent limb and spreading up his leg through the stump to his shoulders and head. Further questioning revealed that he had been living in a residential home away from his wife for several months since the amputation as essential alterations to his house had not been done.

Analgesia was restarted at the bottom of the analgesic ladder with regular paracetamol and codeine if needed. At the same time he was seen by the social worker to look at how to address the social problems. By the next day he reported his pain as improved without the need for any strong opioids, though later it increased again, while his psychosocial issues continued to be addressed. His analgesic requirements were titrated against pain until he achieved satisfactory pain control with a dose of modified release morphine of 20 mg b.d., which is one-quarter as potent as his original dose of fentanyl, and without the necessity to increase it further for several months.

## 8.3.1 Use of analgesics

In 1986, the first edition of *Cancer Pain Relief* was published by the World Health Organization (WHO). This publication proposed a method for relief of cancer pain, based on a small number of relatively inexpensive drugs, including morphine, and introduced the concept of the 'analgesic ladder'. Field-testing in several countries demonstrated the usefulness and efficacy of this method in cancer patients.[29] The second edition, published in 1996,[3] takes into account many of the advances in understanding and practice that have happened since the publication of the first edition, but retained most of the original method. The groundwork for this revision was started in 1989, in the context of the meeting of a WHO Expert Committee on Cancer Pain Relief and Active Supportive Care.[38] These publications stress that pain management should be undertaken as part of comprehensive palliative care. Relief of other symptoms, and of psychological, social, and spiritual problems is paramount. Attempting to relieve pain without addressing the patient's non-physical concerns is unlikely to be successful.[3]

Since then these principles of pain management have become the basis for pain management in other areas of medicine. They can be summarized by five phrases:

- 'by mouth'
- 'by the clock'
- 'by the ladder'
- 'for the individual'
- 'attention to detail'.

### 8.3.1.1 'By mouth'

Whenever possible, drugs should be given orally. Where ingestion or absorption of the medication is uncertain, as in dysphagia or vomiting, or the patient is too weak to swallow, analgesia must be given by an alternative route, usually subcutaneously or rectally.

## 8.3.1.2 'By the clock'

Where pain is continuous, short-acting or normal-release preparations should be prescribed and given regularly. Additional 'breakthrough' or 'rescue' medication should be available on an 'as needed' (prn) basis in addition to the regular dose. This enables the dose to be titrated against need while monitoring toxicity and increasing the dose according to the amount of extra opioid that has been required.

## 8.3.1.3 'By the ladder'

Using the sequence of the WHO analgesic ladder (Fig. 8.1), initial analgesia is selected according to the severity of pain, starting at the lowest appropriate level. The drug should be used at its full tolerated dose before moving to the next level. Only one Step 2 opioid should be used at a time. If ineffective, it is unlikely that another drug from the same step will be effective and generally it is necessary to proceed to a Step 3 analgesic. Step 1 analgesics (NSAIDs and paracetamol) at full dose can be added to Step 2 or 3 drugs. Adjuvant analgesics can be added to all three steps for specific indications.

## 8.3.1.4 'For the individual'

There is no standard dose of strong opioids. The 'right dose' is the dose that relieves the patient's pain without causing unacceptable side-effects. Opioids for mild to moderate pain have a dose limit in practice because of formulation (e.g. combined with aminosalicylic acid or paracetamol) or because of little increase in analgesia above standard doses together with a disproportionate increase in adverse effects at higher doses (e.g. codeine). Doses of opioids for moderate to severe pain have to be titrated against the patient's pain. Only the patient can measure the pain or quantify the side-effects experienced. The clinician must listen to and believe the patient. Sensitivity to different adverse effects is not predictable, and will vary between patients and within the same patient at different times. If an individual finds that a particular strong opioid causes unacceptable side-effects, an alternative has to be sought.

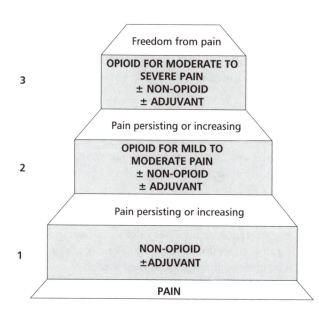

**Fig. 8.1** The WHO analgesic ladder.

### 8.3.1.5 'Attention to detail'

Pain changes over time, thus there is the need for assessment and reassessment until pain relief is achieved. The need for regular administration of pain-relief drugs should be explained to the patient. The first and last doses of the day should be linked to the patient's waking time and bedtime. Side-effects should be explained and actively managed. All patients should have a laxative prescribed if on regular opioids and an antiemetic should be available. Written information about the drug, dosage, reason for using it, and possible side-effects should accompany the prescription.

## 8.3.2 Choice of analgesic

The choice of analgesic will depend on a number of factors including the nature of the pain, the severity of renal impairment, concomitant medication and concurrent illnesses. Special consideration is needed when prescribing for patients with renal insufficiency and a basic knowledge of renal drug handling is required.

### 8.3.2.1 Handling of drugs by the kidney

Many drugs and their metabolites are excreted in the kidney by glomerular filtration, tubular secretion, or both. Renal impairment thus has a significant effect on the clearance of these drugs, with potentially important clinical consequences. These are most obvious in patients with overt renal failure but more subtle forms of renal dysfunction may also be important and are extremely common, most notably as an accompaniment of ageing.

Patients on dialysis are often prescribed multiple drugs.[39] Also, patients with acute and chronic renal failure are likely to be on complex medication regimes. Although in theory changes in dose and dosage interval of all drugs that are affected by renal impairment need to be considered, in practice, dose adjustment is important for relatively few specific drugs with a narrow therapeutic index or adverse effects related to drug or metabolite accumulation.

Although renal impairment has its most important effects upon excretion, other aspects of pharmacokinetics (what the body does to the drug)—absorption, metabolism, distribution (including protein binding) and renal haemodynamics—may be affected, as may pharmacodynamics (what the drug does to the body).

The major determinant of alteration in dosage is the change in drug clearance. This can be estimated from measurements of glomerular filtration rate (GFR), which can be estimated from the serum creatinine concentration using the Cockcroft and Gault formula.[40] However, tubular secretion of drugs[41] and changes in pharmacokinetics due to extrarenal factors[42] do not always change in parallel with GFR.

There are many handbooks that provide guidelines for the adjustment in dosage in renal impairment.[43–45] The data in these are derived from measurement or estimation of changes in clearance, half-life, and volume of distribution. The determination of these pharmacokinetic variables is very model-dependent and their application has limitations.[46–48] Consequently these guidelines should be regarded only as useful approximations.

### 8.3.2.2 Pharmacokinetics

Subcutaneous and intramuscular drug administration may be associated with reduced absorption in patients with acute renal failure or who are critically ill with shock and hypotension.

Protein binding is affected by renal impairment resulting in increased plasma concentrations of a number of acidic compounds that compete with drugs for binding sites on albumin and other plasma proteins.[49,50] Serum albumin concentration is low in patients with nephrotic syndrome and may also decline in cachectic patients and in the elderly, reducing the number of drug-binding sites. As a consequence the proportion of free to bound drug is increased, and there are greater fluctuations in the free drug following the administration of each dose. This could be responsible for an increased susceptibility to adverse drug reactions.[51]

Drugs are excreted by the kidney either as the original (parent) drug or more polar (water-soluble) substances after metabolism in the liver. Uraemia may directly affect liver drug metabolism by affecting hepatic enzyme function.[52] Kidneys also contain many of the enzymes important in hepatic drug metabolism. In experimental uraemia, the metabolism of drugs such as morphine and paracetamol has been shown to be reduced in the diseased kidney.[52] These alterations in metabolism are minor in comparison to active metabolite retention as a direct consequence of renal impairment. Renal failure may also reduce drug activation. For example, the conversion of sulindac to its active sulphide metabolite is reduced in uraemia.[53] This has been invoked as a partial explanation for the lower incidence of side-effects observed with sulindac compared with indomethacin.[54]

## 8.3.3 WHO analgesic ladder. Step 1: non-opioid analgesics ± adjuvants

The non-opioid analgesics include acetylsalicylic acid (ASA, aspirin), other non-steroidal anti-inflammatory drugs (NSAIDs) and paracetamol (acetaminophen). In most countries several NSAIDs will be available and the choice will depend on a number of factors including cost and the physician's experience with the drug.

### 8.3.3.1 Non-steroidal anti-inflammatory drugs (NSAIDs)

NSAIDs, including ASA, inhibit prostaglandin synthesis by inhibition of cyclo-oxygenase, of which there are two main isoforms, cyclo-oxygenase-1 (COX-1) and COX-2. The primary renal prostaglandins in humans are prostaglandin $E_2$ and $I_2$, each of which is a vasodilator and natriuretic.[55] In addition to effects on renal blood flow, the prostaglandins also influence tubular ion transport directly. In healthy individuals the inhibition of cyclo-oxygenase has no detectable effects on renal function, but in patients with decreased effective circulating volume (e.g. patients with cardiac failure, nephrotic syndrome, liver disease, or renal failure) the cyclo-oxygenase inhibitors cause a reduction in GFR that can be severe and irreversible.[56,57] They can also cause sodium and water retention, aggravating hypertension,[58,59] and hyperkalaemia. Inhibition of COX-1 reduces the production of thromboxane and thus impairs platelet aggregation. It also compromises the gastrointestinal mucosa by inhibiting the secretion of cytoprotective mucus. As a result, the major limitation of NSAIDs is their gastrointestinal toxicity.[60] The effectiveness of selective COX-2 inhibitors as analgesics is comparable with COX-1 inhibitors such as naproxen, ibuprofen, and diclofenac with lessened gastric toxicity.[60-62]

Unlike non-selective NSAIDs, selective COX-2 inhibitors do not inhibit platelet aggregation and may affect the haemostatic balance and favour thrombosis. Indeed a large trial with over 8000 patients found myocardial infarctions to be more frequent statistically in patients treated with the selective COX-2 inhibitor rofecoxib than the non-selective NSAID naproxen.[60] However, there is now compelling evidence that patients treated with naproxen have a decreased incidence of myocardial infarction compared with patients treated with other NSAIDs or those not receiving NSAIDs.[63-65] This suggests that naproxen has beneficial cardiovascular protective actions, probably by inhibiting platelet aggregation,[66] rather than rofecoxib increasing cardiovascular risk.[67] However, although naproxen reduces the risk of myocardial infarction it offers less protection than aspirin,[68] therefore low dose aspirin should be considered in patients at risk of cardiovascular disease who are taking naproxen or other NSAIDs.

Hypersensitivity occurs occasionally as an idiosyncratic reaction with NSAIDs. Manifestations of this syndrome may occur within minutes of drug ingestion and symptoms range from vasomotor rhinitis with profuse watery secretion, angioneurotic oedema, urticaria, and bronchial spasm to laryngeal oedema, hypotension, shock, loss of consciousness, and complete vasomotor collapse. A hypersensitivity reaction can occur after ingestion of only a small amount of aspirin or other NSAID. To minimize the risk of an allergic reaction the patient should be asked if they can tolerate aspirin or aspirin-like compounds. If hypersensitivity occurs, aspirin and NSAIDs should not be prescribed and a change made to an alternative non-opioid (e.g. paracetamol). If pain persists they may need an opioid analgesic.

### 8.3.3.2 Paracetamol (acetaminophen)

Paracetamol is a long-established, non-prescription, antipyretic analgesic drug[69–71] with weak anti-inflammatory activity.[72] These effects are thought to be mediated by inhibition of prostaglandin synthesis, although the exact mechanism is still not clear.[72] In therapeutic doses, paracetamol has no other important pharmacological effects and does not adversely affect platelet function and haemostasis.[73]

Paracetamol is extensively metabolized in the liver. Some 2–5% of the therapeutic dose is excreted unchanged in the urine.[73] The kinetics of paracetamol elimination have been investigated in patients with renal, hepatic, thyroid, and gastrointestinal disease. No clinically significant changes have been observed except in patients with severe acute and decompensated chronic liver disease in whom the half-life is considerably prolonged. In patients with chronic renal failure there is a marked accumulation of inactive paracetamol conjugates.[74] Paracetamol is also less likely to cause further deterioration in renal function than NSAIDs[75] in patients with chronic renal failure. It is therefore generally considered safe to give paracetamol at full dose to patients with ESRD although there are concerns that chronic use may hasten the progression of renal failure.[76]

## 8.3.4 WHO analgesic ladder. Step 2: opioid for mild to moderate pain ± non opioid ± adjuvant

The WHO analgesic ladder divides opioids into those used for mild to moderate pain (Step 2; Fig 8.1) and those used for moderate to severe pain (Step 3). Lower doses of drugs used in Step 3 will have a similar analgesic effect as higher doses of those used in Step 2. When pain persists or increases despite non-opioid drugs a Step 2 analgesic should be started. These include codeine, dihydrocodeine, dextropropoxyphene, and tramadol.

### 8.3.4.1 Codeine

Codeine, a naturally occurring opium alkaloid produced by methylation of morphine, is a less potent analgesic than morphine with a ceiling effect.[77] It is metabolized in the liver to form morphine and norcodeine and conjugated to form glucuronides and sulphates of both codeine and its metabolites.[78] Its analgesic action is thought to be in part through binding to the μ and κ opioid receptors in addition to an effect from the morphine produced by metabolism.[79,80] The metabolites of codeine are renally excreted and accumulate in patients with renal impairment.[81–83] Serious dependence is rarely associated with codeine, and withdrawal symptoms develop more slowly than with morphine and are milder.

In normal subjects codeine does not cause appreciable respiratory depression but does have antitussive[84] and constipating effects.[85] However, there have been several case reports of prolonged narcosis in patients with renal impairment following ingestion of codeine.[83,86]

Profound unconsciousness and respiratory depression, which can be delayed, has occurred after trivial doses. This appears to be an idiosyncratic phenomenon. In the authors' experience patients are often still distressed and in pain despite profound central nervous system depression. Some patients with ESRD, however, are able to tolerate regular doses of codeine for a prolonged period without experiencing toxicity.

### 8.3.4.2 Dextropropoxyphene

Dextropropoxyphene is an opioid for mild to moderate pain usually prescribed in combination with paracetamol.[87] Decreased elimination of dextropropoxyphene and its major pharmacologically active metabolite, norpropoxyphene, have been reported in patients with renal failure.[88] Norpropoxyphene accumulation is associated with central nervous system toxicity, respiratory depression, and cardiotoxicity.[89] Dextropropoxyphene is, therefore, not recommended for use in patients with severe renal impairment.

### 8.3.4.3 Tramadol

Tramadol, which is a single-entity, centrally acting analgesic, was originally marketed in Germany in 1977[90] and launched in the UK in 1994 and in the USA in 1995. It exerts its analgesic actions through at least two complementary modes of action; agonism at the $\mu$ opioid receptor and inhibition of noradrenaline and serotonin re-uptake.[91,92] It can be administered orally, rectally, or parenterally.

Good results have been published for cancer pain in a number of studies[93] where it was shown to be effective in different types of moderate to severe pain, including neuropathic pain, though with a ceiling effect and the need to progress to Step 3 analgesics when pain increased.[94]

Tramadol is metabolized in the liver to $O$-desmethyl tramadol (M1) which has a higher affinity for the $\mu$ opioid receptor than the parent drug,[95] but its slow production results in very low and clinically insignificant plasma levels. Ninety percent of tramadol and its metabolites are excreted in the urine, with 30% as unchanged tramadol.[96]

It has been suggested that tramadol induces fewer opioid side-effects for a given level of analgesia compared with traditional opioids.[94,97] Importantly it does not appear to cause significant respiratory depression when recommended doses are used.[93,97–99] This has been attributed to the low affinity of tramadol for the $\mu$ receptor which is 10 times less than codeine and 6000 times less than morphine.[98] Only 30% of the antinociceptive and analgesic actions of tramadol can be antagonized by naloxone.[100]

In those with normal renal function the recommended dose of tramadol is 50–100 mg four times daily with a maximum dose of 400 mg a day. Adjustments are required in patients over 75 years of age and in those with renal or hepatic impairment.[90] Suggested dose adjustments are that patients with a creatinine clearance of <30 ml/min should receive 50–100 mg 12-hourly.[90] In our own practice, up to 200 mg per day of tramadol in divided doses appears to be well tolerated in dialysis patients.

## 8.3.5 WHO analgesic ladder. Step 3: opioid for moderate to severe pain ± non-opioid ± adjuvant

### 8.3.5.1 Tolerance, dependence and addiction—myths and fears

There are many myths surrounding the use of morphine. These may not extend to other strong opioids because many do not appreciate that they have similar mechanisms of action to morphine. Tolerance is defined as the need for increasing doses of a drug in order to achieve the same pharmacological action. It can occur both to unwanted effects such as respiratory depression (see Case study 3) and nausea as well as to the desired pain relief. Incomplete cross-tolerance to unwanted effects is the basis for switching from one opioid to another with the aim of maintaining analgesia while reducing side-effects. Studies of cancer patients taking oral morphine show that patients may continue on the same dose of morphine for months or years without needing to increase the dose. The requirement for dose escalation is usually on account of progression of disease. Fear of tolerance or addiction can lead to reluctance to start appropriate strong opioids for severe pain.

Physical dependence is characterized by withdrawal symptoms if treatment is stopped abruptly or an antagonist given. This does not, however, prevent dose reduction if pain is relieved by other means and in practice it does not prevent the effective use of opioids. Addiction or psychological dependence is a behavioural pattern characterized by craving for the drug and an overwhelming preoccupation with obtaining it. Extensive clinical experience has shown that it occurs extremely rarely or not at all in patients receiving opioids for pain relief.[3,101]

If pain is relieved by other means then a gradual discontinuation of opioids will prevent withdrawal symptoms.[102] After abrupt pain reduction such as a nerve block, the dose will need to be reduced to prevent respiratory depression.[103]

## Case study 3: Tolerance to adverse effects

A 56-year-old Caucasian female with polycystic kidney and liver disease had started haemodialysis at age 53. Eighteen months later she was admitted with severe liver pain, caused by infection in one of the cysts. Analgesia had been gradually increased until she was taking hydromorphone 1.3 mg every 4 h with only partial relief. A fentanyl 25 µg/h transdermal patch was started with excellent pain control at 24 h (when blood levels would still be rising). By 48 h she was toxic with falling oxygen saturation and the patch was removed. Subcutaneous fentanyl was then started at 50% of the 25 µg/h patch (i.e. 300 µg/24 h). This was supplemented with prn fentanyl 25 µg SC. By taking into account the previous days prn doses the dose in the SC syringe driver was gradually increased through 400 µg to 500 to 600 µg/24 h over 5 days. At this time, the transdermal patch was reintroduced (25 µg/h = 600 µg/24 h) without further toxicity.

When pain subsequently escalated the strong opioid dose was titrated upwards using hydromorphone 1.3 mg prn. She was later able to tolerate transdermal fentanyl at doses of 50 µg/h and then 75 µg/h without respiratory depression.

### 8.3.5.2 Initiating strong opioids

The initiation of strong opioids is triggered by the intensity of pain and not the life expectancy of a patient. In view of the potential for severe and unpleasant toxicity, normal-release (short-acting) not modified-release (long-acting) preparations should ideally be used. Breakthrough medication should be available. The key to safety is through use of the oral route and the proper evaluation and recording of benefit and toxicity. The effective analgesic dose of any opioid in patients with normal renal function varies considerably. The correct dose is the dose that relieves the pain without causing unacceptable side-effects. The balance between toxicity and benefit with opioid administration for those with renal impairment or on renal replacement therapy is weighted heavily towards toxicity, hence the need for alternative strong opioids discussed below. The onset of adverse side-effects should trigger a reassessment of analgesic strategy and choice of strong opioid.

### 8.3.5.3 Morphine

Sir William Osler referred to morphine as 'God's own medicine'. It was isolated from an opium extract in 1803 but the chemical structure was not elucidated until 1925 and chemical synthesis was not achieved until 1952.[104] Nevertheless, morphine is still the opioid drug against which all new drugs with suspected opioid activity are compared and it is generally considered to be the 'drug of choice' for the treatment of severe pain in patients with normal renal function.

There are three main opioid receptors: $\mu$, kappa and delta. Morphine is a potent $\mu$ agonist and the $\mu$ receptor, in addition to analgesia, is thought also to mediate some non-analgesic actions such as respiratory depression, euphoria, reduced gastrointestinal motility and physical dependence.[105] Information about kappa receptor effects suggests that in addition to analgesia it mediates dysphoria and psychotomimetic effects[106], while protecting against some of the unpleasant $\mu$ and delta effects.

Morphine has a relatively low oral bioavailability of 20–30%. It is absorbed in the upper small bowel and undergoes extensive first-pass effect with considerable interindividual variability. It is extensively metabolized by hepatic biotransformation and only a small percentage is excreted unchanged in the urine (5–10% of the dose). Despite this, liver disease does not appear to have a marked effect on morphine pharmacokinetics,[107] although the clearance of morphine has been found to be decreased in liver cirrhosis[108] with the consequent risk of accumulation with repeated administration. Lower doses or longer dosage intervals can be used to minimize this risk.

Morphine-3-glucuronide (M3G) is the major metabolite (~45% of a dose). Morphine-6-glucuronide (M6G) is a quantitatively minor (5% of a dose) but important metabolite[109] due to its actions, which are indistinguishable from those of morphine. When given systemically, M6G is approximately twice as potent an analgesic as morphine.[110] It plays a special role in morphine's effects accounting for a significant proportion of morphine's analgesic actions with chronic administration.[110–113] It is excreted by the kidney and therefore M6G accumulates in renal failure,[114–119] probably explaining morphine's toxicity and long duration of action in patients with renal impairment.

It has been postulated that the ratio of M3G and M6G to morphine plays a role in the experience of toxicity, though studies are conflicting. When the drug is administered parentally this ratio is lower than following oral administration.[120] Theoretically, therefore, in renal patients where the progressive accumulation of M6G is greater than that of morphine,[115,121] there may be some therapeutic advantage in administering parenteral morphine or diamorphine.

In our experience, **chronic administration** of morphine is not well tolerated by patients with severe renal failure or by those needing dialysis. It is our practice therefore to use alternative strong opioids such as hydromorphone, alfentanil and fentanyl when starting strong opioids for prolonged use (see section 8.5.1.4 for dose titration methods prior to use of transdermal fentanyl).

### 8.3.5.4 Hydromorphone

Hydromorphone is a potent $\mu$ receptor agonist first synthesized in 1921 and introduced into clinical medicine in 1926. It is an effective analgesic[122] approximately five to seven times more potent than morphine following oral administration. Studies with parenteral patient-controlled analgesia suggest the parenteral potency is about three times that of morphine.[123] It has a similar side-effect profile to morphine[124] though it may cause less pruritus, sedation, and nausea.[125]

Hydromorphone is primarily metabolized in the liver to hydromorphone-3-glucuronide (H3G) and the conjugates excreted in the urine. An approximate four-fold increase in the ratio of H3G to hydromorphone was demonstrated in one patient with renal failure when compared with 18 cancer patients with normal renal function.[126] This led to the postulation that H3G may have been responsible for myoclonus in another patient in renal failure who received 1003 mg of hydromorphone over 24 h parenterally and a further patient who experienced severe agitated delirium at a lower dose of 144 mg hydromorphone orally as she went into acute renal failure.[127] As morphine glucuronides are not cleared by dialysis it is reasonable to assume that H3G also accumulates in patients on dialysis.[126,127]

Despite these theoretical considerations, a recent retrospective audit[128] and our own clinical experience suggest that hydromorphone is better tolerated than morphine by patients with renal impairment. Careful dose titration, with monitoring for potential toxicity, has enabled many patients with ESRD and severe pain to take hydromorphone with adequate pain relief without unacceptable toxicity. This leads us to believe that it can be used safely and effectively in some patients with renal failure, if it is appropriately monitored and its toxicity recorded (see case studies).

### 8.3.5.5 Methadone

Methadone is a synthetic effective opioid analgesic for the treatment of severe pain[129,130] with activity mainly at the μ receptor. In addition there is some evidence that it is able to function as an NMDA receptor antagonist.[131] It has high oral bioavailability and is extensively distributed in the tissues where it accumulates with repeated dosing. Thus, though it has a plasma half-life of 2–3 h, it has prolonged pharmacological action because of slow release from the reservoirs in the tissues, of up to 60 h.[132,133]

Clinically its main use has been as a substitute opioid in the management of dependence. In addition, it is used as an alternative opioid in cancer pain,[134] where some clinicians believe it may be more effective for neuropathic pain than other strong opioids because of its NMDA receptor antagonism.

Methadone is excreted mainly in the faeces, with metabolism into pharmacologically inactive metabolites primarily in the liver, although ~20% is excreted unchanged in the urine.[135] It is not removed by dialysis[136,137] but in anuric patients methadone is exclusively excreted in faeces with no accumulation in plasma.[136] These factors would suggest that methadone may be a safe, effective analgesic for use in patients with renal impairment, if carefully monitored.[136]

### 8.3.5.6 Pethidine (Meperidine)

Pethidine is a synthetic opioid agonist, which is less potent and shorter-acting than morphine, with a similar side-effect profile. When given by the oral route, pethidine is about 25% as potent as when given parenterally and has 12% of the potency of oral morphine in repeated doses. It has a short duration of action.

It is metabolized in the liver mainly to norpethidine, which is pharmacologically active, and other inactive metabolites, with only 5% excreted in the urine unchanged.[138,139] Norpethidine is about half as potent as an analgesic but has twice the proconvulsive activity as its parent compound.[140] It is excreted in the urine[138] and accumulates in patients with renal impairment.[141]

Pethidine is not recommended for use in chronic pain because of its short duration of action and hence need for frequent doses; in addition accumulation of norpethidine can occur even in the presence of normal renal function with neuroexcitatory effects and risk of convulsions.

Pethidine should be avoided in patients with renal failure other than as single doses for acute pain.

### 8.3.5.7 Oxycodone

Oxycodone is a semisynthetic opioid.[142] It has a similar analgesic and side-effect profile to morphine,[143,144] with the possible exception of hallucinations, which may occur less commonly after oxycodone.[145] It is eliminated mainly by metabolism in the liver[146] to noroxycodone[147] and oxymorphone,[148] which one study suggests may contribute to some of its effect.[143] Less than 10% of administered oxycodone is excreted unchanged in the urine.[149] There are few studies of chronic administration in renal failure, but a single-dose study in patients prior to renal transplant demonstrated a prolonged mean elimination half-life of oxycodone and noroxycodone.[150]

Oxycodone is a useful opioid in patients with normal renal function when an 'opioid switch' is required to improve analgesia with fewer adverse effects. In North America low-dose oxycodone is often used as a Step 2 opioid. Despite a lack of published evidence it is used by some clinicians in patients with chronic renal failure and appears to be well tolerated in a proportion.

### 8.3.5.8 Fentanyl (see Case study 3)

Fentanyl is a potent synthetic opioid μ receptor agonist with a short onset time and relatively short half-life (terminal half-life range 1.5–6 h)[151] mainly because of rapid redistribution. Alfentanil and sufentanil are derived from fentanyl citrate.[151] Fentanyl is 50–100 times more potent and 1000 times more lipophilic than morphine.[152] These properties make it suitable for use in a transdermal delivery system.[153] Fentanyl causes less histamine release, has a lower incidence of constipation, and affords greater cardiovascular stability than morphine,[154] and can thus be a useful alternative when morphine's side-effects hamper effective pain management.[152]

Fentanyl has poor oral bioavailability; it is therefore usually administered intravenously or transdermally, the latter only suitable for stable pain or to provide background analgesia while dose titration takes place with a short-acting opioid. It is rapidly metabolized in the liver, with only 5–10% excreted unchanged in the urine.[155] Its metabolites are considered to be inactive. There does not appear to be any clinically significant accumulation of fentanyl when administered to patients with renal impairment.[154,156–158] However, it should be remembered that a subcutaneous depot forms under a transdermal patch so a patient will continue to receive fentanyl for up to 24 h after removal of the patch (see Case study 4). Within palliative care it has been used quite extensively by the subcutaneous route and the authors have found it particularly useful in patients with renal impairment, where toxicity, such as myoclonus or agitation, has been experienced with morphine or parenteral diamorphine but pain is still present. Continuous subcutaneous doses of between 150 and 300 μg/24 h, equivalent to a quarter to a half that in the smallest patch (delivering 25 μg/h) have been found to be effective starting doses. Use of subcutaneous fentanyl boluses prn to titrate the dose against need enable pain control to be achieved.

## Case study 4: Prolonged opioid toxicity following cessation of transdermal fentanyl for a reduction in pain intensity

Z was 61 when he was first diagnosed with myeloma. Over the following 2 years he received many courses of chemotherapy until his disease became refractory to treatment and he was maintained on supportive therapy including regular bisphosphonate infusions. He had been dialysis dependent due to myeloma since its diagnosis. Pain had been a consistent feature of his illness with only a partial response from palliative radiotherapy. Each course had taken 4 to 5 weeks before onset of relief of pain. His analgesia had been titrated upwards using oral hydromorphone and transdermal fentanyl so that by 6 months from diagnosis he required fentanyl 125 μg/h transdermally to achieve acceptable pain control.

He remained on this dose of fentanyl for the next 16 months, at which time he developed severe pain in his wrists due to diffuse infiltration with myeloma, demonstrated on MRI scan. He received further

**Case study 4: Prolonged opioid toxicity following cessation of transdermal fentanyl for a reduction in pain intensity** *(continued)*

palliative radiotherapy and over the following 4 weeks his fentanyl was increased to 200 μg/h. Five weeks after radiotherapy a course of dexamethasone was started as an adjuvant analgesic, and a week later while attending his regular dialysis, he became increasingly drowsy and collapsed with a respiratory rate of six breaths per minute followed by apnoea. His fentanyl patches were removed and he was given naloxone with a good response but this was not sustained and it was necessary to maintain him on a naloxone infusion for the following 24 h. Over the next 48 h he gradually awoke, though he experienced opioid withdrawal symptoms, with crampy abdominal pain, diarrhoea, shaking, and a new feeling of distress. These were treated with short-acting opioids, benzodiazepines, and loperimide. One month following this, his pain was managed with regular paracetamol and tramadol 50 mg prn.

His sudden reduction in pain was likely due to the combination of radiotherapy and steroids. With pain no longer acting as a physiological antagonist to the opioid, he developed opioid toxicity, resulting in respiratory depression. The elimination plasma half-life for transdermal fentanyl is almost 24 h resulting in the need for continuous reversal of narcosis following removal of the patch.

### 8.3.5.9 Alfentanil

Alfentanil, a derivative of fentanyl, is approximately a quarter as potent as fentanyl and 10 times more potent than subcutaneous diamorphine as an analgesic.[151] It is extensively metabolized in the liver to inactive compounds and its clearance may be reduced in patients with hepatic dysfunction. Its pharmacokinetic profile differs from fentanyl by having a smaller volume of distribution and a shorter terminal half-time in plasma leading to less accumulation than with fentanyl.[151] Alfentanil can be administered more easily by subcutaneous infusion[159] because of its greater solubility, leading to a smaller total volume required for equianalgesic doses; this also favours its use for intranasal or buccal administration for breakthrough pain.[160]

### 8.3.5.10 Buprenorphine

Buprenorphine is a semisynthetic opioid with a long duration of action.[161] It is between 30[162] and 60 times as potent as oral morphine when given sublingually.[161] It is a partial agonist at the μ opioid receptor[162,163] and an antagonist at the κ opioid receptor.[164] Despite this, within the analgesic range of less than 10 mg in 24 h, it behaves as a full agonist and can have an additive effect to morphine and other μ agonists. For effects other than analgesia, a ceiling effect has been demonstrated at doses of 16 to 32 mg, well in excess of the analgesic range. For respiratory depression, the curve is bell-shaped.[165,166] Because of the avidity with which buprenorphine binds to the μ opioid receptor, it might be difficult to antagonize the acute effects buprenorphine with opioid antagonists.[167]

Buprenorphine is metabolized by the liver[168] with little unchanged drug found in the urine.[169] The two major metabolites, buprenorphine-3-glucuronide (B3G) and norbuprenorphine, are excreted in the urine and accumulate in patients with renal failure, although the parent compound does not.[169] B3G is inactive and norbuprenorphine is probably a markedly less potent analgesic than buprenorphine as evidenced by its activity in rats.[170] However, B3G is a more potent respiratory depressant than buprenorphine in rats.[171]

Buprenorphine is an effective, long-acting opioid analgesic. It has an apparent ceiling effect on respiration and unchanged kinetics in renal failure. It can be administered effectively sublingually or via a transdermal patch. These properties make it a potentially useful analgesic for use in patients with renal impairment. However, when used for prolonged periods in patients with renal failure there are serious concerns over the accumulation of norbuprenorphine and its effects on respiration. The authors have no experience with this drug in chronic dosing and until there is further evidence cannot recommend its use.

### 8.3.5.11 Adverse effects of strong opioids (Table 8.2)

Of the adverse effects associated with morphine/strong opioid use, constipation is persistent and nearly universal while nausea and vomiting occur in approximately 50% of people, wearing off in most after 7–10 days. The central nervous system effects occur most frequently on initiating strong opioids and when escalating the dose. Patients should be warned of this, as there may be improvement after a few days at a stable dose. Respiratory depression is rare in patients taking strong opioids for pain if oral, short-acting preparations are used. Pain is said to be the physiological antagonist of opioids. The use of long-acting, slow-release, or parenteral preparations in patients with renal failure is more likely to be associated with narcosis and respiratory depression. Hallucinations are a very distressing adverse effect and should be managed either by dose reduction with co-administration of haloperidol, if needed, or by switching to an alternative opioid if possible.

Adverse effects of strong opioids are sufficiently common to prevent effective analgesia and should be vigorously managed. Patients should be warned of these and also informed of the steps that can be taken to prevent or treat them (see drugs to manage opioid side-effects).

## 8.3.6 Naloxone

Naloxone is the first competitive opioid antagonist to be developed that is devoid of agonist activity. It is more potent at the μ receptor than at other opioid receptors.[172] Its observed effects are related to antagonism of endogenous or exogenous opioids and it produces no effects when administered in clinical doses to healthy subjects. When administered to those in pain who have not received exogenous opioids, some studies have demonstrated a biphasic response dependent on the dose used, with low doses producing analgesia and higher doses hyperalgesia.[173,174]

Naloxone will reverse all the effects of exogenous opioids, i.e. analgesia, respiratory depression, pupillary constriction, delayed gastric emptying, dysphoria, coma, and convulsions in

**Table 8.2** Adverse effects of morphine/strong opiods

| | |
|---|---|
| 1. | Occur with sufficient severity in a substantial minority to prevent successful analgesia, and with an increased incidence in patients with renal failure |
| 2. | Include the following common symptoms:<br>Gastrointestinal: nausea and vomiting, constipation<br>Autonomic nervous system: dry mouth, itching, sweating<br>Central nervous system: drowsiness, cognitive impairment, hallucinations, delirium, respiratory depression, myoclonus |
| 3. | Striking interindividual variability in sensitivity to adverse effects |
| 4. | Ageing associated with altered pharmacokinetics and generally lower doses are required |
| 5. | Tolerance to some adverse effects appears to occur after some days |
| 6. | Explanation to the patient and vigorous management (see text) essential |

addition to the analgesia produced by stress, transcutaneous electrical nerve stimulation, acupuncture, and placebo response.[175]

Naloxone is mainly metabolized by conjugation in the liver with little excreted unchanged in urine.[176] No dosage alteration is required in renal impairment. However, it should be remembered that prolonged dosing may be needed to counteract the accumulation of opioid metabolites in renal patients.

Naloxone may be administered by the intravenous, intramuscular, or subcutaneous routes. In opioid overdose, 5–10 μg/kg is the usual initial intravenous dose and may be repeated at 2–3 min intervals until the desired response is seen. At least 2 mg should be used to constitute an adequate trial in overdose of unknown cause. If no response is seen after 150 μg/kg then the diagnosis of opioid overdose should be seriously questioned. The duration of action of long-lasting opioids, particularly those with a long duration of action such as methadone or those administered by the transdermal route where there may be a depot of the drug remaining under the skin, may outlast that of an intravenous dose of naloxone so patients should be carefully monitored for signs of returning opioid depression. Intravenous infusions have been used to overcome this problem starting at 2.5 μg/kg hourly and adjusted according to response (see Case study 4).

Administration of naloxone to postoperative patients who have received buprenorphine as a perioperative analgesic may result in restoration of full analgesia.[177] This effect is thought to be a consequence of the bell-shaped dose–response curve seen with buprenorphine, with diminishing analgesia at high doses.

## 8.3.7 Alternative routes for administration of morphine and other opioids (Table 8.3)

Most patients are able to take strong opioids by mouth. However, it is often necessary to make use of alternative routes for a number of reasons including vomiting, end-of-life weakness, bowel obstruction, and severe adverse effects with oral administration. The transmucosal route may be a useful alternative for rapid effect with short duration of action (see Table 8.3). Where systemically administered opioids are associated with unacceptable toxicity or failure of pain relief then the spinal route may be indicated. Local anaesthetic agents have been shown to be helpful for movement related or incident pain in cancer patients[178] and clonidine,[179] in neuropathic pain when used in conjunction with spinal opioids to enhance their effect. The availability of the expertise necessary for their use may vary from centre to centre.

### 8.3.7.1 Topical analgesia

The potential toxicity of systemic analgesics in patients with renal failure makes the possibility of using drugs topically where applicable very attractive. Most drugs appear to act locally rather than through local systemic absorption, thus it is possible to use lower doses:

◆ **Topical opioids**: in the presence of inflammation, peripheral opioid receptors are recruited very rapidly and have been identified on peripheral cutaneous sensory nerves.[180] The effect of intra-articular morphine is probably mediated in this way, a theory that is supported by the fact that it can be reversed by naloxone. The presence of inflammation appears to be essential for the efficacy of topical morphine and case reports support this.[181] The use of a number of opioids has been described, including morphine, diamorphine, and fentanyl. The opioid is added to a suitable medium, frequently a commercial hydrogel containing carboxymethylcellulose polymer (Intrasite) and spread on the ulcerated area once or twice a day at dressing changes. Benefit appears to occur shortly after the first application and may last 12 or more hours.[181,182]

**Table 8.3** Alternative routes for analgesic administration

| Route | Indications | Advantages | Disadvantages and contraindications | Suitable drugs | Additional comments |
|---|---|---|---|---|---|
| Per rectum | Oral intake not possible. Poor absorption. End of life drowsiness | Simple, effective. Suitable for home use | Immunocompromised patients, diarrhoea, incontinence | Paracetamol, morphine, oxycodone, NSAIDS | Consider patient preference |
| Subcutaneous | Reduced or no oral intake. End-of-life drowsiness or weakness | Simple, non-invasive, effective, portable, safe for home use, cheap | Very low platelets. Widespread oedema | Morphine, diamorphine, hydromorphone (not UK), methadone, fentanyl, alfentanil | Can be combined with other drugs if needed (e.g. antiemetics). Continuous infusion preferable to intermittent dosing |
| Intramuscular | Rapid pain relief required | Simple | Painful | Morphine, hydromorphone, methadone, pethidine | Only use if subcutaneous route not possible or intravenous route not appropriate |
| Intravenous | Rapid pain relief required | Rapid effect. Rapid dose titration | Requires higher level of trained staff. Not suitable for repeated home use | As for subcutaneous | |
| Transdermal | Stable pain. Suitable for strong opioid | Simple. Infrequent patch change | Theoretical risk of increased absorption with pyrexia or sweating | Fentanyl, buprenorphine | Lowest patch size may contain too high a dose for initiation |
| Transmucosal e.g. buccal, intranasal or sublingual | Breakthrough analgesia in conscious patient | Simple. Patient may finely control breakthrough analgesia required | Dry mouth may hinder use | Fentanyl, buprenorphine, alfentanil | |
| Spinal (epidural/ intrathecal) | Severe adverse effects or pain poorly responsive to opioids | Pain relief with few adverse effects | Expensive. Special expertise. Infection | Opioids, local anaesthetics | Selective availability |

◆ **Topical NSAIDs**: it has been shown in a systematic review[183] that topically applied NSAIDs can provide effective pain relief. The review found a number needed to treat (NNT) of 3.1 (2.7–3.8) for 50% pain relief. When applied topically, NSAIDs do not appear to be associated with serious side-effects. Where pain is present in joints or non-ulcerated skin, this may be a useful alternative to oral administration.

◆ **Topical capsaicin**: capsaicin is an alkaloid from chillies that can deplete substance P, which is thought to be associated with the transmission of painful stimuli in local sensory nerve endings and thus may have a part to play in cutaneous analgesia. A meta-analysis by Zhang *et al.*[184] showed that for every four patients with diabetic neuropathy treated with capsaicin one would have the pain relieved who would not otherwise have done so with placebo and one in three with osteoarthritis. Both these conditions are prevalent in patients with ESRD. Though it is not as effective as anticonvulsants, it has lower toxicity.

## 8.4 Adjuvant drugs

An adjuvant drug can be defined as any drug that has a primary indication other than pain, but is analgesic in some situations.[185] It has also come to mean drugs used in combination with analgesics either to enhance their action or manage their side-effects such as antiemetics and laxatives. This is not strictly within the definition and thus it may be necessary to use an alternative classification:

◆ Drugs with a primary indication other than pain management (e.g. antidepressants, corticosteroids).

◆ Drugs to treat the adverse effects of analgesics (e.g. antiemetics, laxatives, and psychotropics).

◆ Drugs to treat concomitant psychological disturbances such as insomnia, anxiety, and depression (e.g. night sedatives, anxiolytics, and antidepressants).

### 8.4.1 Pain syndromes requiring adjuvant drugs

#### 8.4.1.2 Neuropathic pain (Table 8.4)

Many patients with ESRD experience neuropathic pain or mixed neuropathic and nociceptive pain. For **pure neuropathic pain** adjuvant drugs are often used alone or with analgesics from Step 1 or 2 of the WHO analgesic ladder. For **severe mixed pains** they can be used with analgesics from all three steps of the WHO analgesic ladder. Where the pain appears to be sensitive to a weak opioid, continuing on to Step 3 may give added benefit and should be tried. Strong opioids should be titrated upwards in the normal way until maximum or optimal pain relief is achieved or toxicity prohibits further increase. It is important when making changes to do so to one drug at a time so efficacy and causes of toxicity can be accurately determined.

Tricyclic antidepressants (TCA) and anticonvulsants are the two classes of drugs for which there is most evidence of efficacy in neuropathic pain. Although antidepressants have been used in the UK for over 30 years to manage neuropathic pain, no antidepressant has a product licence for this indication. A systematic review of their use found that antidepressants were effective in reducing neuropathic pain. [186] The NNT for at least 50% pain relief compared with placebo in diabetic neuropathy was 3.0 (2.4–4.0). This was similar for other causes of neuropathic pain. In a similar review of anticonvulsants, a NNT of 2.9 (2.4–3.7) was found.[187] Both these classes of drugs have important side-effects; minor events occur in about one-third of

**Table 8.4** Adjuvant drugs in neuropathic pain

| Class of drug | Class of drug | Renal handling | Side-effects | | Contraindications | Dose schedule | Comments |
|---|---|---|---|---|---|---|---|
| | | | Commonly occurring | Less common but important | | | |
| Tricyclic antidepressants | Amitriptyline | Metabolized in the liver (cytochrome P-450). <5% excreted unchanged in the urine. Unaffected by dialysis | Antihistaminic: sedation. Anticholinergic: dry mouth, blurred vision, constipation, urinary retention. Central effects: fatigue, dizziness, weakness, tremor, confusion, postural hypotension | Conduction disturbances, especially tachyarrhythmias. Weight gain. Reduced libido | Glaucoma. Concurrent MAOIs. Recent myocardial infarction. Multiple drug interactions | 10–25 mg nocte, increasing every few days to relief or toxicity (rarely need to use more than 75 mg) | Lowers seizure threshold. Dose alteration not usually necessary in renal failure, though may be poorly tolerated |
| Anticonvulsants | Carbamazepine | Metabolized by liver. Induces microsomal enzymes | Anorexia, nausea, vomiting, ataxia, headaches, dizziness, drowsiness, visual disturbance—may improve with continued treatment | Fluid overload due to antidiuretic action. Interaction with: warfarin, oral contraceptive pill, dextropropoxyphene | Concurrent MAOIs | 200 mg daily increasing weekly to effectiveness or toxicity or a maximum dose of 1600 mg | Effect may occur within 2–3 days Plasma concentrations reduced by other anticonvulsants |
| | Valproic acid | Metabolized by the liver and eliminated via the kidneys | Gastric irritation, nausea, tremor, ataxia, drowsiness, weight gain | Liver toxicity | Acute liver disease, family history of severe hepatic dysfunction, porphyria | 200 mg daily increasing by 200 mg to pain control or a maximum dose of 1000 mg | Well tolerated. Interaction with other anticonvulsants |

**Table 8.4** (continued) Adjuvant drugs in neuropathic pain

| Class of drug | Renal handling | Side-effects | | Contraindications | Dose schedule | Comments |
|---|---|---|---|---|---|---|
| | | Commonly occurring | Less common but important | | | |
| Gabapentin | Excreted unchanged by the kidney. Accumulates in renal impairment | Drowsiness, dizziness, ataxia, fatigue. Need to watch closely for signs of toxicity | Instability of bloodglucose in diabetics. Antacids reduce absorption | Lactation | Creatinine clearance <15 ml/min 300 mg q.o.d. HD 200–300 mg after each 4 h dialysis | Withdraw dose gradually over 1 week. Licensed (UK) for treatment of neuropathic pain |
| Clonazepam | | Sedation | | | 0.5–1mg nocte, gradual increase to a maximum of 2 mg daily | Simple to administer, evidence for efficacy in one study |
| Oral local anaesthetic agents e.g. Mexiletine | | Nausea, ataxia, tremor, dizziness, confusion | Cardiac conduction defects | History of cardiac disease | See text | Should be used with great caution, consult pain specialist |
| NMDA receptor antagonists e.g. Ketamine | See text | | | | | Consult specialist physician |
| Topical agents e.g. Capsaicin | See text | | | | | |

MOAIs, monoamine oxidase inhibitors.

patients. One patient in 22 stopped TCA treatment and 1 in 8 stopped anticonvulsants on account of them. Selective serotonin re-uptake inhibitors (SSRIs) appear to be less effective as adjuvant analgesics but have fewer adverse reactions.[186]

If benefit is to be obtained from an antidepressant it occurs more quickly than the antidepressant effect, typically within 10 days and at lower doses. Usually doses of 75 mg a day or less of amitriptyline are needed.

It is suggested that the mechanism of action of anticonvulsants is similar to that which reduces the risk of seizure, through blocking use-dependent sodium channels (e.g. carbamazepine) or the facilitation of gamma aminobutyric acid (GABA) inhibition (e.g. sodium valproate). Although anticonvulsants are widely used in the treatment of chronic pain, especially for neuropathic pain that is burning or lacinating,[27] surprisingly few trials show analgesic effectiveness.[187] There is no evidence that anticonvulsants are effective for acute pain.[187] Gabapentin is the only anticonvulsant licensed in the UK for use in neuropathic pain and is increasingly being used for its management. However, the evidence suggests that it is not superior to carbamazepine.[187]

Ketamine is a dissociative anaesthetic agent, often used for short painful procedures in children or where there is limited availability of anaesthetists.[188] It is used illegally as a recreational drug. It is a potent NMDA receptor antagonist.[189] Activation of the NMDA receptor is thought to be associated clinically with the phenomenon of 'wind up'.[190] This is a description of prolongation of the pain state with an increase in magnitude out of proportion to the painful stimulus, and is commonly a feature of neuropathic pain. Ketamine has potent analgesic actions at subanaesthetic doses, probably due to this effect.[188] Oral ketamine has low bioavailability, so is usually administered by the intravenous, intramuscular, or subcutaneous routes.[191] The majority of the drug is metabolized to norketamine, which has about a third of the potency of the parent drug. Less than 10% of the drug is excreted unchanged.[191] Norketamine is produced in greater proportions when it is given orally compared with parenteral administration and may contribute to the benefit seen in some patients when used orally in conjunction with strong opioids.[192,193] When used for anaesthesia or analgesia, a significant number of patients experience unpleasant hallucinations and other phenomena which means its use frequently has to be accompanied with either a benzodiazepine or an antipsychotic such as haloperidol.[194,195]

Ketamine may have a role in severe, intractable neuropathic pain, or for short painful procedures, but should be supervised by an experienced practitioner.

Oral local anaesthetics may have a role in severe, resistant neuropathic pain. Some such as mexilitine work by blocking sodium channels. However, all carry the risk of cardiac rhythm disorders and should only be administered and monitored by those experienced in their use.

### 8.4.1.3 Musculoskeletal pain (Table 8.5)

Benzodiazepines,[27] particularly diazepam, can be used for pain caused by muscle spasm. Clonazepam,[196] in addition, has some evidence for its use in neuropathic pain. At the end of life, subcutaneous midazolam may be helpful for agitation and distress, and thus indirectly help pain control. Diazepam has antispasticity efficacy but side-effects are common. However, it may be useful for the pain of muscle spasm, particularly associated with back pain from disc or other spinal lesions. Clonazepam is easy to administer with a once daily oral or subcutaneous nocturnal dose.

Antispasticity activity has been shown for baclofen,[197] a stimulant of GABA receptors, and also for tizanidine, an alpha-2 agonist.[198] These drugs may be tried where muscle spasm is thought to play an important part in the aetiology of pain.

**Table 8.5** Adjuvant drugs

| Class of Drug | Indication | Drug name | Dose adjustment in renal failure | Adverse effects and contraindications | Suggested dose range | Comment |
|---|---|---|---|---|---|---|
| Corticosteroids | Nerve root compression. Raised intracranial pressure | Dexamethasone | No dose change normally necessary | See text | 8–16 mg daily after food | See text |
| Benzodiazepines | Muscle spasm | Diazepam | Start with small doses; increased sensitivity | Drowsiness, weakness | 2–10 mg daily | |
| Benzodiazepines | Myoclonus, agitation | Midazolam | As above | Sedation at high doses. Tolerance if given over long periods | Dose rapidly titrated, usual range 2.5–7.5 mg IV or SC hourly. Continuous infusion, 10–50 mg/24 h | Rapid effect after SC administration. Can be repeated hourly if needed for optimal benefit. If several doses needed advise 24-h infusion |
| Skeletal muscle relaxants | Muscle spasm, hiccups | Baclofen | Renally cleared, dose reduction necessary | Sedation, nausea | 5 mg o.d./b.d. titrated up to a maximum of 10 mg t.i.d. | Must discontinue by gradual dose reduction to avoid serious side-effects |

| Class | Indication | Drug | Dose adjustment | Side effects | Dose | Notes |
|---|---|---|---|---|---|---|
| Alpha-2 agonist | Muscle spasm | Tizanidine | Low initial dose advised | Drowsiness | 2 mg o.d. initially with slow titration up to 36 mg daily in divided doses | Contraindicated in hepatic dysfunction |
| Alpha-2 agonist | Neuropathic pain | Clonidine | | Somnolence, orthostatic hypotension, dry mouth | | Consult pain specialist. Can be given, orally, transdermally, or epidurally |
| Antimalarial | Nocturnal cramps | Quinine | | Tinnitus, headaches | 200–300 mg nocte | Can take 4 weeks for maximum benefit |
| NSAIDS | Renal colic | See text | See text | | | |
| Anticholinergic | Bowel colic or excess secretions | Hyoscine butylbromide | No dose change normally necessary | Dry mouth | 20 mg SC prn or as 24-h infusion 60–160 mg/24 h | Does not cross blood–brain barrier, so not sedative |

### 8.4.1.4 Nerve compression and raised intracranial pressure (Table 8.5)

Corticosteroids have a role in the management of pain associated with nerve compression and headache associated with raised intracranial pressure. For these indications dexamethasone is usually recommended in preference to prednisolone due to its greater potency and reduced mineralocorticoid activity. It has good oral bioavailability and a long duration of action so can be given once daily. Dose reduction is not usually necessary in renal failure.

The dose of dexamethasone for nerve root compression is initially 6–12 mg daily, reducing after 7 to 10 days to as low a dose as can be used to maintain relief. For raised intracranial pressure, doses of up to 16 mg daily will be needed initially, again with gradual dose reduction to prevent the long-term adverse effects relating to its glucocorticoid, mineralocorticoid, and immunosuppressant effects. In the United States and Canada, higher doses are used with a daily dose of 40 mg of dexamethasone being fairly standard. If used in conjunction with an NSAID, the risk of peptic ulceration is greatly increased.

### 8.4.1.5 Renal colic—stones (Table 8.5)

NSAIDs may be particularly useful in some pain syndromes such as renal colic.[199] Acute ureteral obstruction by a stone can increase renal pressure leading to a release of prostaglandins causing vasodilation of the afferent arterioles and inhibition of antidiuretic hormone. This results in diuresis and a further increase in renal pressure establishing a vicious cycle leading to renal colic. Thus, NSAIDs would be seem to be an ideal choice in managing pain from kidney stones. Studies have shown that they are as effective, if not more so, than opioids in providing pain relief from kidney stones.[199,200]

### 8.4.1.6 Colic—bowel obstruction (Table 8.5)

Hyoscine butylbromide (scopolamine butylbromide) has a useful role in the management of severe bowel colic, particularly where it is associated with bowel obstruction.[201] It can provide effective pain relief without the toxicity of opioids.[202] As it is poorly absorbed,[203] it has to be given parenterally. This can be done either by subcutaneous (intermittent or continuous), intramuscular, or intravenous injections. Subcutaneous injections of octreotide, a somatostatin analogue, have also been shown to be effective in controlling gastrointestinal symptoms of bowel obstruction.[201,204]

## 8.4.2 Drugs to manage opioid side-effects

### 8.4.2.1 Antiemetics (Table 8.6)

Antiemetics are needed by between 50 and 75% of patients on strong opioids, some of whom may have additional causes for nausea and vomiting. As this may result in patients not taking medication or interfere with drug absorption, it can hamper successful pain management. Effective management with appropriate antiemetics is therefore important. A methodical approach will enhance this:

- Postulate the cause.
- Select an appropriate antiemetic (Table 8.6).
- Give it regularly by most suitable route at full dose.
- Prescribe a rescue antiemetic, either further doses of the same drug if not at maximum dose or complementary drug (Table 8.6).
- Assess effectiveness and review the cause of vomiting and route and absorption of drug before changing or adding additional drugs.

**Table 8.6** Suggested use of antiemetics

| Cause | Site of action | First choice agent | PRN drug | Second choice agents |
|---|---|---|---|---|
| Uraemia, opioids, sepsis, hypercalcaemia | Chemoreceptor trigger zone (CTZ) | Haloperidol: 1.5–3 mg orally up to 10 mg/24h. 2–10 mg/24 h SC infusion | Haloperidol | Levomepromazine (see text): 6 mg orally nocte or b.d. or 6.25–12.5 mg/24 h SC infusion |
| NSAIDs, opioids, tricyclic antide-pressants. Functional bowel obstruction | Gastric stasis | Metoclopramide: 5–10 mg orally t.i.d. or 30–40 mg/24 h SC infusion | Haloperidol | Haloperidol or levomepromazine |
| Liver distension, gastrointestinal/peritoneal stimulation, raised intracranial pressure, mechanical bowel obstruction | Vomiting centre (VC) | Cyclizine: 50 mg orally t.i.d. or 100–150 mg/ 24h SC | Haloperidol | Haloperidol |
| Bowel obstruction with colic | Gastrointestinal tract | Hyoscine butylbromide: 60–120 mg/24 h SC infusion | Hyoscine butylbromide: 20 mg SC | Octreotide 300–900 µg/24 h SC infusion |
| Chemotherapy, radiotherapy, anaesthesia | Histamine: 5-HT$_3$ receptors in CTZ, VC and vagal afferents in the gut | Ondansetron, tropisetron, granisetron, dolasetron (not UK) | Haloperidol or metoclopamide | |
| Ischaemia | Vestibular apparatus | Hyoscine hydrobromide (1.0 mg/72 h transdermal) or cyclizine | Cyclizine or hyoscine hydrobromide | Cyclizine or hyoscine hydrobromide |

In the authors' experience, if parenteral antiemetics are necessary, a continuous subcutaneous infusion may be more effective than intermittent boluses.

Opioids are thought to cause nausea and vomiting either by stimulation of the chemoreceptor trigger zone or by delayed gastric emptying; thus an appropriate first choice antiemetic is either haloperidol[205] or metoclopramide.[206] Cyclizine, a histamine antagonist with antimuscarinic activity, is also a useful general-purpose antiemetic.[207] Unfortunately, it may contribute to the dry mouth caused by opioids and increase the discomfort for renal patients who may be fluid restricted. In theory, it blocks the prokinetic action of metoclopramide so the two drugs should not be used concurrently.

### 8.4.2.2 Haloperidol

Haloperidol[205,208] is used both as an antiemetic and for relief of hallucinations caused by strong opioids. It is predominantly a dopamine antagonist with some action at histamine H1 receptors. It is extensively metabolized, mainly in the liver, but also in the brain and other tissues.[209] Around 1% is excreted in the urine and renal failure has very little effect on its pharmacokinetics so no dosage adjustment is usually necessary. Liver enzyme inducers (e.g. rifampicin) increase the elimination of haloperidol and the dose may need to be increased by up to 50%. It is absolutely contraindicated in patients with closed-angle glaucoma[210] and should be used with caution in patients with epilepsy as it lowers the seizure threshold.[211] Parkinson's disease can be exacerbated by it,[210] and caution should be exercised in patients at risk of cardiac arrhythmias as they can be precipitated.[212,213] Haloperidol can be prescribed on a regular or as-required basis.

### 8.4.2.3 Metoclopramide

Metoclopramide is a prokinetic agent having effects on the upper gastrointestinal tract to increase lower oesophageal sphincter pressure, gastric emptying, and gastric–duodenal coordination.[214] Its effects on the gut may result from a local action on acetycholine release or be in part related to its actions within the central nervous system, which are mediated primarily via dopamine receptor antagonism.[214] This latter action can result in adverse effects including acute dystonia, akathisia, parkinsonism, tardive dyskinesia, and hyperprolactinaemia.[214]

Metoclopramide is extensively metabolized but the major route of elimination is the urine.[214] In patients with renal impairment the clearance is approximately half of that found in normal subjects.[215] Significantly reduced doses of metoclopramide need to be used in patients with severe renal failure because of the increased risk of extrapyramidal side-effects.

### 8.4.2.4 Cyclizine

Cyclizine is an antihistaminic antiemetic with antmuscarinic effects.[207] The same oral and parenteral doses can be used. Its main disadvantages are due to its sedating and antimuscarinic effects, particularly dry mouth, in patients who have many other causes of dry mouth to contend with. There are no studies on its use in renal failure, so it should be used with care, although in clinical practice dose reduction has not been found to be necessary.[45]

### 8.4.2.5 5-hydroxytryptamine 3 (5-HT₃) receptor antagonists

This group of drugs was developed specifically for the management of chemotherapy-induced vomiting for which there is evidence of benefit as well as for anaesthetic and radiation-induced vomiting.[216–219] Ondansetron was the first to be developed, but this has been followed by other agents with similar efficacy.[220] The elimination of ondansetron is mainly by hepatic metabolism and the renal clearance of is low.[221] No dosage reduction is necessary in renal impairment.[222] Some,[223] but not all,[224] studies have shown an improvement in uraemic pruritus with regular use of ondansetron. Consideration could be given to using this agent if nausea and uraemic pruritus are a problem in the same patient.

### 8.4.2.6 Levomepromazine

Levomepromazine is a broad-spectrum antiemetic, with dopamine, 5-HT$_2$, and alpha$_1$ receptor antagonist properties. It is very sedative at antipsychotic doses but has recently been used extensively at low doses for antiemesis in palliative care patients.[225] It has approximately 50% oral bioavailability. Essentially all the drug is metabolized in the liver though the activity of the metabolites is not fully quantified. Excretion is mainly in the urine and faeces. Reduced doses are suggested because of the risk of increased cerebral sensitivity. However, as the doses suggested for antiemesis are considerably lower than those used for psychosis, it is probably safe in the doses recommended in Table 8.6.

## 8.4.3 Laxatives

As a general rule, a laxative should be prescribed when an opioid is started. Opioids reduce gut mobility and increase electrolyte and water absorption from faeces. Thus most patients need the regular use of a peristaltic stimulant such as senna, and a faecal softener such as sodium docusate. As there is considerable interindividual variation, the doses required will differ between patients. If the patient is severely constipated, rectal measures will be an important first step.

## 8.4.4 Psychotropic drugs

Psychotropic drugs have an important role in managing psychological morbidity that may accompany ESRD and in minimizing the side-effects of analgesics. Haloperidol is the most important, used to alleviate hallucinations and to help the vivid and often unpleasant dreams that can be associated with strong opioids. In addition, they may be needed to manage depression and anxiety which frequently accompany pain in patients with ESRD, or for night sedation to improve overall quality of life.

The concurrent use of two or more drugs that act on the central nervous system is likely to produce a greater sedative effect in ill and malnourished renal patients. The starting dose of any psychotropic drug may need to be less than that used for physically healthy patients.

## 8.4.5 Non-drug measures for pain relief

### 8.4.5.1 Transcutaneous nerve stimulation (TENS), acupuncture

The gate theory of pain[226] provides the rationale for TENS. It postulates that if the spinal cord is bombarded with impulses from the TENS machine then it is distracted from transmitting the pathological pain signal. There is little published evidence that TENS is effective in the treatment of acute pain, although it can be effective in patients with chronic pain.[227] However, even in this field there are few robust studies with which to judge the efficacy of this treatment in specific situations.[228] Attention to detail (e.g. electrode placement) makes considerable difference to the efficacy of TENS.[229] It may have a useful role in neuropathic pain where efficacy of drugs is reduced by the potential for toxicity, for example where the pain is due to vertebral collapse with nerve compression from non-malignant causes.

The data that acupuncture is effective in the management of chronic pain, back pain, or headache are equivocal or contradictory.[230,231] There is, however, evidence that acupuncture is effective for emesis developing after surgery or chemotherapy in adults[231] and it therefore might be considered in refractory nausea. Theories for its mode of action in pain relief include the production of endorphins and other neurohumeral mechanisms for which there is some evidence, particularly in animal models. It is not routinely available in mainstream medicine, but where conventional medicine has failed to relieve symptoms and the patient wishes, it can be explored and used if effective. Fortunately it is not affected by renal function so its side-effect profile remains favourable!

### 8.4.5.2 Physiotherapy and variants

Despite a lack of evidence for the benefits of physiotherapy and manipulation for pain management,[232] many people will try these methods of pain relief where conventional methods have been unsuccessful. Physiotherapists are usually members of pain management programmes, to which patients may be referred with chronic pain. Physiotherapy programmes, particularly in the bed-bound or those with markedly reduced mobility, may improve overall well-being and thus pain relief.

Although it is important to keep an open mind to the potential benefit of physical therapies, the evidence from back pain suggests that on rigorous outcome measures, physiotherapy and other forms of manipulation have only limited success.[232] However, these therapies may provide pain relief for individual patients and that in itself is a strong argument for a trial of therapy where conventional medicine has not relieved symptoms.

### 8.4.5.3 Psychological treatments

Psychological factors are central to the experience of pain, and their management is essential for the delivery of effective analgesia and for the specific treatment of chronic pain in adults.[233] Where it is thought serious psychological distress is impeding good symptom management, particularly pain, then where services are available, it is important to make full use of them as patients on dialysis are known to have a high incidence of psychological illness, particularly anxiety and depression.[35,36] Psychological treatments, when used as an adjunct, may enhance the efficacy of pharmacological measures and improve quality of life, though this may be difficult to prove.

## 8.4.6 Specific pain syndromes in renal patients

The principles of pain management discussed above are common to all causes of pain. However, there are a number of painful syndromes which are encountered almost exclusively in renal patients. These conditions may require very specific measures that will almost certainly involve very specialized skills in pain management and possibly surgery. The two examples given below are not intended to be an exhaustive list but have been chosen as illustrative examples of difficult problems.

### 8.4.6.1 Adult polycystic kidney disease

The pain of bursting renal cysts: 'A quaint little pain this one, it actually had an almost exact time scale of 45 minutes start to finish. Always the same it would proceed thus: vague sensation in the pit of the stomach, not unakin to the feeling of butterflies. Within 5 minutes I would have taken the defensive position. I would then oscillate between trying to relax and losing it to full blown panic, the pain would grow worse as I knew it would, panic would rise as I knew it would and for the next 30 minutes I would be in (literally) unbearable pain'

Acute and chronic pain are common in patients with adult polycystic kidney disease (APKD).[234] It is by far the most common of genetic conditions causing ESRD.[235] APKD patients may suffer complications such as infected cysts, cyst rupture/haemorrhage, and nephrolithiasis that cause severe acute pain.[234,236] Patients with APKD are also commonly afflicted by chronic pain syndromes. Chronic back pain is a common problem caused by increased abdominal girth leading to increased lumbar lordosis that accelerates degenerative change in the spine. As in the general population, the problem of back pain is complex and requires a thorough evaluation to determine the exact cause, which will then need to be treated appropriately. Pain also occurs as a result of compression of cysts on surrounding tissues, traction on the pedicle of the kidney, and distension of the renal capsule. Polycystic liver disease in patients with APKD often causes more disabling pain than renal pain. This appears to be especially true of multiparous women. Liver cysts can become massive and occupy most of the abdominal cavity causing intractable pain.

In addition to the usual pain relief measures discussed in the previous sections there are physical/invasive measures that have been used to control resistant pain related to APKD. Autonomic (coeliac) plexus blockade,[236] spinal cord stimulation by implantable electrodes,[237] neuraxial opioids, and local anaesthetics often given by continuous infusion[238] have been used in problematic cases. Surgical management including cyst decortication and marsupialization, renal denervation, and nephrectomy in patients approaching ESRD have been used with some success.[236] Surgical liver fenestration and combined liver resection–fenestration techniques have been used with some success in problematic liver disease.[239] Liver transplantation has also been tried when all other measures at pain control have failed.[240]

### 8.4.6.2 Calciphylaxis

Calciphylaxis refers to the syndrome of tissue ischaemia due to metastatic calcification of subcutaneous tissue and small arteries, usually occurring as a consequence of hyperparathyroidism in dialysis patients.[241,242] The predominant presentation consists of painful, ischaemic skin ulceration. The pain experienced in the skin and subcutaneous tissues can be very severe and debilitating. Wide areas may be extremely painful to the lightest pressure. Sympathetic blockade has been reported as providing some benefit.[243] However, it is often very difficult to provide adequate pain relief even with expert help.[241] The pain experienced may have features of both nociceptive and neuropathic pain, and a thorough history may guide the clinician to the drugs most likely to help. Psychological issues are paramount too, as with the increasing debility that is experienced comes the realization of the extremely high mortality associated with this condition.[241,242,244]

Hyperbaric oxygen therapy has been reported to cure the cutaneous ulcers of calciphylaxis,[241] although there have been reports of patients experiencing an increase in pain at the end of their period of treatment.[244] However, hyperbaric oxygen is not widely available and is expensive. Supplemental oxygen therapy may improve cutaneous oxygen values and may therefore help cutaneous ulcer healing.[241] It is thought that the supplemental oxygen therapy may also improve the cutaneous hyperaesthesia related to nerve ischaemia.

Most of the mortality occurs as a result of infection in open wounds. This high mortality and the severity of pain associated with calciphylaxis make referral to palliative care services important.

## 8.5 Suggested guidelines for using the WHO analgesic ladder in patients with severe renal failure and ESRD

### Case study 5: pain relief using one neuropathic agent and the step-wise titration of Step 3 analgesia

X is a 72-year-old male who lives alone. He had a right nephroureterectomy in 1990 for a transitional cell carcinoma of the ureter. Eleven years later glomerulonephritis led to renal failure requiring dialysis, complicated by infected discitis the following year. This was managed medically with intravenous antibiotics and drainage. Following treatment, rehabilitation was unsuccessful due to severe pain on movement and during dialysis. He required readmission to hospital for pain control.

His pain was a mixture of nociceptive pain in his back and neuropathic pain going down his leg. Prior to referral he had received tramadol 50 mg t.i.d. and paracetamol 1 g q.i.d. and had moved up the analgesic ladder to hydromorphone 2.6 mg 4-hourly at the time of referral. Although there was partial improvement, he still had a pain score of 5/10 at rest and 8/10 on movement or during dialysis.

A stepwise approach was taken.

### In hospital

A dose of fentanyl (25 µg/h) equivalent to the hydromorphone he had been taking was administered by transdermal patch. Hydromorphone 2.6 mg orally 2-hourly prn was continued for breakthrough pain. There was some improvement when he used 6 prn doses in 24 hs, so the fentanyl patch size was increased to 50 µg/h with a corresponding increase in the prn hydromorphone dose to 5.2 mg. The neuropathic element remained prominent so clonazepam 0.5 mg was started at night and increased to 1 mg after a few days, with benefit, though he was not yet pain free.

### Able to return to rehabilitation unit

Over the following 2 months his analgesic requirements were monitored by a palliative care nurse at his dialysis visits. By increasing the patch size to account for prn doses of hydromorphone for breakthrough pain, a dose of fentanyl 125 µg/h was reached. When on 100 µg/h of fentanyl he was:

### Able to return to his own home with considerable help

As the dose per hour of fentanyl increased there was a corresponding increase in the dose of hydromorphone used for breakthough pain. As pain relief was achieved, fewer doses were needed and currently one dose of 7.8 mg at night is sufficient.

**Twenty weeks from referral he was living independently**, had dispensed with delivered meals because he could cook his own and his mobility had progressed to needing only a walking stick for help.

He is likely to have some back pain for the rest of his life. However, attending physicians should be alert to the risk of opioid toxicity with this long-acting opioid preparation should **his pain diminish**. As the long-acting drug is fentanyl he is not thought to be at risk of toxicity due to retention of active metabolites, but the subcutaneous depot of fentanyl will remain a source of analgesia for at least 24 hours following patch removal.

## 8.5.1 General points (see Case study 5)

- Assess the patient's pain.
- Choose an appropriate step.
- Give the drug regularly.
- Assess the response and toxicity.
- Adjust or move up a step as appropriate.

### 8.5.1.2 Step 1

- Non-opioid analgesic (paracetamol 1 g q.i.d. and/or NSAID).
- Caution needed with NSAID use because of potential detrimental effects on renal function and increased toxicity.
- If NSAID to be used, consider selective COX-2 inhibitor or gastroprotection.
- Consider use of adjuvant drugs for specific indications.

### 8.5.1.3 Step 2. Pain persisting or increasing

- Non-opioid analgesic (paracetamol 1 g q.i.d. and/or NSAID).
- Add codeine 30 mg q.i.d. and 30 mg prn up to a total daily dose of 240 mg (see text).
- Or use tramadol 50 mg b.d./q.i.d. up to a total daily dose of 200 mg.
- Warn patient and monitor carefully for toxicity.
- Consider the use of adjuvant drugs for specific indications.

### 8.5.1.4 Step 3. Pain persisting or increasing

**Patient able to swallow oral medication**

- Non-opioid analgesic (paracetamol 1 g q.i.d. and/or NSAID).
- Stop codeine or tramadol and **substitute**:

   **Hydromorphone 1 to 1.3 mg 6-hourly and prn** (smallest available capsule in UK is 1.3 mg; 0.5 mg capsules are available in the USA and Canada allowing for lower initial doses and more gradual dose titration).

- If tolerated, increase frequency to 4-hourly within 24 h if needed. Titrate dose upwards every 24 to 48 h according to the number of prn doses needed.
- If dose reaches 2.6 mg or greater, 4-hourly, introduce transdermal fentanyl patch (25 μg/h) and continue with hydromorphone 1.3–2.6 mg prn.
- Continue dose titration upwards if needed, remembering to increase the dose of hydromorphone for breakthrough pain if the patch size increases (see Table 8.7).
- Monitor carefully for toxicity: myoclonus, sedation, or agitation.

   Alternatives include:

   **Normal-release morphine 2.5–5 mg four to 6-hourly and prn**. Then as for hydromorphone, with close monitoring. The appearance of toxicity varies but is likely to increase with the duration of treatment, and can be reduced by converting to transdermal fentanyl if the dose reaches 20 mg q.i.d. or above.

**Methadone**. This should only be used following consultation with a physician experienced in its use. There are several ways of switching a patient to methadone; it is suggested the physician becomes familiar with one method and uses it consistently. One technique is to stop all other opioids before switching to methadone; this will usually require inpatient monitoring. An alternative approach is to start patients on a low dose (e.g. 1 mg t.i.d.) and titrate upwards as needed every few days with gradual reduction of previous opioid. Hydromorphone should be available for breakthrough pain. Monitor carefully for signs of toxicity.

**Table 8.7** Comparison of strengths of transdermal fentanyl: may be used to calculate the breakthrough dose remembering that toxicity may be caused by morphine, diamorphine, and hydromorphone

| 4-hourly oral morphine (mg) | 4-hourly oral hydromorphone (mg) | Fentanyl patch strength ($\mu$g/h) | 24-h fentanyl dose ($\mu$g) | 24-h SC diamorphine dose (mg) |
|---|---|---|---|---|
| <20 | <2.6 | 25 | 600 | <45 |
| 25–35 | 2.6–3.9 | 50 | 1200 | 45–75 |
| 40–50 | 5.2 | 75 | 1800 | 75–105 |
| 55–65 | 6.5–7.8 | 100 | 2400 | 105–135 |
| 70–80 | 9.1 | 125 | 3000 | 135–165 |
| 85–90 | | 150 | 3600 | 165–195 |
| 100–110 | | 175 | 4200 | 195–225 |
| 110–125 | | 200 | 4800 | 225–255 |

### Patient unable to swallow

**Patient in continuous pain:**

- Start 24 h SC fentanyl or alfentanil in syringe driver.
- Initial dose depends on previous analgesic use, pain intensity and size/frailty of patient.
- In the opioid naïve patient, fentanyl 150–300 $\mu$g/24 h and fentanyl SC 12.5–25 $\mu$g prn are safe starting doses or 0.6–1.2 mg/24 h of alfentanil with 0.1–0.2 mg prn for pain that breaks through.
- Adjust dose in the syringe driver accordingly depending on toxicity or number of prn doses required.
- In those already taking strong opioids by mouth convert to the appropriate size fentanyl patch using additional SC fentanyl while therapeutic blood levels are reached and for titration. Alternatively, convert to a 24-h SC fentanyl or alfentanil syringe driver with prn drug available as needed, adjusting the dose as above (see Table 8.7 for approximate equivalent doses).

**Patient in intermittent pain:**

- Use as needed SC fentanyl 12.5–25 $\mu$g.
- If more than three doses needed in 24 h, set up continuous 24-h infusion.
- Alfentanil can be substituted for fentanyl at appropriate doses if preferred. It is one quarter as potent (see end-of-life guidelines, Chapter 15).

## 8.5.2 Guidelines for starting a fentanyl patch

◆ A fentanyl patch can be started as treatment for stable pain, or to provide background pain relief while dose titration takes place once the first patch size is reached.

◆ Patch size required can be calculated from Table 8.7.

◆ Apply patch; continue regular normal release strong opioid for first 12 h.

◆ Prescribe a normal-release strong opioid equivalent to the 4-hourly dose for breakthrough pain (Table 8.7).

## 8.5.3 Breakthrough pain, incident or movement related pain

A short-acting preparation that works quickly is required for dose titration, or prior to planned activity:

◆ For **patients who can swallow**: for morphine, hydromorphone, and oxycodone use normal-release preparation at one-sixth of the 24-h dose.

◆ For **patients unable to swallow or vomiting**: if on fentanyl or alfentanil as 24-h SC infusion or fentanyl transdermally, then use the same drug, usually SC but the buccal or intranasal route can also be used.

◆ **Calculation of prn dose**: there is no formula for the dose needed to relieve breakthrough pain when using fentanyl. It is sensible to start with a low dose such as either 12.5 µg or 25 µg, depending on the pain and the patient. If pain is not relieved in 1 h, repeat the dose. If a second dose at 1 h is needed consistently, then increase the breakthrough dose accordingly. The breakthrough dose can be titrated upwards according to the response and background dose of fentanyl. It is suggested that a breakthrough dose of between one-tenth and one-sixth of the 24 hour dose of alfentanil is appropriate but this too can be individually titrated.

## 8.5.4 Alternative routes for prn medication

◆ Oral transmucosal fentanyl. A hardened lozenge on a stick enabling the fentanyl to be delivered buccally. No formula for dose required, so each patient has to go through a dose titration exercise to find which lozenge size is effective. The patient must be able hold the lozenge against the buccal mucosa, which may be less easy if the mouth is dry.

◆ Nasal/buccal sublingual fentanyl, alfentanil, sufentanil. This route can be used for all three of these drugs. There is good bioavailability and clinically effective plasma concentrations are achieved in less than 10 min for all three.[160]

## 8.6 Summary

In this chapter we have described the problem of pain, which often goes unrecognized, and its treatment in patients with renal failure. We have also described some of the difficulties which contribute to poor management in these patients. We have described two examples of painful syndromes, almost exclusively confined to those with renal disease, to illustrate the importance of familiarity with these conditions as well as the need to seek further expert help and advice. Using the WHO analgesic ladder as a template and basic pharmacological principles, we have described a simple method for the assessment and treatment of pain in renal failure patients. There is much still to be learnt about the incidence, prevalence, and severity of pain in this population as well as further information about the handling of opioids for those needing chronic administration. This approach is supported by a recent review of the evidence available for analgesics used in patients with ESRD, it emphasizes a similar method of working and acknowledges the urgent need for further studies of analgesics in these patients.[245] Genetic differences probably explain, in part, the large variation in response, both therapeutic and toxic, between patients. This highlights the importance of a thorough patient assessment with repeated reassessments as well as an individualized plan.

## Ethical case analysis

It has been said that the first ethical responsibility of the physician is to be technically competent in the treatment of patients. This competence includes proficiency in pain and symptom management. Dialysis patients report that pain is their most common symptom and the one symptom that they are most concerned about at the end of life. For these reasons, it is very important for a nephrologist to master the principles of pain assessment and management discussed in this chapter. As Case studies 1 and 2 in this chapter illustrate, pain may be more than physical. In this chapter, the authors describe the concept of 'total pain'. It includes not only physical stimuli but also psychological, social, and spiritual factors. In Case 1, both of the patient's parents had diabetic nephropathy, and her mother had died from it. The initiation of dialysis was associated with excruciating pain. It is certainly possible that some of this pain may have been other than physical in origin. The case history notes that 'anxiety about this pain dominated her feelings'. Her treatment included not only gradually escalating doses of fentanyl but also an anxiolytic, clonazepham, and an antidepressant, amitriptyline. With time and increasing doses of all three medications, the patient's pain gradually subsided. Although it is entirely possible that her pain was due only to the treatment of the infected, loculated fluid on her abdominal wall by the plastic surgeons, it is also possible that her total pain subsided as she became accustomed to being on dialysis and less fearful about it. In Case 2, the patient's pain seemed to resolve when the social worker assisted him in addressing his social problems. This case again emphasizes the ethical responsibility for nephrologists to do a complete pain assessment with attention to psychosocial and spiritual matters as well as physical.

## Acknowledgements

All quotations were contributed by Mr Christopher Wilson-Gleave.

## References

1. Merskey, H., and Bogduk, N. (1994). *Classification of Chronic Pain*, p. 210. Seattle, WA: International Association for the Study of Pain Press.
2. Saunders, C. (1967). *The Management of Terminal Illness*. London: Edward Arnold.
3. WHO (1996). *Cancer Pain Relief*, 2nd edn. Geneva: World Health Organization.
4. Binik, Y.M., Baker, A.G., Kalogeropoulos, D., *et al*. (1982). Pain, control over treatment, and compliance in dialysis and transplant patients. *Kidney Int.,* **21**: 840–8.
5. Parfrey, P.S., Vavasour, H.M., Bullock, S.H.M., *et al*. (1988). Clinical features and severity of non-specific symptoms in dialysis patients. *Nephron,* **50**: 121–8.
6. Brown, E.A., Gower, P.E. (1982). Joint problems in patients on maintenance haemodialysis. *Clin. Nephrol.,* **18**: 247–50.
7. Davison, S.N. (2002). Pain in hemodialysis patients: prevalence, etiology, severity and analgesic use. *J. Am. Soc. Nephrol.,* **13**: 587A.

8. Fortina, F. (1999). Chronic pain during hemodialysis. Pharmacologic therapy and its cost. *Minerva Urol. Nephrol.*, **51**: 85–7.

9. Davison, S.N. (2002). The impact of pain in hemodialysis patients: effects on mood, sleep, daily activities and the desire to withdraw from dialysis. *J. Am. Soc. Nephrol.*, **13**: 589A.

10. US Renal Data system (2001). *Annual Data Report: Atlas of End-stage Renal Disease in the United States.* Bethesda, MD: National Institutes of Health, National Institute of Diabetes and Digestive and Kidney Diseases.

11. Cohen, L.M., Germain, M.J., Poppel, D.M., *et al.* (2000). Dying well after discontinuing the life support treatment of dialysis. *Arch. Intern. Med.*, **160**: 2513–18.

12. Davison, S.N. (2003). Pain in hemodialysis patients: prevalence, cause, severity, and management. *J. Am. Soc. Nephrol.*, **42**: 1239–47.

13. Cohen, L.M., Germain, M., Poppel, D.M., *et al.* (2000). Dialysis discontinuation and withdrawal of dialysis. *Am. J. Kidney Dis.*, **36**: 140–4.

14. Ferrell, B.R., Wisdom, C., Wenzl, C. (1989). Quality of life as an outcome variable in the management of cancer pain. *Cancer* **63**: 2321–7.

15. Becker, N., Thomsen, A.B., Olsen, A.K., *et al.* (1997). Pain epidemiology and health related quality of life in chronic non-malignant pain patients referred to a Danish multidisciplinary pain center. *Pain*, **73**: 393–400.

16. Skevington, S.M. (1998). Investigating the relationship between pain and discomfort and quality of life. *Pain*, **76**: 395–406.

17. Wang, X.S., Cleeland, C.S., Mendoza, T.R., *et al.* (1999). The effects of pain severity on health related quality of life: a study of Chinese cancer patients. *Cancer*, **86**: 1848–55.

18. Poulos, A. (2001). Pain, mood disturbance and quality of life in patients with multiple myeloma. *Oncol. Nursing Forum*, **28**: 1163–71.

19. Nie, J., Liu, S., Di, L. (2000). Cancer pain and its influence on cancer patients' quality of life. *Zhonghua Zhong Liu Za Zhi*, **22**: 432–4.

20. Bajwa, K., Szabo, E., Kjellstrand, C.M. (1996). A prospective study of risk factors and decision making in discontinuation of dialysis. *Arch. Intern. Med.*, **156**: 2571–7.

21. Chochinov, H.M., Wilson, K.G., Enns, M. *et al.* (1995). Desire for death in the terminally ill. *Am. J. Psychiatry* **152**: 1185–91.

22. Seale, C., Addington-Hall, J. (1994). Euthanasia: why people want to die. *Soc. Sci. Med.*, **39**: 647–54.

23. Back, A.L., Wallace, J.I., Starks, H.E., Pearlman, R.A. (1996). Physician-assisted suicide and euthanasia in Washington state: patient request and physician responses. *J. Am. Med. Assoc.*, **275**: 919–25,1996.

24. van der Maas, P.J., van Delden, J.J.M., Pijnenborg, L., Looman, C.W.N. (1991). Euthanasia and other medical decisions concerning the end-of-life. *The Lancet* **338**: 669–74.

25. Wilson, K.G., Scott, J.F., Graham, I.D. *et al.* (2000). Attitudes of terminally ill patients toward euthanasia and physician-assisted suicide. *Arch. Intern. Med.*, **160**: 2454–60.

26. Devins, G.M., Armstrong, S.J., Mandin, H., *et al.* (1990). Recurrent pain, illness intrusiveness and quality of life in end stage renal disease. *Pain* **42**: 279–85.

27. McQuay, H., Carroll, D., Jadad, A.R., *et al.* (1995). Anticonvulsant drugs for management of pain: a systematic review. *Br. Med. J.*, **311**: 1047–52.

28. McQuay, H., Moore, A. (1998). *An Evidence-based Resource for Pain Relief.* Oxford: Oxford University Press.

29. Zech, D.F.J., Grond, S., Lynch, J., *et al.*, Validation of World Health Organization Guidelines for cancer pain relief: a 10-year prospective study. *Pain* 63:65–76,1995.

30. Cleeland, C., Gonin, R., Hatfield, A.K., *et al.* (1994). Pain and its treatment in outpatients with metastatic cancer. *New Engl. J. Med.*, **330**: 592–6.

31. Anderson, K.O., Mendoza, T.R., Valero, V. *et al.* (2001). Minority cancer patients and their providers: pain management attitudes and practice. *Cancer* **88**: 1929–38.

32. Melzack, R. (1975). The McGill Pain Questionnaire: major properties and scoring methods. *Pain* **1**: 277–99.

33. Daut, R.L., Cleeland, G.S., Flanery, R.C. (1983). Development of the Wisconsin Brief Pain Questionnaire to assess pain in cancer and other diseases. *Pain,* **17**: 197–210.

34. Caraceni, A., Cherny, N., Fainsinger, R. *et al.* (2002). Pain measurement tools and methods in clinical research and palliative care: recommendations of an expert working group of the European Association of Palliative Care. *J. Pain Symptom Manage.,* **23**: 239–55.

35. Wuerth, D., Finkelstein, S.H., Ciarcia, J., *et al.* (2001). Identification and treatment of depression in a cohort of patients maintained on chronic peritoneal dialysis. *Nephron,* **37**: 1011–17.

36. Kimmel, P.L. (2001). Psychosocial factors in dialysis patients. *Kidney Int.,* **59**: 1599–613.

37. Dworkin, R.H., Gitlin, M.J. (1991). Clinical aspects of depression in chronic pain. *Clin. J. Pain* **7**: 79–94.

38. WHO (1990). *Cancer Pain Relief and Palliative Care: Report of a WHO Expert Committee.* Geneva: World Health Organization.

39. Anderson, R.J., Gambertoglio, J.G., Schrier, R.W. (1982). Prescriber medication in long term dialysis units. *Arch. Intern. Med.,* **142**: 1305–8.

40. Cockcroft, D.W., Gault, M.H. (1976). Prediction of creatinine clearance from serum creatinine. *Nephron,* **16**: 31–41.

41. Reidenberg, M.M. (1985). Kidney function and drug action. *New Engl. J. Med.,* **313**: 816–18.

42. Gibaldi, M. (1977). Drug distribution in renal failure. *Am. J. Med.,* **62**: 471–4.

43. British Medical Association and Royal Pharmaceutical Society of Great Britain (2002). *British National Formulary.*

44. Aronoff, G.R., Berns, J.S., Brier, M.E. *et al.* (1998). *Drug Prescribing in Renal Failure,* 4th edn. Philadelphia, PA: American College of Physicians.

45. Ashley, C., Bunn, R. (ed.) (1999). *The Renal Drug Handbook.* Oxford: Radcliffe Medical Press.

46. Chennevasin, P., Brater, D.C. (1981). Normograms for drug use in renal disease. *Clin. Pharmacokinet.,* **6**: 193–214.

47. Michael, K.A., Mohler, J.L., Blouin, R.A., *et al.* (1985). Failure of creatinine clearance to predict gentamycin half-life in a renal transplant with diabetes mellitus. *Clin. Pharm.,* **4**: 572–5.

48. Maderazo, E., Sun, H., Jay, G. (1992). Simplification of antibiotic dose adjustment in renal insuficiency: the DREM system. *The Lancet* **340**: 767–70.

49. Gulyassay, P.F., Depner, T.A. (1983). Impaired binding of drugs and ligands in renal diseases. *Am. J. Kidney Dis.,* **2**: 578–601.

50. Vanholder, R., van Landschoot, N., de Sweet, R., *et al.* (1988). Drug protein binding in chronic renal failure: evaluation of nine drugs. *Kidney Int.,* **33**: 996–1004.

51. Lewis, G.P., Jusko, W.J., Burke, C.W. (1971). Prednisolone side-effects and serum protein levels. *The Lancet* **ii**: 778–80.

52. Gibson, T.P. (1986). Renal disease and drug metabolism: an overview. *Am. J. Kidney Dis.,* **8**: 7–17.

53. Gibson, T.P., Dobrinska, M.R., Estwhistle, L.A., *et al.* (1987). Biotransformation of sulindac in end-stage renal disease. *Clin. Pharmacol. Ther.,* **42**: 82–8.

54. Berg, J.K., Talseth, T. (1985). Acute renal effects of sulindac and indomethacin in chronic renal failure. *Clin. Pharmacol. Ther.,* **37**: 325–9.

55. Hart, D., Lifschitz, M.D. (1987). Renal physiology of the prostaglandins and the effects of non-steroidal anti-inflammatory agents on the kidney. *Am. J. Nephrol.,* **7**: 408–18.

56. Kleinknecht, D., Landais, P., Goldfarb, B. (1986). Analgesic and non-steroidal anti-inflammatory drug-associated acute renal failure: a prospective collaborative study. *Clin. Nephrol.,* **25**: 275–81.

57. Shankel, S.W., Johnson, D.C., Clark, P.S., *et al.* (1992). Acute renal failure and glomerulopathy caused by non-steroidal anti-inflammatory drugs. *Arch. Intern. Med.,* **152**: 986–90.

58. Minuz, P., Barrow, S.E., Cockcroft, J.R., *et al.* (1990). Effects of non-steroidal anti-inflammatory drugs on prostacyclin and thromboxane biosynthesis in patients with essential hypertension. *Br. J. Clin. Pharmacol.,* **30**: 519–26.

59. Farrell, B., Godwin, J., Richards, S., *et al.* (1991). The United Kingdom ischaemic transient attack (UK TIA) aspirin trial: final results. *J. Neurol. Neurosurg. Psych.,* **54**: 1044–54.

60. Bombardier, C., Laine, L., Reicin, A., *et al.* (2000). Comparison of upper gastrointestinal toxicity of rofecoxib and naproxen in patients with rheumatoid arthritis. *New Engl. J. Med.,* **343**: 1520–8.

61. Silverstein, F.E., Faich, G., Goldstein, J.L., *et al.* (2000). Gastrointestinal toxicity with celecoxib vs non-steroidal anti-inflammatory drugs for osteoarthritis and rheumatoid arthritis: the CLASS study: a randomised control trial. *J. Am. Med. Assoc.,* **284**: 1247–55.

62. Lanas, A. (2002). Clinical experience with cyclooxygenase-2 inhibitors. *Rheumatology* **41**(Suppl. 1): 35–42.

63. Solomon, D.H., Glynn, R.J., Levin, R., *et al.* (2002). Nonsteroidal anti-inflammatory drug use and acute myocardial infarction. *Arch. Intern. Med.,* **162**: 1099–104.

64. Watson, D.J., Rhodes, T., Cai, B., *et al.* (2002). Lower risk of thromboembolic cardiovascular effects with naproxen among patients with rheumatoid arthritis. *Arch. Intern. Med.,* **162**: 1105–10.

65. Rahme, E., Pilote, L., LeLorier, J. (2002). Association between naproxen use and protection against acute myocardial infarction. *Arch. Intern. Med.,* **162**: 1111–15.

66. Van Hecken, A., Schwartz, J.L., Depre, M., *et al.* (2000). Comparative activity of rofecoxib, meloxicam, diclofenac, ibuprofen and naproxen on COX-2 versus COX-1 in healthy volunteers. *J. Clin. Pharmacol.,* **40**: 1109–20.

67. Dalen, J.E. (2002). Selective COX-2 inhibitors, NSAIDs, aspirin, and myocardial infarction. *Arch. Intern. Med.,* **162**: 1091–2.

68. Herbert, P.R., Hennekens, C.H. (2000). An overview of the 4 randomized trials of aspirin therapy in the primary prevention of vascular disease. *Arch. Intern. Med.,* **160**: 3123–7.

69. Eden, A.N., Kaufman, A. (1967). Clinical comparison of three antipyretic agents. *Am. J. Dis. Child.,* **114**: 284–7.

70. Brewer, E.J. (1968). A comparative evaluation of indomethacin, acetaminophen and placebo as antipyretic agents in children. *Arthritis Rheum.,* **11**: 645–51.

71. Skjelbred, P., Lokken, P. (1979). Paracetamol versus placebo: effects on postoperative course. *Eur. J. Clin. Pharmacol.,* **15**: 27–33.

72. Botting, R. (2000). Paracetamol-inhibitable COX-2. *J. Physiol. Pharmacol.,* **51**: 609–18.

73. Koch-Wesser, J. (1976). Acetaminophen. *New Engl. J. Med.,* **295**: 1297–300.

74. Forrest, J.A.H., Clements, J.A., Prescott, L.F. (1982). Clinical pharmacokinetics of paracetamol. *Clin. Pharmacokinet.,* **7**: 420–31.

75. Prescott, L.F. (1982). Analgesic nephropathy; a reassessment of the role of phenacetin and other analgesics. *Drugs,* **23**: 75–149.

76. Fored, M., Ejerblad, E., Lindblad, P., *et al.* (2001). Acetaminophen, aspirin, and chronic renal failure. *New Engl. J. Med.,* **345**: 1801–8.

77. Lasagna, L. (1964). The clinical evaluation of morphine and its substitutes as analgesics. *Pharmacol. Rev.,* **16**: 47–83.

78. Boeruer, U., Abbott, S., Roe, R.L. (1975). The metabolism of morphine and heroin in man. *Drug Metab. Rev.,* **4**: 39–73.

79. Desmueles, J., Gascon, M.P., Dayer, P. *et al.* (1991). Impact of environmental and genetic factors on codeine analgesia. *Eur. J. Clin. Pharmacol.,* **41**: 23–6.

80. Sindrup, S.H., Poulsen, L., Brozen, K., *et al.* (1993). Are poor metabolizers of sparteine/debrisoquine less pain tolerant than extensive metabolizers? *Pain* **53**: 335–49.

81. Barnes, J.N., Williams, A.J., Tomson, M.J., *et al.* (1985). Dihydrocodeine in renal failure: further evidence for an important role of the kidney in the handling of opioid drugs. *Br. Med. J.,* **290**: 740–2.

82. Guay, D.R., Awni, W.M., Findlay, J.W., *et al.* (1988). Pharmacokinetics and pharmacodynamics of codeine in end-stage renal disease. *Clin. Pharmacol. Ther.,* **43**: 63–71.

83. Davies, G., Kingswood, C., Street, M. (1996). Pharmacokinetics of opioids in renal dysfunction. *Clin. Pharmacokinet.,* **31**: 410–22.

84. Empey, D.W., Laitman, L.A., Young, G.A., *et al.* (1979). Comparison of the antitussive effects of codeine phosphate 20 mg, dextromethorphan 30 mg and noscapine 30 mg using citric acid-induced cough in normal subjects. *Eur. J. Clin. Pharmacol.,* **16**: 393–7.

85. Bradshaw, M.J., Harvey, R.F. (1982). Antidiarrhoeal agents—clinical pharmacology and therapeutic use. *Drugs,* **24**: 440–51.

86. Barnes, J.N., Goodwin, F.J. (1983). Dihydrocodeine narcosis in renal failure. *Br. Med. J.,* **286**: 438–9.

87. Messick, R.T. (1979). Evaluation of acetaminophen, propoxyphene, and their combination in office practice. *J. Clin. Pharmacol.,* **19**: 227–30.

88. Gibson, T.P., Giacomini, K.M., Briggs, W.A., *et al.* (1980). Propoxyphene and norpropoxyphene concentrations in the anephric patient. *Clin. Pharmacol. Ther.,* **27**: 665–70.

89. Nickander, R.C., Emmerson, J.L., Hynes, M.D., *et al.* (1984). Pharmacologic and toxic effects in animals of dextropropoxyphene and its major metabolite norpropoxyphene: a review. *Human Toxicol.,* **3**: 13S–36S.

90. Gibson, T.P. (1996). Pharmacokinetics, efficacy, and safety of analgesia with a focus on tramadol HCl. *Am. J. Med.,* **101**(Suppl. 1A): 47S–53S.

91. Raffa, R.B., Friderichs, E., Reimann, W., *et al.* (1992). Opioid and nonopioid components independently contribute to the mechanism of action of tramadol, an 'atypical' opioid analgesic. *J. Pharmacol. Exp. Ther.,* **260**: 275–85.

92. Raffa, R.B., Friderichs, E., Reimann, W., *et al.* (1993). Complementary and synergistic antinociceptive interaction between the enantiomers of tramadol. *J. Pharmacol. Exp. Ther.,* **267**: 331–40.

93. Radbruch, L., Grond, S., Lehmann, K.A. (1996). A risk–benefit assessment of tramadol in the management of pain. *Drug Safety,* **15**: 8–29.

94. Desmeules, J.A. (2000). The tramadol option. *Eur. J. Pain* **4**(Suppl. A): 15–21.

95. Sevcik, J., Nieber, K., Driessen, B., *et al.* (1993). Effects of the central analgesic tramadol and its main metabolite, O-desmethyltramadol, on rat locus coeruleus neurones. *Br. J. Pharmacol.,* **110**: 169–76.

96. Lintz, W., Erlacin, S., Trankus, E., *et al.* (1981). Biotransformation of tramadol in man and animals. *Arzneimittelforschung* **31**: 1932–43.

97. Scott, L.J., Perry, C.M. (2000). Tramadol: a review of its use in perioperative pain. *Drugs,* **60**: 139–76.

98. Bamigbade, T.A., Langford, R.M. (1998). Tramadol hydrochloride—an overview of current use. *Hosp. Med.,* **59**: 373–6.

99. Shipton, E.A. (2000). Tramadol—present and future. *Anaesth. Intensive Care,* **28**: 363–74.

100. Desmules, J.A., Piguet, V., Collart, L., *et al.* (1996). Contribution of monoaminergic modulation to the analgesic effect of tramadol. *Br. J. Clin. Pharmacol.,* **41**: 7–12.

101. Foley, K.M. (1993). Opioid analgesics in clinical pain management. In: *Handbook of Experimental Pharmacology,* ed. A. Herz, pp. 697–743. Berlin: Springer-Verlag.

102. Messahel, F.M., Tomlin, P.J. (1981). Narcotic withdrawal syndrome after intrathecal administration of morphine. *Br. Med. J.,* **283**: 471–2.

103. Cousins, M.J., Cherry, D.A. (1988). Acute and chronic pain: use of spinal opioids. In: *Neural Blockade in Clinical Anesthesia and Management of Pain,* ed. M.J. Cousins, pp. 955–1029. Philadelphia, PA: Lippincott.

104. Gates, M., Tschudi, G. (1952). The synthesis of morphine. *J. Am. Chem. Soc.,* **74**: 1109–10.

105. Narita, M., Funada, M., Suzuki, T. (2001). Regulation of opioid dependence by opioid receptor types. *Pharmacol. Ther.,* **89**: 1–15.

106. Gutstein, H.B., Akil, H. Opioid analgesics and antagonists. In: Hardman J.G., Limbird, L.E., eds *Goodman and Gilman's The Pharmacological Basis of Therapeutics.* 10th edn. New York, McGraw-Hill, 2001: 569–619.

107. Patwardhan, R.V., Johnson, R.F., Hoyumpa, A., Jr., *et al.* (1981). Normal metabolism of morphine in cirrhosis. *Gastroenterology* **81**: 1006–11.

108. Tegeder, I., Lotsch, J., Geisslinger, G. (1999). Pharmacokinetics of opioids in liver disease. *Clin. Pharmacokinet.,* **37**: 17–40.

109. Yeh, S.Y., Gorodetzky, C.W., Krebs, H.A. (1977). Isolation and identification of morphine 3- and 6-glucuronides, morphine-3,6-diglucuronide, morphine-3-ethereal sulphate, normorphine, and normorphine-6-glucuronide as morphine metabolites in humans. *J. Pharm. Sci.,* **66**: 1288–93.

110. Osborne, R.J., Joel, S.P., Trew, D., *et al.* (1988). The analgesic activity of morhine-6-glucuronide. *The Lancet* **i**: 828.

111. Osborne, R.J., Joel, S.P., Trew, D., *et al.* (1990). Morphine and metabolite behaviour and different routes of morphine administration: demonstration of the active metabolite morphine-6-glucuronide. *Clin. Pharmacol. Ther.,* **47**: 12–19.

112. Portenoy, R.K. (1990). Chronic opioid therapy in nonmalignant pain. *J. Pain Symptom Manage.,* **5**: S46–S62.

113. Portenoy, R.K., Khan, E., Layman, M., *et al.* (1991). Chronic morphine therapy for pain for cancer pain: plasma and cerebrospinal fluid morphine and morphine-6-glucuronide concentrations. *Neurology,* **41**: 1457–61.

114. Sawe, J., Odar-Cederlof, I. (1987). Kinetics of morphine in patients with renal failure. *Eur. J. Clin. Pharmacol.,* **32**: 377–82.

115. Sear, J.W., Hand, C.W., Moore, R.A., *et al.* (1989). Studies on morphine disposition: influence of renal failure on the kinetics of morphine and its metabolites. *Br. J. Anaesth.,* **62**: 28–32.

116. Chauvin, M., Sandouk, P., Scherrmann, J.M., *et al.* (1987). Morphine pharmacokinetics in renal failure. *Anesthesiology* **66**: 327–31.

117. Osborne, R.J., Joel, S.P., Slevin, M.L. (1986). Morphine intoxication in renal failure: the role of morphine-6-glucuronide. *Br. Med. J.,* **292**: 1548–9.

118. Wolff, J., Bigler, D., Broen Christensen, C., *et al.* (1988). Influence of renal function on the elimination of morphine and morphine glucuronides. *Eur. J. Pharmacol.,* **34**: 353–7.

119. Hanna, M.H., D'Costa, F., Peat, S.J., *et al.* (1993). Morphine-6-glucuronide disposition in renal impairment. *Br. J. Anaesth.,* **70**: 511–14.

120. Faura, C.C., Collins, S.L., Moore, R.A., *et al.* (1998). Systematic review of factors affecting the ratios of morphine and its major metabolites. *Pain* **74**: 43–53.

121. Pauli-Magnus, C., Hofmann, U., Mikus, G., *et al.* (1999). Pharmacokinetics of morphine and its glucuronides following intravenous administration of morphine in patients undergoing continuous ambulatory peritoneal dialysis. *Nephrol. Dial. Transpl.,* **14**: 903–9.

122. Bruera, E., Sloan, P., Mount, B., *et al.* (1996). A randomized, double-blind, double-dummy, crossover trial comparing the safety and efficacy of oral sustained-release hydromorphone with immediate-release hydromorphone in patients with cancer pain. *J. Clin. Oncol.,* **14**: 1713–17.

123. Dunbar, P.J., Chapman, C.R., Buckley, F.P., *et al.* (1996). Clinical analgesic equivalence for morphine and hydromorphone with prolonged PCA. *Pain,* **68**: 265–70.

124. Quigley, C. (2002). Hydromorphone for acute and chronic pain. *Cochrane Database Syst. Rev.* CD003447.

125. Sarhill, N., Walsh, D., Nelson, K.A. (2001). Hydromorphone: pharmacology and clinical applications in cancer patients. *Support Care Cancer,* **9**: 84–96.

126. Babul, N., Darke, A.C., Hagen, N. (1995). Hydromorphone metabolite accumulation in renal failure. *J. Pain Symptom Manage.,* **10**(3): 184–6.

127. Fainsinger, R., Schoeller, T., Boiskin, M., *et al.* (1993). Palliative care round: cognitive failure and coma after renal failure in a patient receiving captopril and hydromorphone. *J. Palliative Care,* **9**: 53–5.

128. Lee, M.A., Leng, M.E., Tiernan, E.J. (2001). Retrospective study of the use of hydromorphone in palliative care patients with normal and abnormal urea and creatinine. *Palliative Med.,* **15**: 26–34.

129. Morrison, J.D., Loan, W.B., Dundee, J.W. (1971). Controlled comparison of of the efficacy of four-teen preparations in the relief of post-operative pain. *Br. Med., J.* **2**: 287–90.

130. Gourlay, G.K., Cherry, D.A., Cousins, M.J. (1986). A comparative study of the efficacy and pharma-cokinetics of oral methadone and morphine in the treatment of severe pain in patients with cancer pain. *Pain,* **25**: 297–312.

131. Davies, A.M., Inturrisi, J. (1999). D-Methadone blocks morphine tolerance and N-methyl-D-aspartate-induced hyperalgesia. *J. Pharmacol. Exp. Ther.,* **289**: 1048–53.

132. Fainsinger, R., Schoeller, R., Bruera, E. (1993). Methadone in the management of cancer pain. *Pain,* **52**: 137–47.

133. Dole, V.P., Kreek, M.J. (1973). Methadone plasma level: sustained by a reservoir of drug. *Proc. Natl. Acad. Sci. USA,* **70**: 10–15.

134. Bruera, E., Neumann, C.M. (1999). Role of methadone in the management of pain in cancer patients. *Oncology,* **13**: 1275–88.

135. Pohland, A., Boaz, H.E., Sullivan, H.R. (1971). Synthesis and identification of metabolites resulting from the biotransformation of D,L-methadone in man and in the rat. *J. Med. Chem.,* **14**: 194–7.

136. Kreek, M.J., Schecter, A.J., Gutjahr, C.L., *et al.* (1980). Methadone use in patients with chronic renal disease. *Drug Alcohol Depend.,* **5**: 197–205.

137. Furlan, V., Hafi, A., Dessalles, M.C., *et al.* (1999). Methadone is poorly removed by haemodialysis. *Nephrol. Dial. Transpl.,* **14**: 254–5.

138. Mather, L.E., Meffin, L.E. (1978). Clinical pharmacokinetics pethidine. *Clin. Pharmacokinet.,* **3**: 352–68.

139. MacDonald, A.D., Wolfe, A.G., Bergel, F., *et al.* (1946). Analgesic actions of pethidine derivatives and related compounds. *Br. J. Pharmacol.,* **1**: 4–14.

140. Miller, J.W., Anderson, H.H. (1954). The effect of N-demethylation on certain pharmacologic actions of morphine, codeine and meperidine in the mouse. *J. Pharmacol. Exp. Ther.,* **112**: 191–6.

141. Szeto, H.H., Inturrisi, C.E., Houde, R., *et al.* (1977). Accumulation of normeperidine, an active metabolite of meperidine, in patients with renal failure or cancer. *Ann. Intern. Med.,* **86**: 738–41.

142. Ripamonti, C., Dickerson, E.D. (2001). Strategies for the treatment of cancer pain in the new millennium. *Drugs,* **61**: 955–77.

143. Kalso, E., Vamio, A., Mattula, M.J., *et al.* (1990). Morphine and oxycodone in the management of cancer pain: plasma levels determined by chemical and radioreceptor assays. *Pharmacol. Toxicol.,* **67**: 322–8.

144. Rischitelli, D.G., Karbowicz, S.H. (2002). Safety and efficacy of controlled-release oxycodone: a sys-tematic literature review. *Pharmacotherapy* **22**: 898–904.

145. Poyhia, R., Vainio, A., Kalso, E. (1993). A review of oxycodone's clinical pharmacokinetics and pharmacodynamics. *J. Pain Symptom Manage.,* **8**: 63–7.

146. Leow, K., Smith, M.T., Watt, J.A., *et al.* (1992). Comparative oxycodone pharmacokinetics in humans after intravenous, oral and rectal administration. *Ther. Drug Monit.,* **14**: 479–84.

147. Weinstein, S.H., Gaylord, J.C. (1979). Determination of oxycodone in plasma and identification of a major metabolite. *J. Pharm. Sci.,* **68**: 527–8.

148. Baselt, R.C., Stewart, C.B. (1978). Determination of oxycodone and a major metabolite in urine by electron-capture GLC. *J. Anal. Toxicol.,* **2**: 107–9.

149. Poyhia, R., Okkola, K.T., Seppala, T., *et al.* (1992). The pharmacokinetics of oxycodone after intravenous injection in adults. *Br. J. Clin. Pharmacol.,* **32**: 516–18.

150. Kirvela, M., Lindgren, L., Seppala, T., *et al.* (1996). The pharmacokinetics of oxycodone in uremic patients undergoing renal transplantation. *J. Clin. Anesth.,* **8**: 13–18.

151. Clotz, M.A., Nahata, M.C. (1991). Clinical uses of fentanyl, sufentanil and alfentanil. *Clin. Pharm.,* **10**: 581–93.

152. Paix, A., Coleman, A., Lees, J., *et al.* (1995). Subcutaneous fentanyl and sufentanil infusion substitution for morphine intolerance in cancer management. *Pain,* **63**: 263–9.

153. Zech, D.F.J., Grond, S.U.A., Lynch, J., *et al.* (1992). Transdermal fentanyl and initial dose-finding with patient-controlled analgesia in cancer pain. A pilot study with 20 terminally ill cancer patients. *Pain,* **50**: 293–301.

154. Koren, G., Crean, P., Goresky, G.V., *et al.* (1984). Pharmacokinetics of fentanyl in children with renal disease. *Res. Comm. Chem. Pathol. Pharmacol.,* **46**: 371–9.

155. McClain, D.A., Hug, C.C., Jr., (1980). Intravenous fentanyl kinetics. *Clin. Pharmacol. Ther.,* **28**: 106–14.

156. Koehntop, D.E., Rodman, J.H. (1997). Fentanyl pharmacokinetics in patients undergoing renal transplantation. *Pharmacotherapy* **17**: 746–52.

157. Bower, S. (1982). Plasma protein binding of fentanyl: the effect of hyperlipoproteinaemia and chronic renal failure. *J. Pharm. Pharmacol.,* **34**: 102–6.

158. Mercadante, S., Caligara, M., Sapio, M., *et al.* (1997). Subcutaneous fentanyl infusion in a patient with bowel obstruction and renal failure. *J. Pain Symptom Manage.,* **13**: 241–4.

159. Geerts, P., Noorduin, G., Vanden Bussche, G., *et al.* (1987). Practical aspects of alfentanil infusion. *Eur. J. Anaesthesiol.,* **4**(Suppl. 1): 3–12.

160. Dale, O., Hjortkjaer, R., Kharasch, E.D. (2002). Nasal administration of opioids for pain management in adults. *Acta Anaesthesiol. Scand.,* **46**: 759–70.

161. McQuay, H.J., Moore, R.A., Bullingham, R.E.S. (1986). Buprenorphine kinetics. In: *Opioid Analgesics in the Management of Clinical Pain*, ed. K.M. Foley, C.E. Inturrisi, pp. 271–8. New York: Raven Press.

162. Martin, W.R., Eades, C.G., Thompson, J.A., *et al.* (1976). The effects of morphine- and nalorphine-like drugs in the nondependent and morphine-dependent chronic spinal dog. *J. Pharmacol. Exp. Ther.,* **197**: 517–32.

163. Lewis, J.W. (1985). Buprenorphine. *Drug Alcohol Depend.,* **14**: 363–74.

164. Arner, S., Meyerson, B.A. (1988). Lack of analgesic effect of opioids on neuropathic and idiopathic forms of pain. *Pain* **33**: 11–231988.

165. Budd, K. (1981). High dose buprenorphine for postoperative analgesia. *Anaesthesia* **36**: 900–3.

166. Walsh, S.L., Preston, K.L., Stitzer, M.L., *et al.* (1994). Clinical pharmacology of buprenorphine: ceiling effect at high doses. *Clin. Pharmacol. Ther.,* **55**: 569–80.

167. Bullingham, R.E.S., McQuay, H.J., Moore, R.A., *et al.* (1981). Oral buprenorphine and paracetamol combination compared with paracetamol alone: a single dose double-blind postoperative study. *Br. J. Clin. Pharmacol.,* **12**: 863–7.

168. Armstrong, S.C., Cozza, K.L. (2003). Pharmacokinetic drug interactions of morphine, codeine, and their derivatives: theory and clinical reality. *Psychosomantics* **44**: 515–20.

169. Hand, C.W., Sear, J.R., Uppington, J., *et al.* (1990). Buprenorphine disposition in patients with renal impairment: single and continuous dosing, with special reference to metabolites. *Br. J. Anaesth.,* **64**: 276–82.

170. Ohtani, M., Kotaki, H., Sawada, Y., *et al.* (1995). Comparative analysis of buprenorphine- and norbuprenorphine-induced analgesic effects based on pharmacokinetic-pharmacodynamic modeling. *J. Pharmacol. Exp. Ther.,* **272**: 505–10.

171. Ohtani, M., Kotaki, H., Nishitateno, K., *et al.* (1997). Kinetics of respiratory depression in rats induced by buprenorphine and its metabolite, norbuprenorphine. *J. Pharmacol. Exp. Ther.,* **281**: 428–33.

172. Kosterlitz, H.W., Watt, A.J. (1968). Kinetic parameters of narcotic agonists and antagonists with particular reference to *N*-allynoroxymorphone (naloxone). *Br. J. Pharmacol. Chemother.,* **33**: 266–76.

173. Levine, J.D., Gordon, N.C., Fields, H.L. (1979). Naloxone dose dependently produces analgesia and hyperalgesia in postoperative pain. *Nature,* **278**: 740–1.

174. Lasagna, L. (1965). Drug interactions in the field of analgesic drugs. *Proc. R. Soc. Med.,* **58**: 978–83.

175. Kenyon, J.N., Knight, C.J., Wells, C. (1983). Randomised double-blind trial on the immediate effects of naloxone on classical Chinese acupuncture therapy for chronic pain. *Acupuncture Electrotherapeutic Res.,* **8**: 17–24.

176. Weinstein, P.C., Pfeffer, M., Schor, J.M., *et al.* (1971). Metabolites of naloxone in human urine. *J. Pharm. Sci.,* **60**: 1567–8.

177. Berkowitz, B.A., Ngai, S.H., Hempstead, J., *et al.* (1975). Disposition of naloxone: use of a new radioimmunoassay. *J. Pharmacol. Exp. Ther.,* **195**: 499–504.

178. Mercadente, S. (1999). Problems of long-term spinal opioid treatment in advanced cancer patients. *Pain,* **79**: 1–13.

179. Uhle, E.I., Becker, R., Gatscher, S., *et al.* (2000). Continuous intrathecal clonidine administration for the treatment of neuropathic pain. *Stereotact. Funct. Neurosurg.,* **75**: 167–75.

180. Stein, C., Machelska, H., Schafer, M. (2001). Peripheral analgesic and antiinflammatory effects of opioids. *Z. Rheumatol.,* **60**: 410–24.

181. Twillman, R.K., Long, T.D., Cathers, T.A., *et al.* (1999). Treatment of painful skin ulcers with topical opioids. *J. Pain Symptom Manage.,* **17**: 288–92.

182. Back, I.N., Finlay, I. (1995). Analgesic effect of topical opioids on painful skin ulcers. *J. Pain Symptom Manage.,* **10**: 493.

183. Moore, R.A., Tramer, M.R., Carroll, D., *et al.* (1998). Quantitative systematic review of topically applied non-steroidal anti-inflammatory drugs. *Br. Med. J.,* **316**: 333–8.

184. Zhang, W.Y., Li Wan Po, A. (1994). The effectiveness of topically applied capsaicin. A meta-analysis. *Eur. J. Clin. Pharmacol.,* **46**: 517–22.

185. Doyle, D., Hanks, G.W., MacDonald, N. (ed.) (1997). *Oxford Textbook of Palliative Medicine.* Oxford: Oxford University Press.

186. McQuay, H.J., Tramer, M., Nye, B.A., *et al.* (1996). A systematic review of antidepressants in neuropathic pain. *Pain,* **68**: 217–27.

187. Wiffen, P.A., Collins, S., McQuay, H., *et al.* (2000). Anticonvulsant drugs for acute and chronic pain. *Cochrane Database Syst. Rev.,* **2**: CD001133.

188. Fallon, M.T., Welsh, J. (1996). The role of ketamine in pain control. *Eur. J. Palliative Care,* **3**: 143–6.

189. Oye, I. (1998). Ketamine analgesia, NMDA receptors and the gates of perception. *Acta Anaesthesiol. Scand.,* **42**: 747–9.

190. Hughes, A.M., Rhodes, J., Fisher, G., *et al.* (2002). Assessment of the effect of dextromethorphan and ketamine on the acute nociceptive threshold and wind-up of the second pain response in healthy male volunteers. *Br. J. Clin. Pharmacol.,* **53**: 604–12.

191. Clements, J.A., Nimmo, W.S., Grant, I.S. (1982). Bioavailability, pharmacokinetics, and analgesic acitvity of ketamine in humans. *J. Pharm. Sci.,* **71**: 539–42.

192. Grant, I.S., Nimmo, W.S., Clements, J.A. (1981). Pharmacokinetics and analgesic effects of i.m. and oral ketamine. *Br. J. Anaesth.,* **53**: 805–10.

193. Enarson, M.C., Hays, H., Woodroffe, M.A (1999). Clinical experience with oral ketamine. *J. Pain Symptom Manage.,* **17**: 384–6.

194. Mercadante, S., Arcuri, E., Tirelli, W., *et al.* (2000). Analgesic effect of intravenous ketamine in cancer patients on morphine therapy: a randomized, controlled, double-blind, crossover, double-dose-study. *J. Pain Symptom Manage.*, **20**: 246–52.

195. Giannini, A.J., Underwood, N.A., Condon, M. (2000). Acute ketamine intoxication treated by haloperidol: a preliminary study. *Am. J. Ther.*, **7**: 389–91.

196. Sindrup, S.H., Jensen, T.S. (2002). Pharmacotherapy of trigeminal neuralgia. *Clin. J., Pain*, **18**: 22–7.

197. Young, R.R. (1981). Drug therapy: spasticity. *New Engl. J. Med.*, **304**: 96–9.

198. Groves, L., Shellenberger, M.K., Davis, C.S. (1998). Tizanidine treatment of spasticity: a meta-analysis of controlled, double-blind, comparative studies with baclofen and diazepam. *Adv. Ther.*, **15**: 241–51.

199. Hetherington, J.W., Philp, N.H. (1986). Diclofenac sodium versus pethidine in acute renal pain. *Br. Med. J.*, **292**: 237–8.

200. Oosterlinck, W., Philp, N.H., Charig, C., *et al.* (1990). A double-blind single dose comparison of intramuscular ketrolac tromethamine and pethidine in the treatment of renal colic. *J. Clin. Pharmacol.*, **30**: 336–41.

201. Mystakidou, K., Tsilika, E., Kalaidopoulou, O., *et al.* (2002). Comparison of octeotide administration vs conservative treatment in the management of inoperable bowel obstruction in patients with far advanced cancer: a randomized, double-blind, controlled clinical trial. *Anticancer Res.*, **22**: 1187–92.

202. Ventafridda, V., Ripamonti, C., Caraceni, A. *et al.* (1990). The management of inoperable gastrointestinal obstruction in terminal cancer patients. *Tumori*, **76**: 389–93.

203. Hellstrom, K.A., Rosen, A., Soderlund, K. (1970). Gastrointestinal absorption and excretion of 3H-butylscopolamine (hyoscine butylbromide) in man. *Scand. J. Gastroenterol.*, **5**: 585–92.

204. Mercadante, S., Ripamonti, C., Casuccio, A., *et al.* (2000). Comparison of octrotide and hyoscine butylbromide in controlling gastrointestinal symptoms due to malignant inoperable bowel obstruction. *Support. Care Cancer*, **8**: 188–91.

205. Critchley, P., Plach, N., Grantham, M., *et al.* (2001). Efficacy of haloperidol in the treatment of nausea and vomiting in the palliative patient: a systematic review. *J. Pain Symptom Manage.*, **22**: 631–4.

206. Pinder, R.M., Brogden, R.N., Sawyer, P.R., *et al.* (1976). Metoclopramide: a review of its pharmacological properties and clinical use. *Drugs*, **12**: 81–131.

207. Dundee, J.W., Loan, W.B., Morrison, J.D. (1975). A comparison of the efficacy of cyclizine and perhenazine in reducing the emetic effects of morphine and pethidine. *Br. J. Clin. Pharmacol.*, **2**: 81–5.

208. Davis, M.P., Walsh, D. (2000). Treatment of nausea and vomiting in advanced cancer. *Support. Care Cancer*, **8**: 444–52.

209. Pakes, G.E. (1982). Haloperidol: pharmacokinetic properties. In: *Haloperidol Decanoate in the Treatment of Chronic Schizophrenia*, ed. P Johnson, pp. 41–7. New York: Adis Press.

210. Shader, R.I., Dimascio, A., (1970). *Psychotropic Drugs Side Effects: Chemical and Theoretical Perspectives*. Baltimore, MD: Williams and Wilkins.

211. Pisani, F., Oteri, G., Costa, C., *et al.* (2002). Effects of psychotropic drugs on seizure threshold. *Drug Saf.*, **25**: 91–110.

212. Metzger, E., Friedman, R. (1993). Prolongation of the corrected QT and torsades de pointes cardiac arrhythmia associated with intravenous haloperidol in the medically ill. *J. Clin. Psychopharmacol.*, **13**: 128–32.

213. DiSalvo, T.G., O'Gara, P.T. (1995). Torsade de pointes caused by high dose intravenous haloperidol. *Clin. Cardiol.*, **18**: 285–90.

214. Harrington, R.A., Hamilton, C.W., Brogden, R.W., *et al.* (1983). Metoclopramide—an updated review of its pharmacological properties and clinical use. *Drugs*, **25**: 451–94.

215. Bateman, D., Gokal, N., Dodd, T.R.P., *et al.* (1981). The pharmacokinetics of single doses of metoclopramide in renal failure. *Eur. J. Clin. Pharmacol.*, **19**: 437–41.

216. Marty, M., Pouillart, P., Scholl, S., *et al.* (1990). Comparison of the 5-HT3 (serotonin) antagonist ondansetron (G468 032F) with high dose metoclopramide in the control of cisplatin-induced emesis. *New Engl. J. Med.,* **322**: 816–21.

217. Baber, N., Palmer, J.L., Frazer, N.M., *et al.* (1992). Clinical pharmacology of ondansetron in postoperative nausea and vomiting. *Eur. J. Anaesthesiol.,* **9**(Suppl. 6): 11–18.

218. Priestman, T.J. (1989). Clinical studies with ondansetron in control of radiation-induced emesis. *Eur. J. Cancer,* **25**(Suppl. 1): S29–S33.

219. Roberts, J.T., Priestman, T.J. (1993). A review of ondansetron in the management of radiotherapy-induced emesis. *Oncology* **50**: 173–9.

220. Walton, S.M. (2000). Advances in the use of 5-HT3 receptor antagonists. *Expert Opin. Pharmacother.,* **1**: 207–23.

221. Saynor, D.A., Dixon, C.M. (1989). The metabolism of ondansetron. *Eur. J. Cancer Clin. Oncol.,* **25**(Suppl.): S75–S77.

222. Wilde, M., Markham, A. (1996). Ondansetron. *Drugs,* **52**: 773–94.

223. Balaskas, E.V., Bamihas, G.I., Karamouzis, M. *et al.* (1998). Histamine and serotonin in uremic pruritus: effect of ondansetron in CAPD-pruritus patients. *Nephron,* **78**: 395–402.

224. Ashmore, S.D., Jones, C.H., Newstead, C.G., *et al.* (2000). Ondansetron therapy for uremic pruritus in hemodialysis patients. *Am. J. Kidney Dis.,* **35**: 827–31.

225. Twycross, R.G., Barkby, G.D., Hallwood, P.M. (1997). The use of low dose levomepromazine (methotrimeprazine) in the management of nausea and vomiting. *Prog. Palliative Care,* **5**: 49–53.

226. Melzack, R., Wall, P.D. (1965). Pain mechanisms: a new theory. *Science,* **150**: 971–8.

227. Rushton, D.N. (2002). Electrical stimulation in the treatment of pain. *Disabil. Rehabil.,* **24**: 407–15.

228. Brosseau, L., Milne, S., Robinson, V., *et al.* (2002). Efficacy of transcutaneous nerve stimulation for the treatment of low back pain: a metaanalysis. *Spine* **27**: 596–603.

229. Johnson, M.I., Ashton, C.H., Thompson, J.W. (1992). Long term use of transcutaneous electrical nerve stimulation at Newcastle Pain Relief Clinic. *J. R. Soc. Med.,* **85**: 267–8.

230. Linde, K., Vickers, A., Hondras, M., *et al.* (2001). Systemic reviews of complementary therapies—an annotated bibliography. Part 1: Acupuncture. *BMC Complement. Altern. Med.,* **1**: 3.

231. Kaptchuk, T.J. (2002). Acupuncture: theory, efficacy and practice. *Ann. Intern. Med.,* **136**: 374–83.

232. Furlan, A.D., Brosseau, L., Imamura, M., *et al.* (2002). Massage for low back pain. *Cochrane Database Syst. Rev.,* **2**: CD001929.

233. Eccleston, C. (2001). Role of psychology in pain management. *Br. J. Anaesth.,* **87**: 144–52.

234. Steinman, T.I. (2000). Pain management in polycystic kidney disease. *Am. J. Kidney Dis.,* **35**: 770–2.

235. Gabow, P.A. (1990). Autosomal dominant polycystic kidney disease, more than a renal disease. *Am. J. Kidney Dis.,* **16**: 403–13.

236. Bajwa, Z., Gupta, S., Warfield, C., *et al.* (2001). Pain management in polycystic kidney disease. *Kidney Int.,* **60**: 1631–44.

237. Meglio, M., Cioni, B., Rossi, G.F. (1989). Spinal cord stimulation in the management of chronic pain. A 9-year experience. *J. Neurosurg.,* **70**: 519–24.

238. Staats, P.S. (1999). Neuraxial infusion for pain control. *Oncology* **13**: 58–62.

239. Soravia, C., Mentha, G., Giostra, E. *et al.* (1995). Surgery for adult polycystic liver disease. *Surgery,* **117**: 272–5.

240. Swenson, K., Seu, P., Kinkhabwala, M., *et al.* (1998). Liver transplantation for adult polycystic liver disease. *Hepatology,* **28**: 412–15.

241. Wilmer, W.A., Magro, C.M. (2002). Calciphylaxis: emerging concepts in prevention, diagnosis, and treatment. *Semin. Dial.,* **15**: 172–86.

242. Mathur, R.V., Shortland, J.R., El Nahas, A.M. (2001). Calciphylaxis. *Postgrad. Med. J.,* **77**: 557–61.

243. Green, J.A., Green, C.R., Minott, S.D. (2000). Calciphylaxis treated with neurolytic lumbar sympathetic block: case report and review of the literature. *Reg. Anesth. Pain Med.,* **25**: 310–12.

244. Wilmer, W.A., Voroshilova, O., Singh, I., *et al.* (2001). Transcutaneous oxygen tension in patients with calciphylaxis. *Am. J. Kidney Dis.,* **37**: 797–806.

245. Kurella, M., Bennett, W.M., Chertow, G.M. (2003). Analgesia in patients with ESRD: a review of available evidence. *Am. J. Kidney Dis.,* **42**: 217–28.

Chapter 9

# Psychological and psychiatric considerations in patients with advanced renal disease

Jean Hooper and Lewis M. Cohen

The onset of advanced renal disease is difficult to identify. At what point does the medical care become palliative? Who identifies this—the patient or the health worker? On the patient's journey through the condition, when does the care change from treatment for life to preparation for dying? Is there a difference?

There are no definitive answers to these questions. On the other hand, there are some things that are clear in the management of this population. For example, the healthcare, however it is described, should begin at the time of the diagnosis of renal failure—irrespective of the age of the patient or how advanced the condition at that time.

What is offered should depend on a variety of factors both medical and personal, in a combination that is unique to each patient. Individual differences occur as a result of biological, physical, cognitive, emotional, environmental, social, historical, educational, and familial factors. And luck.

In order to offer effective care, social and psychological aspects of the patient's condition should be addressed as well as the medical markers indicating current physiological status. While the latter help to maintain the existence of life, the former are essential for the quality of the lived experience. This chapter outlines the major psychological reactions known to affect patients with a chronic condition such as end-stage renal disease (ESRD) and suggests approaches for optimum holistic care. It also briefly summarizes treatment issues in the management of common co-morbid psychiatric disorders.

## Case study

John was in his late 30s when he came to the attention of the renal care staff. He was articulate, had a business degree, and worked in a senior position in the high-quality hotel/leisure industry. His own leisure time was spent in several energetic sports, particularly skiing black runs, motor racing, and hang-gliding. He was not married, in fact had never had a close personal relationship with anybody. He always attended clinic appointments alone saying that he had no particular friends. His lifestyle revealed expensive tastes in accommodation, wine, food, vacations, and entertainment. There was no indication of any psychological pathology, and he reported that his quality of life was highly satisfactory and described himself as actively content.

His medical history revealed that he had lived in the shadow of renal failure all his life, knowing from late childhood that his kidneys were failing and that he would eventually need dialysis to keep him alive. His renal function was regularly checked but never discussed within his family.

**Case study** *(continued)*

When active treatment could no longer be delayed he opted for haemodialysis at a local hospital, and during the thrice-weekly sessions would use his laptop and mobile phone to maintain his work schedule. He gave up his sporting activities. While always pleasant, he never made friends with any of his fellow patients. He was very popular with the staff and frequently brought sweets and chocolates for them as well as providing reduced rates for their social functions in one of the chain of hotels he managed. He was known to disregard the fluid and dietary limitations regularly. This was well tolerated because the staff believed that he was intelligent enough to know what he was doing and would come to no harm. In all other respects he was regarded as a model patient and they were genuinely pleased when he received a successful transplant.

He immediately resumed his former active lifestyle, focusing on solo rather than team sports, and practised hard to regain his former levels of skill. He accepted a more senior position in the company.

Within 5 years it became apparent that the transplanted kidney was failing. His presentation to the haemodialysis staff during this time was much the same, but perceptive ones among them observed that his good spirits seemed very fragile and false. To the psychologist in a routine predialysis interview he admitted that he hated being unable to influence the course of his disease, and was working and playing harder to maximize his experiences in the limited time he still had available before dialysis. He was unable to disclose his bleak feelings to the staff, as they were so encouraging and positive. They still thought of him as he had been when he had high expectations of a successful transplant.

It seemed to him that there was no alternative but once again to give up his sporting activities. He was concerned that his very senior management position would be compromised by his need for treatment. A fistula was formed in his dominant arm and a date set for his return to dialysis. As these arrangements progressed he planned a skiing holiday and talked enthusiastically about it with the staff, proudly showing them the black runs he planned to ski.

He never returned.

## 9.1 Initial reactions

The psychological effects of receiving bad news are well documented.[1] They include shock, encounter reaction, and retreat before an uneasy acceptance. Patients experience these states in apparent random order for varying lengths of time and may visit each many times in sequence or concurrently. There is nothing neat and organized about reactions to news of a terminal condition.

The initial reaction of **shock** occurs as a response to any kind of bad news, but will be more extreme if the news is unexpected. The patient appears stunned and uses well-rehearsed living skills to behave in an automatic fashion: 'I don't know how I drove home after the doctor told me'. They also feel detached from ordinary life and often from their closest family members. There is the beginning of a sense of isolation which brings with it the belief that they have to manage this alone, that no one can understand what they are experiencing, that they must not burden others with this dreadful experience. While we do not know from the records how John reacted initially to the news of his renal failure, his avoidance of close relationships/friendships may indicate this sense of isolation from an early stage.

**Encounter reaction** is characterized by disorganized thinking, and a range of feelings including loss, grief, despair, and helplessness. The patient is overwhelmed by the enormity of the news and may behave uncharacteristically, make strange plans, or withdraw from decision-making altogether. It is during this phase that the behaviour labelled as 'denial' often emerges.

Much has been written about denial, with some misrepresentation of this coping strategy as a negative response to be immediately eliminated therapeutically. It is certainly misinterpreted as such by large numbers of healthcare workers. Denial is one of many defence mechanisms identified by Freud. Others often utilized in chronic conditions include intellectualization, where the news is dealt with on an abstract and intellectual level to avoid the painful emotions engendered, and suppression, where the news is not permitted to be remembered at all and the patient continues with the ordinary activities of daily living.

Denial has been described as an effective coping mechanism for mediating the impact of dialysis-related stress. It is not limited to the period of diagnosis but may also be evident at other critical milestones in a renal career.[2] Denial is regarded as a form of avoidance coping. This contrasts with approach coping such as taking pills, going to the doctor, resting, changing the diet, etc. which is more highly valued and encouraged by care staff. However, for the patient there are many advantages in adopting an avoidance coping strategy:

◆ It allows time for information to be assimilated. Most patients have very little understanding of the nature, process, and consequences of renal failure.

◆ It is certainly easier to maintain the existing relationships and roles within the family.

◆ It minimizes the risk of pity and avoidance from friends and colleagues.

◆ It sustains the sense of self-worth and personal identity which are often lost in accepting the patient role.

◆ There may well be a reduction in symptom perception, a decrease in any negative emotions, and a shift in the perception of the illness. For example: 'This nauseous headache is not bad [denial] now I feel less anxious about completing the report [emotions], and the condition does not stop me from working [illness cognition]'.

◆ It takes little effort to maintain and is well-rehearsed (think of your customary response to the enquiry 'How are you?').

Denial may also be seen as a positive interpretation of an unpleasant reality. One of the strongest models of health behaviour posits that patients form a representation of their illness in order to manage it.[3] In the same way that people have beliefs about health, they also have beliefs about illness. Such beliefs are often called 'illness cognitions' or 'illness representations'. Individuals deal with their illness by processing information from a variety of sources. This information is not always processed rationally and the cognitions may be constructed from erroneous as well as valid material. This personal illness representation is idiosyncratic and may bear no relation to the medical view, so may be seen as a denial of the medical facts. Another model to assist in understanding the patient's behaviour at this time is the theory of cognitive adaptation.[4] This proposes that following a threatening event such as the diagnosis of renal failure, individuals are motivated to search for meaning, for mastery, and for increase in their self-esteem. It is suggested that these processes involve developing illusions and that these illusions are a necessary and essential component of cognitive adaptation and that reality orientation (as suggested by other coping models) may actually be detrimental to adjustment.

So denial may be a rejection of the medical description, rather than a negation of suffering from renal failure. It is part of the process for patients to assimilate a whole range of new information and behaviours. As there is as yet no standardized objectively validated instrument to measure defence mechanisms such as denial, and the hypotheses of its function are always proposed *post hoc*, it remains an often misinterpreted behaviour. It is more helpful for healthcare staff to name it 'minimizing the problems'. John's life was full of examples of this: his choice of sports—very challenging but solo; his pursuit of a high profile job that focused on giving people a good time; pushing himself to high achievements in his work; never discussing the renal issue with the family; managing the dietary and fluid restrictions himself etc.

During the **retreat phase** Shontz describes patients as denying either the existence of the health problem or its implications. This is such a negative view of one section of a continuous difficult process of adapting to and managing a terminal condition. He describes the phase as ending because reality intrudes, there is no spontaneous recovery; further meetings with health staff confirm the diagnosis, and the symptoms worsen. There is no sense that the patient has any control over the process. He assumes that the patient is merely reacting badly at first and then contacting reality a little at a time until there is full adjustment to the health problem and its implications. The patient is described as someone to whom things happen or are done—as in the old medical model of patient–doctor interaction. In this approach there is very little to encourage the healthcare worker to work in constructive cooperation with the patient.

Throughout the process of dealing with the diagnosis patients frequently use avoidance strategies to control their emotions, particularly when they can see no way of influencing the course of the condition. There has long been evidence to indicate that this helps the patients early in the process of coping with the condition.[5] It enables them to maintain their sense of self as a person rather than a condition, assists them to live a life outside renal failure, and this coping mechanism can be maintained until they die. However, if there is continuous total inability to attend to information and treatment advice, the strategy becomes maladaptive and prevents the development of more constructive approaches.

It should be remembered that patients move in and out of these phases for much of their treatment. It is a dangerous mistake for the healthcare worker to assume that a patient has reached the end of the process, 'come to terms' or 'is able to cope' with the condition. Dealing with symptoms, absorbing information, living through emotional responses, learning about personal coping strategies, adopting treatment advice, adapting family and social life to accommodate dialysis, forming relationships with health professionals, and all the other aspects of managing renal failure constitute a continuing process.

One constant feature of managing renal failure is the ever-changing nature of the demands on the patient, depending on the progress of the condition and medical fashion. The patient's ability to manage the treatment well will fluctuate over time for a number of reasons—some completely divorced from the renal failure. A holistic approach will facilitate appropriate support for the patient who is experiencing difficulties.

## 9.2 Co-morbid mental health issues

There are a number of major psychiatric disorders that can be present before renal failure becomes apparent, or which become evident during the course of dialysis treatment. Nephrologists frequently have to address the mental health requirements of this population as well as coordinate primary and other secondary care in addition to their specialist role. Certain disorders, such as substance abuse, are more common in ESRD, because alcoholic cirrhosis can lead to renal failure, and intravenous drug abuse may lead to AIDS, hepatitis C, or glomerulonephritis with renal failure as a complication. Dementia-like behaviour and delirium are also frequently encountered, both as uraemic encephalopathy and as sequelae of co-morbid diabetes and hypertension. By contrast, co-morbid affective and anxiety disorders are probably no more common than in the general or other chronically ill populations.

### 9.2.1 Depression

#### 9.2.1.1 Definition

Depression is considered to be the most common psychiatric complication of dialysis treatment. In general terms it is defined as a mood state characterized by a sense of inadequacy, a feeling of despondency, a decrease in activity or reactivity, pessimism, sadness, and related symptoms. These will differ with each individual but may include any or all of the following: anhedonia, sleep disturbances, lethargy, feelings of worthlessness, morbid thoughts, and possibly (though not necessarily) suicide attempts. As in the case of ESRD, it may be secondary to another disorder. Depression may take many forms and presentations depending on factors such as inherited susceptibility, precipitating circumstances, personal coping strategies, and co-morbid conditions such as anxiety.

### 9.2.1.2 Reported prevalence/incidence

Despite the observation that for many ESRD patients the various symptoms of depression become chronic, there is no certainty about the prevalence of this disorder in these patients. Examination of the ESRD literature suggests that subsyndromal depression is likely in about 25% of patients, and major depression in 5–22% of patients.[6] The reported incidence may be overestimated because symptoms of uraemic origin are so similar to those of depression. There are also problems with interpretation of the results from research studies because of the differences in the definitions and criteria used for depression.[7] The range of diagnostic instruments reported included clinical impression, self-reports, Beck Depression Inventory, the multiple affect adjective checklist, and the American Diagnostic and Statistical Manual III. Generalizations are also difficult because of differences in patient mix in terms of background, type of therapy, time in treatment, co-morbidity, gender, ethnicity, and age. Nevertheless, clinical depressions are widespread, and unfortunately they are often unrecognized and untreated by nephrologists.[8]

It may be possible to measure the prevalence (and severity) of depression by the extreme outcome of suicide although this has been minimally studied.[9] Despite the claims for a high incidence of suicide among patients, it is difficult to judge their accuracy. The many readily available avenues for parasuicidal behaviour, e.g. overdosing on potassium-rich foods and overt non-compliance with the medical regimens, are also possible outcomes of inadequacy, misunderstanding, and poor management ability. The proportion of patients whose withdrawal from dialysis represents suicide is unknown, with reports providing conflicting evidence. One recent and comprehensive study determined that low depressive indices predict survival at 1 year, and that higher levels of depressive affect are associated with increased mortality.[10] In the United States, this association has led to recent activity on the part of the National Institute of Health, and future research will likely recommend more vigorous detection and treatment. Other studies fail to confirm this apparent association and indicate that most patients who discontinued treatment were not impaired by clinical depression. For the patients who have become unable to make such treatment choices for themselves, e.g. those with advanced dementia, the burden of responsibility for treatment length often falls to the family and loved ones. They find themselves in the position of making a substantial number of decisions on behalf of the patient.[11] Even when the actual responsibility for terminating care rests legally with the consultant (as in the UK) those closest to the patient bear the psychological burden of such decisions.

### 9.2.1.3 Precipitating factors

The wide range in documented levels of depression suggests that it is likely to be influenced by a variety of aspects of the individual's social context such as job loss or death of a family member and not merely by the presence of ESRD itself. However, there are times of increased likelihood of a depressive episode linked directly to renal failure or its treatment. These include the first year of treatment, the period leading to the failure of a transplanted kidney, and non-selection having completed the work-up for a transplant. Early in their renal career patients are required to make decisions regarding their treatment modality that impact on their occupation, their familial role, their leisure activities, and their relationships. They are expected to assimilate information that is foreign as well as frightening. Being in receipt of this information in its many forms does not mean a full understanding of that information or its implications. Many patients take decisions for which they feel totally unprepared. They experience feelings of inadequacy and inferiority and are overwhelmed by the enormity of the situation. These feelings of helplessness and deep personal loss can easily develop further into a severe depressive episode. In periods when their transplanted kidney is failing, or following non-selection for transplant the strong feelings of rejection and worthlessness experienced can again lead to depression.

Depression, like denial, can be viewed as a coping strategy at a time when fundamental beliefs in self and health are being seriously challenged. It is a period of withdrawal from the usual activities of daily living and the relationships therein, to begin to appreciate the enormous change in life expectancy. Such existential challenges are rarely addressed by individuals in full health. Those with the diagnosis of ESRD need time to adjust their image of themselves and to assimilate the implications of organ failure. As this is at a time when their physical health and resources are severely compromised the process of adjustment from self-image as *healthy* to self as *sick and dying* can take some time.

### 9.2.1.4 Presentation

The presentation of an episode of depression will vary with each patient and even with the same patient over time. There is variation in length and fluctuating intensity of all episodes. Of those patients identified as experiencing depression, the majority require psychotherapeutic support. Other family members may also present with similar symptoms and influence the course of both psychotherapeutic and medical treatment.

### 9.2.1.5 Assessment

There are several instruments to measure depression in the general population which are helpful in the initial diagnosis and for assessing change over time. However, their suitability for use in ESRD is not secure, since the common somatic symptoms such as fatigue, anorexia, and changes in sleep and bowel patterns in depression mimic those found in a typical dialysis patient—falsely elevating the depression scores. For example, the complete Beck Depression Inventory (BDI)[12] that taps affective cognitive motivational and physiological symptoms of depression has considerable difficulty in discriminating depressed from non-depressed patients in renal failure, giving a very high rate of false positives. However, the section of the BDI measuring guilt, sadness, and difficulty in making decisions known as the Cognitive Depression Inventory (CDI) is less confounded by the effects of physical illness and may be more helpful as a screening tool prior to fuller diagnostic interviewing in the renal unit.

### 9.2.1.6 Treatment

Effective interventions will support the individual through the episode, helping them to maintain contact with reality and regain a sense of well-being despite the rigours of the treatment and the life changes enforced by the condition. Appropriate carefully monitored antidepressive medication may be effective, as may individual psychotherapy. The optimum approach for depression in the general public is that of concomitant psychological therapy and medication. The following information is a brief summary of current approaches to psychopharmacological treatment. A more detailed explication with tables is available elsewhere.[13]

Reviews of antidepressant management of ESRD have consistently found both selective serotonin re-uptake inhibitors (SSRIs) and tricyclic antidepressants (TCAs) to be beneficial.[13] Although the greatest body of experience is on the TCAs, these have largely been supplanted by the newer generation of antidepressants. Tricyclic antidepressants ought to be reserved for treatment-resistant depression, or where there are additional indications, such as painful peripheral neuropathy. The hydroxylated metabolites of TCAs contribute to both the therapeutic and toxic effects in ESRD. Imipramine and amitriptyline continue to be used for analgesia in neuropathic pain, while trazodone is commonly used in low doses as a sedative–hypnotic for insomnia.

SSRIs are often used in ESRD, but have not been systematically or adequately researched. Fluoxetine is the best-studied medication in this class, and appears to be both non-toxic and efficacious.[14] The kinetic profile of single doses of fluoxetine is unchanged even in anephric patients. A study of multiple doses concludes that renal function does not significantly alter either fluoxetine or norfluoxetine serum levels. Sertraline has not been as intensively studied in this population, but it is also widely prescribed. Like fluoxetine, it is metabolized hepatically and excretion of the unchanged drug in urine is an insignificant route of elimination. Pharmacokinetic investigations in people with mild to severe renal impairment and matched controls show no significant differences. Sertraline has been utilized to help prevent sudden haemodialysis-related hypotension.[15]

Like sertraline and fluoxetine, citalopram kinetics are minimally changed in patients with ESRD and dose adjustment is probably not necessary.[16] Interestingly, plasma concentrations of paroxetine hydrochloride are increased in people with renal impairment, and the recommended initial dose for patients with severe renal insufficiency (10 mg) is one-half that of normal adults.

There are several non-SSRI antidepressant medications that should be used with caution or avoided.[13] For example, little is known about the pharmacokinetics of nefazodone hydrochloride in patients who have chronically impaired renal function. Careful dose adjustment is also necessary with venlafaxine, which is chiefly eliminated in urine along with its metabolites.[17] Its elimination half-life is prolonged and clearance is reduced in people who have chronic renal insufficiency or ESRD. Regular monitoring of blood pressure is recommended for those taking this drug. Bupropion hydrochloride has active metabolites, which are almost completely excreted through the kidney; these metabolites may accumulate in dialysis patients and predispose to seizures.

Care must be taken with patients receiving concurrent drugs metabolized by cytochrome P-450 3A4 (e.g. tacrolimus, cyclosporin, sildenafil) when using antidepressants which are inhibitors of this isoenzyme. These inhibitors include nefazodone, fluoxetine/norfluoxetine, fluvoxamine, paroxetine (a weak inhibitor), sertraline, and valproic acid (a weak inhibitor). For many years, lithium has been the primary pharmacological treatment of bipolar affective disorder. It has efficacy in acute episodes and in prevention of relapses. It is being replaced by classic anticonvulsant medications, such as depakote, carbamazepine, and gabapentin, which also significantly help these patients. For the relatively few bipolar patients with ESRD who require lithium (and do not respond to the anticonvulsants), treatment involves administration of a single dose (usually 600 mg) after each dialysis run. Because it is a small molecule that is readily dialysed, lithium is eliminated by dialysis. A single dose will result in a steady serum level.[18] Serum lithium levels obtained before and after dialysis sessions are used to establish the therapeutic dose. Ideally, these levels should be obtained immediately before dialysis and 2 h after completion; the level obtained immediately after dialysis will often be lower than that observed later due to a post-dialysis redistribution effect. A smaller dose (300 mg) may be given to augment its therapeutic effect in treatment-resistant unipolar depression. Lithium can be nephrotoxic. Efforts should be made to substitute other drugs in patients with renal insufficiency. A long-term follow-up study has found that when the drug is discontinued, renal function will often improve.[19]

### 9.2.1.7 Treatment barriers

In dialysis facilities, major depression is often unrecognized and untreated.[20] It is unfortunately likely that renal care staff influence this lack of care provision for a number of reasons. The most obvious is their lack of training and experience in psychiatric care. A second factor is their reaction to a personal episode of lowered mood. This experience is common to most people, including healthcare staff. They can usually identify its antecedents and after a relatively short period of time in which their usual activities are restricted or modified, the symptoms disappear spontaneously. Because of these personal experiences the healthcare staff often fail to appreciate the difficulty renal patients experience in overcoming a more major episode of depression related to personal health and their very existence. Another important factor is that it is also difficult for some staff (medical and nursing) to acknowledge that their skill and interventions are insufficient to maintain the health and well-being of all their patients. They regard the failure of a patient to be happy in treatment as a critical reflection of their ability to care, and so to protect themselves they enter a process of denial, and fail to appreciate the severity of the mood disorder in any of their patients.

### 9.2.1.8 Conclusion

Periods of depression for patients with end-stage renal failure may have a role in the process of acceptance of the changes enforced by the condition and its treatment. Incidence and prevalence are difficult to gauge, since some symptoms of depression and renal failure have the same presentation. Within the course of treatment it is possible to identify periods of increased risk for depression. A combination of medication and psychological therapy offers the best chance of successful treatment. There may well be under-recognition of the condition by healthcare staff.

Recommended treatment for depression—a diagnostic approach that entails:

◆ describing the criteria for major depression.
◆ eliciting patients' opinion as to whether they believe themselves to be depressed.
◆ obtaining their cooperation in completing a formal assessment such as the CDI.
◆ documenting the existence of associated factors, such as depressive episodes prior to the onset of renal failure, a family history of depression, and past suicide attempts.
◆ combining medication and psychological therapy, monitored with phased withdrawal as the patient recovers.

## 9.2.2 Anxiety and stress

### 9.2.2.1 Definition

Anxiety is probably the most common and pervasive emotion of people who receive hospital treatment. Renal patients are concerned about the severity and variation in their symptoms, and the restrictions the condition imposes on their life and plans for their future. They worry about what the treatment will be like, the degree to which it will be successful, and their ability to manage its complexities. This concern will pervade all aspects of their life. John's reluctance to commit to a close relationship with anyone may well have been a manifestation of his chronic concerns about the condition and the demands he feared it would impose on a close friend or partner. Excessive anxiety, like depression, often goes unrecognized and requires treatment.

Stress is typically described in one of two ways. It can be viewed is a cause/trigger for a behavioural/emotional response—for example John may have felt that the requirement to manage the treatment for renal failure was one stress too many in his life. Alternatively it can be seen as the effect of one or more external factors that make adaptive demands on a person—for example John may have felt stressed by the need to manage his treatment. This stress response is made up of a relatively stereotypical set of psychological and biological patterns. In reality neither stressors nor the stress response exists in isolation—both feed on each other to produce the stress experience. This experience may be defined as the individual's perception that they have insufficient resources to respond adequately to the demands made on them and that this shortfall endangers their well-being.

The effects of chronic stress have been well documented but not well understood or integrated into physical medicine, being viewed separately as an aspect of mental health. This division results in the disregard of significant biological and psychological aspects of the renal patient's condition and their interaction with the treatment regimen. The mechanisms relating to the stress experience have been described by Selye[21] in the general adaptation syndrome (GAS) (Table 9.1). This syndrome evolves through three stages and for each stage posits behavioural and physiological responses. These physiological responses to stress may have a major impact on the renal treatment, and they should be taken into consideration when reviewing the prescribed drugs and dialysis treatment.

**Table 9.1** The general adaptation syndrome

| Stage | Behavioural response | Physiological response |
|---|---|---|
| 1. Alarm reaction | Increased sensitivity to changes in intensity of demands | Enlargement of adrenal cortex |
| | Increased susceptibility to illness | Enlargement of lymphatic system Increase in hormones such as epinephrine |
| | | High arousal |
| 2. Resistance | Increasing sensitivity to demands | Shrinkage of adrenal cortex |
| | Attempts to manage the demands | Lymph nodes return to normal |
| | Resistance to debilitating effects | High hormone levels maintained Parasympathetic branch of autonomic nervous system counteracts high arousal Eventual hormone depletion |
| 3. Exhaustion | Reduction of resistance to demands | Hormone levels maintained or further increased |
| | Onset of depression | Lymphatic structures becoming enlarged or dysfunctional or both |
| | Onset of physical illness that can become severe and even fatal | Adaptive hormones depleted |

### 9.2.2.2 Prevalence/incidence

For a couple of decades it has been acknowledged in research, for example that by Levy,[22] that generalized anxiety disorders are a prominent feature of ESRD with anxiety being more commonly manifested during treatment and during the earlier phase of training and home dialysis. It is likely that the majority of dialysis patients experience episodes of anxiety and stress at some stage in their treatment and that some patients will experience these conditions throughout their dialysis life. Some studies[23,24] report that about one-third of patients experience episodes of moderate anxiety in their first year of treatment, with up to 6% of patients at mild phobic levels. The mode of renal treatment seems to make little difference to the incidence of anxiety/stress experience.

### 9.2.2.3 Effects of anxiety and stress on end-stage renal failure

The effects of the physiological consequences of the stress experience on ESRD and its treatment are little understood. Treatment traditionally focuses on the renal system itself, and those patients who do not respond well to the regimen are frequently made to feel responsible for the problems they encounter. This increases their anxiety and enhances the stress experience, making an interaction between the two conditions more pronounced.

Some of the manifestations of anxiety/stress are shared with those of ESRD, for example fatigue and restlessness, making it more difficult to correctly identify their cause.

### 9.2.2.4 Precipitating factors

The major sources of anxiety or stress experience for the person in ESRD are similar to those that can provoke an episode of depression. They include the following:

◆ Consciousness of the life threat from kidney failure—the mortality rate is high and patients witness others dying. They become aware of the many possible physical complications as they meet more patients with ESRD during their own treatment.

◆ Impaired bodily and cognitive functioning—kidney failure is a urological, nephrological, and endocrinological disease and people on dialysis vary greatly in their sense of well-being. Fluctuating uraemia causes a severe reduction in physical energy, and constant feelings of illness, including nausea, dizziness, restlessness, sleep difficulties, itching, fatigue, and inability to concentrate. They are also made aware of the deterioration of their bones and nerves through regular routine monitoring.

◆ The experience of being a patient:

  ◆ The patient has to meet numerous new people with influence over different aspects of their care. Names, personalities, and interactions for each member of staff have to be learned and remembered.

  ◆ In ESRD, patients contribute little to their own management and exist in a state of helpless dependency that involves the loss of adult status and power. They find themselves in the stressful experience of being required to be compliant and dependent on the medical processes while actively pursuing a normal lifestyle.

  ◆ The exigencies of the dialysis regimen: adherence to diet, fluid restrictions, and attendance at time-consuming treatments.

  ◆ Interpersonal confusion resulting from high staff turnover and inconsistencies in self-care tuition causes stress.

- The dialysis/hospital setting. Because it is their workplace, populated with known colleagues and friends, the members of staff often fail to appreciate the stress experience of the patient who is separated from his/her known security-giving places, people, and roles at a time when extreme pressures have to be managed. This can lead to a form of separation anxiety further reducing the ability to cope.

- Many anxieties stem from a lack of information. Often the paucity of information stems from the care professionals' desire to protect the patient from unpleasant facts. However, this factual confusion may reinforce patients' beliefs that they cannot control the situation, increase their dependency on staff, and interfere with successful treatment.

- Secondary consequences such as loss of employment, financial stringencies, and restrictions on travel and leisure may reduce coping resources and give rise to stress. Descriptive studies such as those by De Nour[25] showed a severe decrease in interest in social life and in participation in leisure activities, with half the participants reporting no social life at all. The dialysis patient experiences the stress associated with a marginal person who has lost full integration into society.

- Any change involves some degree of stress experience. For the renal patient they are legion and include changes in relationships, quality of life, employment, management, and the acquisition of a new language and new skills.

- Adult illness or disability is also a source of stress for the whole family. The inevitable strain on financial resources restricts the family's time and personal freedom and produces very important changes in interpersonal relationships. The roles of family members have to change, often with the spouse and older children adopting the responsibilities previously undertaken by the sick person. The spouse generally experiences stress from fears that the condition will be life-threatening and also from the patient's increased irritability and dependency. Although spouses tend to show increased affection for one another their sexual relations are usually curtailed.

- We cannot ignore the stress experience of the members of staff in regular contact with patients on dialysis. As a routine part of their daily work they are exposed to intrateam tensions, patient deaths, slow deterioration in the health of many patients, time pressures, and the need to respond sensitively to patients about their insurmountable problems and concerns. It has long been recognized that staff–patient interaction is a source of stress for staff. A further study by De Nour[26] showed that high levels of skill and devotion on the part of staff led them to hold high expectations of their patients in terms of compliance with fluids and dietary restrictions, effort at rehabilitation, positive outlook and mood, punctuality, etc. However, the disability induced by uraemia together with the high prevalence of psychopathology caused the staff expectations to be frustrated. This raised tension in staff and provoked a counter-aggression that in turn was seen as provoking psychodynamic defences in the staff—denial, displacement, withdrawal, etc.

## 9.2.2.5 Presentation

Some patients with ESRD will present with a pre-existing high level of anxiety or stress experience. This is likely to be exacerbated by the need for renal treatment. The aetiology of any pre-morbid condition needs to be investigated, but it is unrealistic to suppose that such anxiety/stress can be easily resolved. Patients with previous or current psychiatric illness and prominent anxiety reactions to treatment will be at risk of dropping out of treatment.

It has long been known that a majority of haemodialysis patients will present with shallowness of affect, concrete thinking, little flexibility in response to stress, and a coping style marked by a high degree of passive behaviour and little inclination to deal actively with any problem situations.

The patients at highest risk of developing acute anxiety or stress experience relating to ESRD treatment are those with a high incidence of existing emotional problems in the absence of a confiding relationship. Some patients develop such high levels of anxiety about components of the treatment, such as needling for haemodialysis, that they are unable to continue dialysis without psychological/psychiatric intervention. Their presentation is often referred to as phobic, though they rarely develop behaviours associated with a diagnosis of phobia. Other patients exhibit lower levels of chronic anxiety that result in concurrent symptoms such as tension headaches and nausea.

The effects of the stress experience are mediated by a number of factors including pre-morbid adjustment, length of time on dialysis, and the patient's characteristic style of stress management or psychological defence. Adaptability to previous life changes is significantly related to positive dialysis adjustment, and such adjustment improves for most patients as time progresses.

### 9.2.2.6 Assessment of anxiety

Unfortunately the symptoms considered to indicate pathological levels of anxiety and stress experience are also those commonly found as consequences of ESRD, so reliably accurate assessment is not readily available. The State Trait Anxiety Inventory (STAI)[27] is a widely used measure of state (i.e. situation specific) and trait (i.e. enduring personality style) anxiety with good evidence for its reliability and validity in both general population and chronic illness patient groups. It is a 40-item measure that is simple to administer in about 10 min and score. However, further studies on its clinical usefulness in the renal failure setting are needed, including evaluations of the potential confounding effects of the physical impact of renal failure and its treatment on the STAI scores. Asking the patient if they consider themselves to be experiencing unmanageable levels of anxiety or stress experience is probably the most effective and reliable assessment available to care staff.

### 9.2.2.7 Treatment

There is a significant shortage of literature relating to the psychological treatment of patients with ESRD, with many of the reported studies being descriptive in nature. This reflects the general lack of psychological care in renal units and the statistically insignificant numbers that have been recorded in individual studies. Scanning the literature over the last 30 years, it is apparent that the myriad of stressors impinging on the dialysis patient makes it difficult to advocate a specific treatment for successful adjustment. Each patient will need an accurate and perhaps lengthy assessment and intervention programme. It is also unrealistic to expect patients to be entirely free of anxiety/stress response given their medical/social situation. Optimum interventions should aim to rationalize their experiences and find ways of managing them in keeping with the patient's current lifestyle.

Generally effective treatment interventions include provision of training at pre-dialysis clinics, facilitated interaction with other patients, and the inclusion of a partner/significant other in training and/or treatment sessions.

Pharmacological management is either directed at acute episodes of anxiety and panic, or at more generalized nervousness.[13] Since benzodiazepines are metabolized in the liver, dosage reduction is generally not necessary in ESRD. Exceptions include midazolam and chlordiazepoxide. It is not unusual to give ordinary doses of diazepam, ativan, alprazolam, and clonazepam before or during dialysis sessions. SSRIs are being used increasingly to treat panic and generalized anxiety disorders.

Traditional insight-oriented interpretative psychotherapy groups have been shown to be unsuccessful. Reasons suggested include patients failing to identify with their illness and finding insight into their reactions too threatening. So group patient education and self-help groups that depend on patient observations, education, and cognitive learning are advocated.[28]

Behavioural and cognitive therapies have been used with varying degrees of success to address anxiety/stress reactions related to dialysis treatment and the responsibilities involved in its maintenance. Progressive and deep muscle relaxation and biofeedback techniques have been used to control panic attacks, generalized anxiety, and tension headaches in individuals. For biofeedback to be successful the patient first develops an awareness of the maladaptive nature of the stress/anxiety response and that it can be influenced by his/her thoughts and bodily events. Using visual and auditory biofeedback signals in a protected therapeutic environment, they can begin to control the anxiety/stress response. They can then learn to transfer this control to everyday situations that previously provoked the maladaptive response. Systematic desensitization, fading of stimulus control and social reinforcement, relaxation training, aversive conditioning, contingency management, and goal setting have been shown to be helpful in limited numbers of patients with phobias and unwanted behaviours such as vomiting. Aerobic exercise training, mental imagery, and social support enrichment are also thought to be useful techniques for managing the anxiety/stress experience.

## 9.2.2.8 Treatment barriers

There are many impediments to the delivery of psychological treatment for the anxiety/stress experience, including the resistance of staff and patients and the treatment setting itself:

◆ Significant numbers of staff are unwilling and/or untrained to identify conditions requiring specialist psychological care for their patients. For some this referral represents a failure on their part to adequately care for the patient with whom they have developed a meaningful relationship. Others may view the patient's needs as a rejection of their care and develop defensive mechanisms that prevent them from referring to others.

◆ Many dialysis patients bristle at the suggestion that they should receive psychological/ psychiatric help. Typically they do not interpret their behaviour as indicative of psychological disability and resent the inference that it is 'all in their mind'. They think of themselves as being understandably distressed, anxious, and disturbed and baulk at the psychiatric label.

◆ The practical and psychological adaptations that dialysis necessitates leave many patients with a feeling of resentment and displacement towards a psychologist or hostility towards the nephrologist or dialysis nurse. A referral for this type of care isolates the patient from the dialysis peer group and can increase the stress experience.

◆ Many patients are afraid to express even minimally negative feelings towards someone on whom they feel dependent and whose affections they are frightened of alienating.

◆ The patient may resist open discussion with the psychologist if they are seen as acting in a liaison capacity to help nursing and medical staff understand individual reactions more clearly.

◆ Agreeing with the staff diagnosis of psychological difficulties may lead to questions about their stability/suitability for desired alternative treatments (transplantation, ambulatory peritoneal dialysis (APD)).

- A general atmosphere of no 'permission' or false bonhomie in the unit may intimidate patients so they cannot be overtly anxious/stressed or express strong feelings.
- Learning disability caused by the condition—chronic fatigue, confusion, muzzy head.
- Language—both in terms of new concepts and words and also the fact that for increasing numbers of patients English is not their first language.

### 9.2.2.9 Conclusion

An overwhelming majority of patients will experience episodes of anxiety/stress relating to their treatment or its effects on their lifestyle and relationships. It is not possible to accurately predict the onset of such episodes, although during the first year of treatment there is a high reported incidence. Incidence and prevalence are difficult to gauge. Some manifestations of anxiety/stress experience and renal failure have the same presentation. The therapeutic environment in the renal care setting should tolerate and support patients in an open fashion without being judgmental. There are many barriers to therapeutic interventions.

Recommended treatment for anxiety/stress experience—a diagnostic approach that entails:

- describing the anxiety/stress in terms of its debilitating effect on the patient.
- eliciting patients' opinion as to whether they believe themselves to be so stressed or anxious that their life is disrupted.
- obtaining their cooperation in referring to a specialist for a formal assessment.
- documenting the existence of associated factors, such as pre-morbid management experiences and strategies.
- combining medication and psychological therapy, monitored with planned withdrawal as recovery progresses.

## 9.2.3 Other presentations

### 9.2.3.1 Steroid psychosis

This occurs infrequently as a reaction to high levels of steroids, for example following transplantation. It is corrected by adjusting the dose of steroids. A steroid-induced psychotic episode can cause the patient to lose contact with reality and require intervention for both the individual and the family concerned and also support for the staff who are not psychiatrically trained. It is important to give patients information about possible negative outcomes of interventions so they have the opportunity to monitor their reactions and report any adverse outcomes.

### 9.2.3.2 Lack/loss of motivation

This is noted frequently in patients at all stages of their treatment. It can indicate a number of possible psychological problems including anxiety, depression, stress experience, and cognitive decline. It can also indicate a rational wish to discontinue treatment. Careful assessment is required before any intervention.

### 9.2.3.3 Lowered self-image

Unintentional depersonalization by medical/nursing staff is frequent in the treatment of patients with ESRD. The focus of care is on alleviating the symptoms of the condition and often this takes obvious precedence over the person being treated—for example the blood measures of dialysis efficiency are more important than the reported well-being of the patient.

### 9.2.3.4 Lowered efficacy levels

Two types of efficacy beliefs are important in renal care:

- **Outcome efficacy** relates to beliefs about the likely positive outcome of following a regimen or taking medication, e.g. John may have believed that the proposed second episode of haemodialysis treatment would not be successful in sustaining the quality of life he desired.

- **Self-efficacy** relates to the patient's beliefs about their ability to sustain the treatment regimen in its entirety. For example, John may have believed that he would not be successful in managing the diet/fluid restrictions for a second period knowing the difficulties and deprivations he had suffered during his first treatment period on haemodialysis. Efficacy and control beliefs are strongly influenced by the individual's past experience of success or failure in specific health-related domains.

### 9.2.3.5 Personality disorders

This is most frequently a misdiagnosis of behaviours more correctly attributed to fear, anxiety, and inability to manage the treatment regimen as prescribed by the care staff. The strong desire to conform and not disrupt the healthcare system or upset the staff means that the patient may attempt to instigate changes in a defensive manner with a certain amount of ineptitude and irritation. This can be easily but incorrectly interpreted in terms of a personality disorder, and the issues raised may be dismissed as unimportant. This overestimation of the role of personality and underestimation of the situational factors is an example of a fundamental attribution error on the part of the staff. Personality disorders are likely to be well-documented by the mental health services before the patient is referred for care by renal staff. Good communication and liaison with mental health colleagues is essential for patient, family, and staff.

## 9.2.4 Cognitive ability

Research over the last 30 years relating to the effects of uraemia on the central nervous system has shown deficits in concentration, alertness, flexibility in thinking, and decreased speed of mental manipulation as assessed by the Weschler Adult Intelligence Scale.[29] Patients with chronic kidney disease frequently manifest neurological symptoms even when they are considered to be adequately dialysed. For patients over 65 years who are maintained with dialysis, organic brain syndromes are a leading cause of hospitalization. As renal function worsens, it is increasingly likely that subtle or overt neurological symptoms will occur. Aetiological factors include medication side-effects that are worsened by diminished renal drug clearance, effects of the uraemic milieu, dialysis and transplantation treatment effects, other co-morbid conditions, and electrolyte disturbances.

Memory was also shown to be impaired in patients with high serum creatinine levels, although the research on memory has been criticised for its lack of solid theoretical framework.[30] Improvements on all cognitive measures were noted following the onset of maintenance dialysis and further improvement was found following successful kidney transplantation. However, dialysis itself has been implicated as a causal factor in the dementia-like memory deficits observed in some patients.

Dialysis dementia, or dialysis encephalopathy, is a distinct, progressive, neurological disorder whose aetiology remains controversial. It has been divided into three categories including an epidemic form that is often associated with aluminium, sporadic cases in which aluminium is not a factor, and a type that is associated with congenital or early-childhood renal disease.

Dialysis dementia caused by aluminium toxicity can be treated with deferoxamine, large-surface-area dialysers, or charcoal haemoperfusion.

The wide use of recombinant human erythropoietin has improved many of the negative cognitive consequences previously associated with chronic anaemia, but patients with chronic mild or fluctuating anaemia still report impaired cognitive function.

Maintaining the level of cognitive function enjoyed prior to renal failure is important for all aspects of the patient's sense of self-esteem, confidence, efficacy, and identity. It is also a prerequisite for successful adaptation to dialysis. Referral to a professional qualified to administer and interpret specialized cognitive assessments is essential if either the patient or others notice changes in cognitive functioning.

## 9.3 Psychosocial issues

### 9.3.1 Ageing and mortality

Most of us can avoid examining the ageing process and the increasing closeness of our own death. Unlike most people, the patient with ESRD is forced to confront his or her own mortality every time treatment is required. There is a constant reminder of the dependency on manufactured mechanical aids in order to stay alive. The awareness of relentless increasing frailty is heightened by constant physiological checks. Feelings of hopelessness leading to depression can ensue, or periods of chronic anxiety in response to the sense of helplessness, or a mixture of both. It is difficult for staff to perceive the seriousness or enormity of this lived experience.

### 9.3.2 Communication

This is a major factor in any condition requiring medical treatment. Accurate and open communication between care professionals is essential, but is often minimal and influenced by political and personal factors. The relationship between care professional and patient is unequal and often confuses the communication between them. Interpersonal communication between staff and patients and staff and staff is a significant determinant of harmony and morale in a unit. For instance inadequate information exchange by consultants to patients will result in patients turning to the nurses for the information. Having no brief to give information on medical issues, the nurses feel powerless to respond appropriately although they do say something to reduce the patient's distress. They can then be overtly or covertly resentful towards the medical staff who can respond by reducing the time spent discussing patients and inadvertently exacerbating the communication problem.

Communication between the patient and his or her family and friends is also affected by ESRD. The familial and friendship roles alter, requiring adjustment from everyone concerned at a time when the patient's abilities are compromised by the condition and its treatment. It is also impossible for most patients to find words to express the emotions and thoughts they now have regarding themselves and their relationships. An isolating silence develops.

### 9.3.3 Sexuality

Despite claims that the majority of patients on dialysis experience diminished frequency of or interest in sex, and the number of references to it in the renal literature suggesting that this is a major concern for most patients, the issue of sexual activity is not widely discussed between patients and care staff. Reports focus on the physiological and mechanical aspects since these are more readily observed and measured, and for this reason more has been written about the male performance than the female. Levy, for example, has observed that approximately 70% of men have partial or total impotence, and the majority of women are amenorrhoeic or infertile.[22] He has also reported that even a successful kidney transplant does not always restore a patient's sexual function to that experienced before renal failure.

The subject of sexual performance is complex with cultural, age, gender, racial, religious, and emotional factors to consider before including the impact of any physical disability. Sexual activity has traditionally been performed in private with little or no instruction. Individuals with ESRD do not know if their pre-morbid sexual activity is normal, abnormal, excessive, or infrequent when compared with their peers. Unfortunately the most accessible instruction people can receive is the increasingly detailed portrayal of sexual foreplay and intercourse on the television and in cinemas. However, this gives at best an idealistic representation of the physical act and often leaves people feeling inadequate, deprived, and disappointed when they contrast their own experiences with this celluloid fantasy. Because the norms for sexual behaviour are not openly stated there is a tendency for people to believe that they are underperforming or unacceptably abnormal in their sexual activity. They are reluctant to share details of the activity with others for fear of censure. Discussions about sex are frequently protected with the use of humour and exaggeration, and there is little opportunity to be open about difficulties.

There are many assumptions and prejudices relating to sexual relationships. The following examples are common but not exhaustive:

- Usually there are two people involved in the activity, but any partnership is more than just the sum of two people. Each person will have a complex pattern of beliefs, expectations, emotional responses, and abilities. Their interaction in an intimate relationship results in a complex multifactorial experience regarded in most societies as important for the maintenance of good quality of life and self-esteem. However, there are partnerships of more than two people. In these cases the complexity of interacting factors will increase exponentially and there may be elements of defensiveness in the presentation. Sometimes there is only one person and the difficulties relate to their ability to achieve sexual satisfaction from self-masturbation. Self-pleasuring is not a subject easily discussed since for a majority of people the experience is linked with shame and embarrassment.

- Usually the participants will be of opposite genders. However, it is now becoming increasingly possible that the relationship will be between people of the same gender. In addition to the complexities involved in heterosexual relationships the individuals may have received adverse pressures associated with perceived societal deviance and perhaps traumatic sexual experiences.

- Usually both participants will be consenting adults. The concept of consent is generally assumed in a marriage. However, instances of enforced sexual intercourse within a marriage are not uncommon. In ESRD, for instance, the patient may agree to continuing sexual intercourse to prevent marital discord or from a sense of guilt because they perceive themselves as burdensome to their partner. Honest disclosure of emotions and sexual desires may be too stressful for a patient already burdened with managing the condition and treatment.

- Usually the person is in an enduring supportive relationship. This is an easy assumption to make if the couple have been married for a number of years, but even here the concept of support needs to be explored and confirmed. Many relationships are not sufficiently robust to survive major changes such as management of a terminal condition. There will be many people without a supportive partner, either because they are living alone or because they live in a household where they are feeling increasingly unsupported and isolated. Those without partners who have either never formed an intimate relationship or have experienced the pain and destruction of divorce, may be more concerned about attracting life-partners or about having brief relationships with a number of others.

These and many other assumptions and prejudices about the sexual behaviour of others make it likely that any advice/counselling by unqualified staff will be detrimental rather than helpful. Beliefs and behaviours relating to sexuality and intercourse are not generally well discussed by sexual partners prior to the diagnosis of ESRD. It is likely that their sexual congress has become less satisfying in the time leading up to the diagnosis because of the effects of increasing ill-health. The change may be erroneously attributed to deterioration in the intimacy of the relationship. After the diagnosis the importance of their sexual relationship is overshadowed by concerns relating to the condition, treatment, and lifestyle expectancy. It is only when at least some of these have been resolved and the solutions to the practical problems are in place that the individuals can begin to reconsider the physical and emotional aspects of their relationship.

There are gender-related factors in response to the diagnosis of ESRD. Masculinity and penis function are very closely linked. The ability to create and maintain a hard erect penis is essential to the male self-image. When a man's erectile potency is compromised or destroyed by illness, there is a corresponding effect on his self-confidence and self-efficacy. This outcome is usually subliminal and becomes apparent only through changes in behaviour. He may become withdrawn, unwilling to pursue previously enjoyed activities such as sports, socializing, DIY, and sexual intercourse. These manifestations are so similar to those occurring as a direct result of the symptoms associated with ESRD that it is very difficult to identify the root cause. Fear of failing to achieve penetration and ejaculation will further inhibit performance. One episode of failure will raise anxieties about the reliability of future performances and discourage the man from engaging in any form of intimacy. Such concerns may explain John's determined bachelorhood, as he was not a person to tolerate failure.

Femininity and looks are linked with sexual desirability in Western societies. A youthful female shape and facial appearance, clear skin, and slim silhouette are valued highly. Significant loss of hair, nail discoloration, and changes in skin colour and body shape have a great impact on the woman's sense of femininity and feelings of being sexually attractive. It becomes increasingly difficult for her to maintain the desirable image defined by Western media. She too may become withdrawn and unwilling to expose herself to critical appraisal by her peers. The menstrual cycle, thought by some to be integral to womanhood, is disrupted or even destroyed by the condition. For some women the knowledge that they may never be able to conceive and bear a child reduces sexual intercourse to a physical act devoid of meaning and emotion. The abnormal endocrine function that causes menstrual and fertility changes and swings in hormonal balance are documented elsewhere in this book, but the psychological meaning of these changes to individual women is not well researched.

Both men and women in the end stages of renal disease have body scarring and other major changes in appearance such as unsightly blood vessels and/or a plastic catheter emerging from their distended abdomen to remind them of their disability and lack of control over the condition. Many patients feel they are no longer sexually attractive people because of these disfiguring treatments and their dependency on machines, medication, and the close supervision of others. There is a growing disparity between their pre-morbid and current self-image. Because perceptions of sexual desire and sexual satisfaction originate in the brain, positive self-attribution is an important factor in the enjoyment of sexual intercourse. Levels of libido drop as the beliefs in self as self-determining, viable, influential, attractive, sensual, and valuable diminish.

Further items associated with the condition such as boxes of dialysate, APD machine, and bottles of tablets are frequently located or stored in the bedroom, the traditional venue for intimacy. They are reminders of the inadequacy, impending mortality, and reliance on others. For some this inhibits the desire for any sexual congress. Even the help from care staff can be a deterrent since it emphasizes their dependence, effectively destroys spontaneity, and can encourage performance ratings.

The relationship between depressed mood and loss of libido has long been recognized, but anxiety, low self-esteem, and preoccupation with illness may also affect the capacity to function sexually. While generalized anxiety associated with all aspects of life-threatening conditions will reduce levels of libido, the more specific concerns relating to damaging or dislodging the fistula, shunt, or catheter inhibits close physical contact and makes intercourse difficult. Feeling sick, somnolent, or confused is inconsistent with feeling sexual. Since the effects of anaemia can include malaise, weakness, nausea, dizziness, confusion, disorientation, and depression, low libido levels should be expected in patients suffering from this condition. Neuronal changes can lead to sensory and motor changes, particularly in the lower extremities, leading to concerns about performance reliability and diminishing sensory excitement.

The importance of the marital relationship in supporting the patient through the difficulties associated with the treatment and in managing the changes to their family and social life is assumed by most care staff and supported by anecdotal evidence in most renal units. Less emphasis is placed on the quality of the intimate relationship between patient and spouse. The shift in family role enforced by the condition may impact disastrously on the desire for sex. Although the focus is generally on patient-related factors, the partner's beliefs and emotions should not be overlooked. It is quite possible that regarding the partner as sick and in need of care precludes any feelings of arousal or desire for intimacy. The status of the partnership has to be reviewed and roles changed to suit the new circumstances. Many patients are abandoned or divorced because their partner could not adjust to the role changes required. The newly-single patient has even more skills to learn at a time when psychological resources are low. Any new relationship starts with the unequal carer–patient roles. The advice in a 1979 publication that a ' relaxed, undemanding, un-expectant, tender, warm, affectionate, considerate and intimate manner on the part of the partner works wonders with almost all patients'[22] sounds very simplistic and patient-centred compared with the more holistic approach espoused today. There was not much change 10 years later when the patient was advised to 'substitute social contacts [and] affectionate close personal relationship' for sexual intercourse, and to 'seek alternate activities that sustain the partnership aspects of the relationship'.[28]

Adverse changes are also caused by some of the medication necessary to control the condition and prolong life. Some medications have masculinizing effects, and oral antihypertensive medication is prone to affect sexual function because of its interaction with one or more of the systems involved in sexual activity and performance. Consequences include loss of or decrease in libido, menstrual irregularities, decrease in vaginal lubrication, breast enlargement/tenderness, and various orgasmic difficulties.[31] These aspects are addressed fully in Chapter 10.

This brief overview of the psychological effects of ESRD on the sexuality and intimate relationships of patients cannot conclude without a mention of difficulties encountered by renal care staff. They are not usually trained sexual counsellors. They need to overcome their own embarrassment, acknowledge their own sexuality, prejudices, and beliefs about normal sex, and examine their current and past sexual relationships—not a requirement of renal nursing, but essential for managing their own emotional responses when assessing and counselling renal patients. They may be asked for advice on sexual positions and how to achieve satisfying penetration or orgasm—situations much more intimate and challenging than discussing blood results. Many staff manage this difficulty by adopting a group teaching approach—they offer sexuality as part of their training in dialysis management techniques, usually as a lecture (with handouts, not illustrated) to a number of patients at a similar stage of the disease. However, patients are much more likely to talk about intimate difficulties when they are semi-dressed in the relative privacy of an examination room and when the focus of their difficulties is exposed. Staff need to be aware and prepared to deal with questions as they arise. Staff need knowledge of how ESRD can affect sexual performance, familiarity with all forms of coital and non-coital expressions of physical love, a non-judgemental attitude, genuine sensitivity and warmth for others, and awareness of their own sexuality. Although care staff are not sex therapists they need to be able to broach the subject and identify and deal appropriately with the problem. They must be able to say 'penis' and 'orgasm' in words that the patient will be comfortable with and understand the complexities of the multifactorial intimate relationship. As if this wasn't difficult enough, they should also be aware of the intrusive nature of their attempts to support the renal patient, even with the best of intentions and sensitive approaches. Few non-renal patients have their intimate relationships exposed in the same way. The simplest information and advice can be interpreted as offensive or even salacious. Identifying the salient factors contributing to sexual difficulties and designing effective interventions requires specialist training. Staff will need to acknowledge the limitations of their expertise in this aspect of care, learn when to refer the patient for more specialist interventions, and when to seek support/supervision for the support they are already offering.

### 9.3.4 Family and social relationships

The practical demands of renal failure can tax the most stable families and cause marital rifts. There are severe disruptions to work and social life. The patient tends to become the focus of family attention, and the resulting imbalance of the status quo can prove ultimately destructive of the family unit. The chronically ill may have a greater than average need for various forms of social support. For example, a person who is no longer able to meet certain responsibilities within the home may need more help from caregivers and housekeepers. Although the chronically ill may experience needs for many kinds of social support they may encounter difficulties obtaining adequate support. Chronic illnesses may produce feelings of alienation and estrangement from family members and friends. Frequently, misconceptions about the infectious nature of a condition can reduce the amount of available support.

## 9.4 Managing the condition

End-stage renal failure presents the patient with a shifting set of symptoms and treatments. It is difficult to gain a sense of mastery/control over such a fickle condition. At one hospital appointment the advice may be to severely restrict protein intake with no recommendations regarding fluid levels, and at the next the patient may be told that the fluid intake must be reduced and there is no longer any need to restrict the protein. All this at a time when the patient feels tired and possibly not able to meet the challenge of the condition or its treatment.

Finally … The effort and psychological stamina required to be a 'good' patient are considerable and little understood. The importance of a working partnership between care staff and patient is acknowledged but not always practised. There is an assumption that if patients have the details of their condition and the treatment required they will be able to conform to the medical model of care espoused by most renal teams. Their failure to match this expectation at all times creates difficulties in addition to those they already experience because of the condition. Greater tolerance and flexibility in the treatment may follow from increased understanding of the psychological and psychiatric factors in advanced renal disease. Once members of staff are given the encouragement and opportunity to become more familiar with the psychological and psychiatric considerations in this challenging condition, there is every hope that their partnership with the patient can become more effective and rewarding. It is not possible to be truly effective without such understanding.

## Ethical analysis

The case of John is a tragic one. It raises the ethical question, 'What is the responsibility of the nephrologist and renal team for identifying dialysis patients who are depressed?' At first glance, it would appear that the renal team should have minimal responsibility because mental health issues are outside the scope of practice of nephrologists. Yet the nephrologist and the dialysis staff see dialysis patients more often than any other healthcare provider. If anyone has the opportunity to detect depression in a dialysis patient, surely it should be the dialysis staff. Because of frequent contact with dialysis nurses, technicians, and social workers, it is hard for patients to hide their true feelings for long. What is ethically required of dialysis staff is sensitivity to the increased frequency of a major depressive disorder in dialysis patients and training on how to detect it. As dialysis units become increasingly familiar with providing palliative care, screening of patients for depression should become a standard part of orientation for new patient-care employees and a regular topic in in-service continuing education. Timely referral and intervention can make a difference in the care of depressed dialysis patients.

## References

1. Shontz, F. (1975). *The Psychological Aspects of Physical Illness and Disability*. New York: Macmillan.
2. Devins, G.M., Binik, Y.M., Mandin, H., *et al.* (1986). Denial as a defence against depression in end-stage renal disease: an empirical test. *Int. J. Psychiat. Med.*, **16**(2): 151–63.
3. Leventhal, H., Nerenz, D. (1985). The assessment of illness cognition. In: *Measurement Strategies in Health Psychology*, ed., P Karoly, pp. 517–55. New York.:Wiley.
4. Taylor, S.E. (1983). Adjustment to threatening events: a theory of cognitive adaptation. *Am. Psychol.*, **38**: 1161–73.
5. Suls, J., Fletcher, B. (1985). The relative efficacy of avoidant and non-avoidant coping strategies: a meta-analysis. Health Psychol., **4**: 249–88.
6. O'Donnell, K., Chung, Y. (1997). The diagnosis of major depression in end-stage renal disease. *Psychother Psychosom.*, **66**: 38–43.
7. Levenson, J.L., Glocheski, S. (1991). Psychological factors affecting end-stage renal disease: a review. *Psychosomatics*, **32**: 382–9.
8. Finkelstein, F.O., Finkelstein, S.H. (2000). Depression in chronic dialysis patients: assessment and treatment. *Nephrol. Dial. Transpl.*, **15**: 191–2.
9. Cohen, L.M., Steinberg, M.D., Hails, K.C., *et al.* (2000). The psychiatric evaluation of death-hastening requests: lessons from dialysis discontinuation. *Psychosomatics*, **41**: 195–203.

10. Kimmel, P.L. (2002). Depression in patients with chronic renal disease: what we know and what we need to know. *J. Psychosom. Res.*, **53**: 951–6.

11. Cohen, L.M., Germain, M.J., Poppel, D.M. (2003). Practical considerations in dialysis withdrawal: 'To have the option is a blessing.' *J. Am. Med. Assoc.*, **289**: 2113–19.

12. Beck, A.T. (1987). *Beck Depression Inventory*. San Antonio, TX: The Psychological Corporation.

13. Cohen, L.M., Germain, M.J., Tessier, E.G. (2003). Neuropsychiatric complications and psychopharmacology of end-stage renal disease. In: *Therapy of Nephrology and Hypertension: A Companion to Brenner's The Kidney*, 2nd edn, ed. HR Brady, CS Wilcox, pp. 731–46. Philadelphia, PA: Elsevier Science.

14 Blumenfield, M., Levy, N.B., Spinowitz, B., *et al.* (1997). Fluoxetine in depressed patients on dialysis. *Int. J. Psychiat. Med.*, **27**: 71–80.

15. Dheenan, S., Venketesan, J., Grubb, B.P., *et al.* (1998). Effect of sertraline hydrochloride on dialysis hypotension. *Am. J. Kidney Dis.*, **31**: 624–30.

16. Joffe, P., Larsen, F.S., Pedersen, V., *et al.* (1998). Single-dose pharmacokinetics of citalopram in patients with moderate renal insufficiency or hepatic cirrhosis compared with health subjects. *Eur. J. Clin. Pharmacol.*, **54**: 237–42.

17. Troy, S.M., Schultz, R.W., Parker, V.D., *et al.* (1994). The effect of renal disease on the disposition of venlafaxine. *Clin. Pharmacol. Ther.*, **56**: 14–21.

18. Port, F.K., Kroll, P.D., Rosenzweig, J. (1979). Lithium therapy during maintenance hemodialysis. *Psychosomatics* **20**: 130–2.

19. Braden, G.L. (2001). Lithium-induced renal disease. In: *Primer on Kidney Disease*, 3rd edn, ed. A. Greenberg, pp. 322–4. San Diego, CA: Academic Press.

20. Chen, Y.S., Wu, S.C., Wang, S.Y., *et al.* (2003). Depression in chronic haemodialysed patients. *Nephrology*, **8**(3): 121–6.

21. Seyle, H. (1980). The stress concept today. In: *Handbook on Stress and Anxiety*, ed. I.L. Kutaxxh, L.B. Schlesinger, *et al.*, pp. 127–9. San Francisco, CA: Jossey-Bass.

22. Levy, N.B. (1985). Psychological problems of patients on dialysis. In: *Proceedings of the European Dialysis and Transplant Nurses Association–European Renal Care Association*, Vol. 14, ed. E. Stevens, P. Monkhouse, pp. 177–84. London: Baillière Tindall.

23. Nichols, K.A., Springford, B. (1984). The psycho-social stressors associated with survival in dialysis. *Behav. Res. Ther.*, **22**(5): 563–74.

24. De Nour, A.K. (1981). Prediction of adjustment to haemodialysis. In: *Psychonephrology 1*, ed. N.B. Levy, pp. 117–33. New York: Plenum Press.

25. De Nour, A.K. (1982). Psychosocial adjustment to illness scale (PAIS): a study of chronic dialysis patients. *J. Psychosom. Res.*, **26**: 11–22.

26 De Nour, A.K. (1983). Staff–patient interaction. In: *Psychonephrology 2*, ed. N.B. Levy, pp. 113–116. New York: Plenum.

27. Spielberver, C.D., Gorsuch, R.I., Lushene, R.E. (1970). *Manual for the State-Trait Anxiety Inventory*. Palo Alto: Consulting Psychologists Press.

28. Levy, N.B. (1999). Renal failure, dialysis and transplantation. In: *Psychiatric Treatment of the Medically Ill*, ed. R.G. Robinson, pp. 141–53. New York: Marcel Dekker.

29. Wechsler, D. (1991). *Wechsler Adult Intelligence Scale—III*. New York: Psychological Corporation.

30. Hill, C., Fox, E., Neale, T.J. (1992). Uraemia and working memory. Unpublished manuscript, Victoria University of Wellington.

31. Wartman, S. (1983). Sexual side effects of antihypertensive drugs. *Post Graduate Med.*, **73**(2): 133–5, 138.

# Chapter 10

# Sexual dysfunction in patients with chronic kidney disease

Shirin Shirani and Fredric O. Finkelstein

## 10.1 Introduction

Sexual dysfunction is a common problem in patients with chronic kidney disease (CKD). The most frequently reported symptoms of sexual dysfunction in male patients include problems with decreased libido, difficulty with sexual arousal, erectile dysfunction (ED), premature or delayed ejaculation, and difficulty achieving orgasm.[1] These symptoms are associated with testicular damage and impaired spermatogenesis that may lead to infertility. Less attention, however, has been paid to sexual problems experienced by women with kidney disease. Female patients with advanced renal failure commonly report menstrual irregularities and infertility. Symptoms of sexual dysfunction in female patients include reduced libido, difficulty with sexual arousal, lack of vaginal lubrication, pain during intercourse, and difficulty achieving orgasm. By the time women reach end-stage renal disease (ESRD), most are amenorrhoeic and infertile.[2]

It has been noted for many years that symptoms of sexual dysfunction in patients with CKD begin to occur early in the disease process, well before the need for renal replacement therapy.[3] In addition, the sexual experience of patients with CKD tends to worsen in parallel with deteriorating kidney function. The prevalence of sexual dysfunction in both genders increases as kidney function deteriorates; sexual dysfunction has been reported to occur in about 9% in patients with moderate abnormalities of renal function and in up to 60–70% in patients maintained on dialysis.[3] Several studies have shown that if one examines the prevalence of sexual dysfunction in patients on dialysis, about 65% of male patients report difficulty getting and maintaining an erection and 55% of female patients report difficulty with sexual arousal.[1] In addition, 40% of male dialysis patients and 55% of the female patients report difficulty achieving orgasm. It is interesting that the degree of sexual dysfunction does not correlate with the length of chronic renal failure.[2] Sexual dysfunction occurs with the same frequency in patients maintained on haemodialysis and peritoneal dialysis.[4]

It is important to consider the problems of sexual dysfunction of both male and female patients with CKD in the context of their overall medical and psychological condition. A variety of medical illnesses can directly impact on the sexual experience of the dialysis patient. For example, diabetes and vascular disease can both interfere with the ability of the male patient to achieve an erection. Various psychological factors can have a significant impact on sexual issues for both genders. For example, depression, the most commonly encountered psychological problem in patients with CKD, can interfere with libido and the willingness to engage in sexual activity. Moreover, the sexual problems encountered by patients can in turn contribute to feelings of guilt, sadness, helplessness, and hopelessness.

## 10.2 Aetiology of sexual dysfunction in male patients

### 10.2.1 Hormonal abnormalities

Sexual dysfunction should be thought of as a multifactorial disease that is affected by a variety of both physiological and psychological factors. Male patients with CKD exhibit a variety of abnormalities in endocrine function. Perhaps the most striking changes occur in testicular function with associated changes of androgen synthesis and metabolism that begin to appear early after the onset of renal insufficiency. Reduced testosterone levels are commonly noted that may be related to primary hypogonadism, disturbances of the hypothalamic–pituitary axis, co-morbid conditions, and concomitant drug administration.[5]

Patients with chronic renal insufficiency develop a decrease in testicular size associated with histological changes within the testes.[6] These histological findings include abnormalities of the seminiferous tubules, interstitial fibrosis, calcifications, thickening of the basement membrane, and maturation arrest of the germinal epithelium.[7] These histological changes in patients with CKD are associated with impaired spermatogenesis; semen analyses show decreased volume of ejaculate, either low or complete azoospermia, and a low percentage of sperm motility.[2] These findings are probably the major reason for the infertility often noted in this patient population.

Reductions in plasma testosterone levels in men with chronic renal failure have been well documented. For example, a study conducted by Tourkantonis *et al.*[8] has shown that plasma testosterone levels are significantly lower than levels in normal men; these low levels were attributed to deficient Leydig cell function. This observation was supported by the diminished response in testosterone secretion after human chorionic gonadotrophin (HCG) stimulation in patients with renal failure. Plasma luteinizing hormone (LH) levels are elevated despite low plasma testosterone levels, suggesting that the feedback mechanism between Leydig cells and the hypophysis continues to operate in male dialysis patients. High plasma levels of follicle-stimulating hormone (FSH) in males with impaired spermatogenesis also suggest a continued feedback loop between testes and pituitary.[8]

Abnormalities in pituitary function are also an important feature of the disordered endocrine status of patients with CKD. In male patients with chronic kidney disease, plasma LH levels are often high in association with low plasma testosterone levels. These high levels of LH are observed even in the very early phases of renal insufficiency. The reason for the increase in LH levels is in large part due to stimulation of the pituitary by the diminished release of testosterone from Leydig cells, implying an intact feedback loop between testes and pituitary. There is also an impaired removal rate of LH due to reduced renal clearance of LH.[3] Furthermore, there are abnormalities of secretion of LH in patients with chronic renal disease. In healthy individuals LH is normally secreted in a pulsatile manner, but in patients with kidney disease, although the number of impulses of LH release remains the same, the amount of LH released per impulse is significantly reduced. These abnormalities in the patterns of LH secretion may in turn contribute to the abnormalities in testicular functioning.[1]

However, it is important to note that the elevated levels of LH may not reflect true increases in biologically active hormone. There are increases in both bioactive LH (B-LH) and immunoreactive LH (I-LH); the ratio of B-LH to I-LH, however, is reduced.[9] The LH subtypes that increase in patients with renal failure are more acidic; the basic subtypes are the more biologically active. Thus, there is a reduction in the B-LH/I-LH ratio. This raises the question of whether there is true resistance of the testes to gonadotrophins. However, the resistance of Leydig cells to gonadotrophins is confirmed by studies using HCG administration. These studies have shown that in patients with low testosterone levels, stimulation with HCG results in a suboptimal increase in plasma testosterone level, confirming the presence of abnormalities of Leydig cell function in patients with chronic kidney disease.[9]

The presence of testosterone deficiency has a significant impact on patients. Androgen deficiency probably contributes to the impaired libido and sexual dysfunction of these patients.[5] In addition, androgen deficiency in adults leads to changes in body composition. Snyder et al.,[10] examining the effect of administration of testosterone to hypogonadal males, observed that within 6 months of the start of testosterone replacement, fat-free body mass increased by 5.8% and fat mass decreased. The subjects in this study also reported a general increase in energy and sexual functioning during testosterone treatment. It is interesting to consider whether such a response would be experienced by patients with chronic renal failure.

FSH secretion is largely regulated by inhibin, a peptide produced by Sertoli cells, via a negative-feedback loop. In patients with CKD, there is damage to the seminferous tubules, which leads to damage to Sertoli cells and reduction of inhibin secretion; this in turn results in increased levels of FSH. Thus, with testicular damage from a variety of causes, plasma levels of FSH increase in parallel with impaired spermatogenesis.[11] Thus, the greater the elevation of FSH levels, the more severe the damage to seminiferous tubules and the higher the rate of infertility. In patients with chronic renal disease, the degree of elevation of FSH has been associated with a reduced likelihood of testicular recovery after renal transplantation.[2]

Hyperprolactinaemia is noted frequently in patients with renal disease. Hyperprolactinaemia has been reported in 25–75% of male patients with CKD. Elevated levels appear in the early stages of renal insufficiency and increase in frequency up to an incidence of 80% in patients maintained on haemodialysis.[12] Elevated prolactin levels in individuals on chronic haemodialysis are unchanged by dialysis treatments and are corrected by renal transplantation.[12] Hyperprolactinaemia may well be an important contributory factor to the sexual dysfunction of patients with kidney disease. It is well documented that hyperprolactinaemia interferes with gonadal responses to gonadotrophins resulting in reductions of sexual steroid secretion and circulating testosterone levels. Hyperprolactinaemia has also been associated with decreased libido and sexual dysfunction in patients with normal renal function.

The cause of the elevated prolactin levels in patients with renal disease is uncertain. Hyperprolactinaemia could be due to an impaired renal excretion or degradation of prolactin, or an altered central nervous system inhibitory control due to either decreased secretion of prolactin-inhibiting releasing factor, or an altered responsiveness of the pituitary lactotropes to central regulation. A primary role for the kidney in prolactin metabolism has been supported by the finding of a 16% decrease in prolactin levels between the renal artery and renal vein in subjects with normal renal function.

It is possible that renal failure and maintenance dialysis may constitute a chronic stressful state, and hyperprolactinaemia may be an adaptive phenomenon. Although this could explain the high basal level, it would not explain the autonomous nature of prolactin secretion. Prolactin release is normally under dopaminergic inhibitory control; however, in patients with chronic renal failure prolactin release appears to be autonomous.[2] For example, dopamine infusion or oral L-dopa, which should suppress prolactin levels, fails to decrease the high basal prolactin level in patients with renal failure. Moreover, thyrothropin-releasing hormone infusion or insulin-induced hypoglycemia, that normally cause an increase in prolactin levels, elicit no response or only a blunted response in patients with chronic renal disease.[2,12]

Co-morbid conditions not uncommonly encountered in patients with chronic kidney disease, such as malnutrition, obesity, diabetes mellitus, and hypertension, have been associated with low testosterone levels. In addition, a variety of medications can have an impact on gonadal function and need to be considered in patients with chronic renal disease with sexual difficulties, who are frequently receiving a large number of diverse medications (see below).

## 10.2.2 Erectile dysfunction

Erectile dysfunction (ED) is defined as the persistent inability to achieve and/or maintain a sufficient erection for satisfactory sexual activity.[13] It is a not uncommon condition in middle-aged and older men and frequently occurs in association with various illnesses, such as cardiovascular, hepatic, and also renal disease. The incidence of ED in patients with chronic renal failure is higher than in the general population.[13] The causes of ED are frequently a combination of both organic and psychological factors.[14]

Numerous sexual stimuli are processed by the brain and transmitted to the penis by parasympathetic impulses that pass through the nervi erigentes to the penis. This results in vasodilatation of the arteries, relaxation of the smooth layer, and compression of the veins against the rigid tunica albuginea, thus allowing blood to build up under high pressure in the erectile tissue of the penis. ED is often the result of multisystem disease processes involving the hypothalamic–pituitary–gonadal axis, autonomic nervous system, vascular supply to the penis, and damage to the penile tissue from either infection or trauma. Psychological factors such as depression, fatigue, anxiety, and stress may result from chronic illness and contribute further to the patient's loss of erectile functioning.[14]

ED is a common problem in patients with chronic renal failure. About 65% of male dialysis patients report difficulty getting and maintaining an erection and 40% report difficulty in achieving orgasm.[15] About 40% of married patients on dialysis report never having intercourse. Numerous factors have been implicated as contributing factors for ED in patients with chronic renal failure. As noted above, CKD causes imbalances in the hypothalamic–pituitary–gonadal axis in men, resulting in abnormalities in testicular function and testosterone, FSH, LH, and prolactin secretion; these problems may all contribute to the ED of male patients with CKD.

Accelerated vascular disease, which is well documented in patients with kidney disease, may lead to an impaired arterial blood supply and venous drainage of pelvic organs. A histological study of renal and hypogastric arterial sections in patients with renal failure undergoing renal transplantation found fibroelastic intimal thickening and calcification of internal elastic lamella; these vascular alterations were related to the duration of chronic renal failure.[16] Complete or partial occlusion of large vessels and their arterial tributaries supplying the penis can play an important role in ED. An interesting study evaluating patients with renal failure using pharmaco-cavernosometry and pharmaco-cavernosography has suggested that 78% of patients with ESRD have significant cavernosal artery occlusive disease; corporeal veno-occlusive dysfunction was found in 90% of patients.[17] The vascular disease of the penis noted in these renal failure patients was found to occur at a higher rate than predicted by the presence of known systemic atherosclerotic vascular risk factors.

Anaemia has been reported to be associated with erectile dysfunction. Altered erythropoietin synthesis in patients with kidney disease frequently leads to anaemia with low oxygen delivery to the corpora cavernosa; this has been shown to decrease nitric oxide synthesis and increase endothelium-derived contracting factor, resulting in increased smooth muscle tone and inhibiting erectile capabilities.[14] The reduced oxygen-carrying capacity secondary to anaemia can exacerbate the hypoxia and tissue damage caused by vascular disease to further compromise sexual function.[2] Furthermore, treatment of anaemia with recombinant erythropoietin has been shown to improve erectile functioning in patients with ESRD, as discussed below.

Medication frequently used in the setting of CRF such as diuretics, antihypertensive medications, antidepressant medications, and H2 blockers can contribute to ED. Several drugs are also known to interfere directly with the synthesis of sexual hormones and their effects. Spironolactone and cimetidine block androgen receptors. Moreover, spironolactone and ketoconazole reduce 17$\alpha$-hydroxylase/C17–20lyase activity leading to reduced testosterone biosynthesis. Glucocorticoids reduce testosterone synthesis directly via gonadal steroid receptors and centrally at the hypothalamic level. Tricyclic antidepressants, benzodiazepines, and opiates may induce secondary hypogonadism through central mechanisms.[5]

Sildenafil improves erectile functioning in men with ED by sustaining guanosine 3′,5′-cyclic monophosphate (cGMP)-mediated smooth muscle relaxation in the corpus cavernosum. It also induces systemic vasodilatation, resulting in a minor decrease in blood pressure. The effect of sildenafil has been evaluated in patients with ED of different aetiologies. Goldstein *et al.*[17] demonstrated improvement of ED in men caused by both psychogenic and organic causes. Sildenafil has been reported to result in an improvement of ED in patients with diabetes. However, there are limited studies in patients with CKD and the results of these studies are not in agreement. In a study conducted in male patients with ESRD on peritoneal dialysis, who were screened for ED, only 50% of patients with ED were willing to consider a trial with sildenafil. Of those who agreed to treatment, only a minority completed the full course of treatment and only 33% of the patients reported a satisfactory response to sildenafil.[15] However, other studies, examining patients with ED maintained on haemodialysis and peritoneal dialysis, showed a 60 to 80% response rate to sildenafil, as assessed by scores on the International Index of Erectile Function (IIEF-5).[13,18] Since the aetiology of ED is multifactorial, further investigations regarding the use and efficacy of sildenafil in patients with CKD with ED are needed.

## 10.2.3 Zinc deficiency

Several investigators have evaluated the potential contribution of zinc deficiency to sexual dysfunction. Animal studies have shown that zinc deficiency can result in testicular failure, and studies in children have suggested that zinc deficiency may delay sexual development.[19] Antoniou *et al.*[20] suggested that the sexual dysfunction in patients on dialysis might also result from zinc deficiency. In contrast, Brook *et al.*[21] and Joven *et al.*,[22] in two independent studies, showed that in patients with sexual dysfunction and low zinc serum levels, replacement of zinc failed to result in any significant improvement in the sexual experience of their patients. Lim[23] has recommended that if zinc deficiency is documented a trial of zinc therapy be administrated, either orally as zinc acetate or mixed in dialysate as zinc chloride. There seems to be a need for further investigation the role of zinc deficiency in sexual dysfunction in the ESRD population.

## 10.2.4 Autonomic meuropathy

Dysfunction of the autonomic nervous system is a frequent finding in patients with chronic renal failure; the integrity of this system is essential for normal sexual activity. Autonomic neuropathy contributes to a variety of problems for patients maintained on dialysis, such as dialysis-associated hypotension. It can also have a significant impact on sexual functioning in both male and female patients with CKD. Abnormalities in the pelvic autonomic nervous system can decrease sensation and arousal stimuli during sexual activity. In addition, autonomic neuropathy can interfere with the complex neurological axis that is necessary for the achievement of an adequate erection. The relationship between ED and autonomic dysfunction in patients with chronic renal failure was examined in an interesting study by Campese.[24] In this study, ED was examined by measuring nocturnal penile tumescence (NPT) and autonomic dysfunction was assessed by responses to the Valsalva manoeuvre.[24] Forty-four per cent of patients in this study had markedly reduced NPT and 48% had abnormal responses to the Valsalva manoeuvre. There was a significant correlation between the NPT and autonomic dysfunction in these patients. Furthermore, this study also demonstrated a correlation between both the abnormalities in responses to the Valsalva manoeuvre and NPT and the frequency of intercourse, thus providing support for the role of autonomic disturbances in sexual dysfunction in patients with CKD. The pathogenesis of autonomic neuropathy is not fully understood. It has been shown that parasympathetic neuropathy appears more frequent than sympathetic dysfunction.[25] The presence and severity of autonomic neuropathy do not seem to be related to either the duration of dialysis or renal failure.

### 10.2.5 Anaemia

Anaemia develops in the early stages of renal failure, primarily due to a decrease in production of erythropoietin by the kidney. Symptoms of anaemia may include, in addition to chronic fatigue and weakness, reduction of libido and sexual dysfunction. Recombinant human erythropoietin (rHuEpo) therapy in patients with CKD has led to a correction of anaemia with improved quality of life, decreased fatigue, increased exercise tolerance, and improved overall general well-being. Furthermore, correction of anaemia with rHuEpo has been shown to improve sexual desire and performance in some, but not all, patients.[14,15] rHuEpo therapy has also been shown to improve erectile function in some male dialysis patients.[26] Several authors have evaluated the mechanisms of the improvement of sexual functioning in patients with CKD with erythropoietin supplementation. These studies have shown that there is not only an increase in general well-being but also an improvement in some of the abnormalities in sex hormones levels. For example, Schaefer et al.[27] observed a normalization of elevated prolactin levels associated with an improvement of sexual functioning in patients maintained on haemodialysis. Correction of anaemia with rHuEpo in patients with renal failure has resulted in significant changes in LH secretion. Studies in male dialysis patients have demonstrated a significant decreases in the plasma half-life of B-LH and quantitative and qualitative increases of LH signal strength with correction of anaemia with rHuEpo.[27] In addition, many studies evaluating the changes in quality of life in response to rHuEpo therapy in patients with renal failure have noted significant improvements in not only physical and social functioning and overall mental health, but also in satisfaction with sexual activity.[28,29]

## 10.3 Sexual dysfunction in women with CKD

The normal menstrual cycle is divided into a follicular or proliferative phase and a luteal or secretory phase. Normal follicular maturation and subsequent ovulation require appropriately timed secretion of the pituitary gonadotrophins. FSH secretion exhibits typical negative feedback with hormone levels falling as the plasma oestrogen concentration rises. In contrast, LH secretion is suppressed maximally by low concentrations of oestrogen but exhibits positive-feedback control in response to a rising and sustained elevation of oestradiol. Thus, high levels of oestradiol in the late follicular phase trigger a surging elevation in LH secretion, which is responsible for ovulation. After ovulation, progesterone levels increase due to production by the corpus luteum. Progesterone is responsible for the transformation of the endometrium into the luteal phase.

Women with kidney disease suffer from multiple abnormalities in their menstrual cycle, ranging from amenorrhoea, menorrhagia, and infertility. The menstrual cycle is typically irregular in women with CKD and remains so after initiation of dialysis. It has been suggested that less than 10% of premenopausal female dialysis patients have regular menses and about 40% are totally amenorrhoeic. Many female patients with CKD are anovulatory. Some patients have difficulty with menorrhagia, which can cause significant blood loss and contribute to anaemia. Pregnancy rarely occurs in patients with advanced renal failure, and if it does there is high rate of miscarriage.

Surprisingly, there are limited studies carefully examining ovarian function in women with CRF despite the high prevalence of ovarian dysfunction. The lack of information about ovarian dysfunction in women with kidney disease is likely due to difficulties in studying such a complex cyclical system. It is also partly because women generally do not seek medical attention for symptoms related to ovarian dysfunction. Problems with ovarian dysfunction in patients with CKD generally persist after the start of dialysis; in fact, many patients who had either regular or irregular menses at the beginning of dialysis often ultimately become amenorrhoeic.

The cause of ovarian failure in women with CKD may involve abnormalities at several sites in the hypothalamic–pituitary–ovarian axis. The most detailed study of hormonal functioning in uraemic women was performed by Lim.[23] This work involved the measurement of baseline levels of plasma LH, FSH, estradiol, progesterone, and prolactin in both pre- and postmenopausal women maintained on dialysis. These hormone levels were then measured after clomifene (an antioestrogenic agent), ethinylestradiol (oestrogen stimulation test), and bromocriptine.

The baseline plasma estradiol, progesterone, and FSH were comparable between premenopausal patients with kidney disease and normal women during the follicular phase of the ovarian cycle. However, the LH levels were significantly higher during the follicular phase in pre-menopausal women with kidney disease; but the LH levels were far below the levels observed in normal women during the midcyle LH surge. The plasma prolactin levels were significantly higher in women with kidney disease than normal women. After clomifene administration, which was given to evaluate the responsiveness of the hypothalamic–pituitary axis in uraemic patients, plasma LH and FSH increased significantly, suggesting an intact negative-feedback effect of oestrogen on the hypothalamus and the storage and release of pituitary gonadotrophins. Gonadotrophin-releasing hormone (GHRH) secretion has both a tonic and a cyclic component. The tonic component regulates the basal gonadotrophin secretion and is controlled by a negative estradiol feedback mechanism. The cyclic component is dependent on oestrogen secretion; the increase in oestrogen levels in midcycle is responsible for increased secretion of GHRH and the subsequent LH surge. After the oestrogen stimulation test, normal subjects experienced a surge in plasma LH levels; plasma FSH levels also increase but to a lesser extent. In contrast, in women with CKD, after the administration of oestrogen, plasma LH level did not rise and the plasma FSH levels were suppressed. The absence of an increase in LH levels strongly suggests a defect in the positive hypothalamic feedback mechanism.

Post-menopausal women with kidney disease have elevated gonadotrophin levels. Clomifene administration results in increased secretion of both gonadotrophins.

Eighty per cent of women with kidney disease also demonstrate high levels of serum prolactin. This hyperprolactinaemia may be a contributory factor to ovulatory dysfunction. The administration of bromocriptine reduces the prolactin level to within the normal range, but results in a variable response in the gonadotrophin levels. Ovarian function improved in response to bromocriptine only in those patients whose gonadotrophin secretion resumed cyclicity, suggesting that the predominant action of hyperprolactinaemia in contributing to ovarian dysfunction was an inhibitory effect on GHRH secretion. Taken together, these findings suggest that the pituitary–ovarian axis remains intact in women with renal failure and the primary defect in sex hormone dysfunction is due to absence of the cyclic release of gonadotrophins.

In pre- and post-menopausal women, low levels of estradiol can lead to vaginal atrophy and dryness and dyspareunia, which can affect the sexual function in these women.

The elevated levels of prolactin can also contribute to sexual dysfunction by decreasing libido, in addition to interfering with ovarian function. Women with kidney disease who have hyperprolactinaemia not infrequently also have galactorrhoea.

## 10.4 Psychosocial concerns

Psychosocial factors may have a significant impact on the sexual functioning of patients with kidney disease. Depression is the most common psychological problem presented by dialysis patients. In various studies; it has been noted that 20–30% of patients with renal failure suffer from clinical depression.[1,14] Patients maintained on dialysis frequently exhibit a depressive affect (pessimism, anhedonia, sadness, complaints of feeling helpless and hopeless, suicidal ideation) accompanied by changes in sleep, appetite, activity level, and libido. This depression can have an adverse impact on the functioning of patients in a variety of areas, including marital and family relationships and occupational activity.

The impact of depression on sexual functioning is well-documented. Depression can contribute to problems with interpersonal relationships and reduce libido. It has been suggested that amongst dialysis patients, those patients who are the most depressed are the ones with the most severe degrees of sexual dysfunction.[1] The relationship between depression and sexual dysfunction is important, particularly in view of recent reports commenting on the effective use of antidepressant medication to treat depression in patients maintained on dialysis.[14]

Marital discord is commonly encountered in the marriages of dialysis patients. Over 40% of married couples where one spouse is a dialysis patient experience moderate to severe degrees of discord. Stress in relationships is often caused by role changes, loss of employment, decrease in income, inability to maintain a household, and reduced recreational and social activity. These losses can contribute to couples withdrawing from sexual intimacy. A close correlation has been noted between the degree of marital discord and the level of sexual functioning in dialysis marriages.[30] When dialysis couples are asked to identify areas of marital difficulty, sexual issues are cited as a problem area by nearly 60% of couples.[30]

Problems with body image are also a source of concern for many patients maintained on dialysis. For example, having a catheter or fistula, gaining weight from excess fluid or dextrose loads with peritoneal dialysis, being connected to a machine, and eventual cessation of urination negatively impact on patients' relationship to their body. This may, in turn, result in feeling less desirable and more self-conscious and therefore have a negative impact on sexual functioning.

In addition, there are a variety of other stressors that affect the life of a dialysis patient. These stressors may include dietary issues, time constraints, functional limitations, loss of employment, changes in self-perception, perceived effects of illness, medications used to treat the illness, and fear of disability and death. Adaptive coping mechanisms are needed to deal with these complex changes in patients' lives. In the absence of adequate coping strategies, interpersonal difficulties can occur, accompanied by depression and anxiety, loss of libido, and reduced sexual activity.[31]

## 10.5 Assessment of sexual function

An important first step is to systematically elicit from the patient a detailed sexual history and assessment of current sexual functioning. Often the medical staff are uncomfortable initiating a frank discussion regarding sexuality. Patients are similarly reluctant or embarrassed to raise concerns about their sexual functioning. The medical team needs to develop a strategy to assess patients' sexual functioning as a routine part of care. A standardized protocol for assessing sexual dysfunction should be developed that is built into the routine assessment plans of the dialysis facility. This assessment can be done by the physician, nurse, or social worker.

The initial step in this evaluation should be an assessment of a patient's current experience with sexual function and a comparison of this experience with his/her functioning prior to the onset of illness. If sexual difficulties are present, it is important to determine the timing of the onset of these problems in relationship to the patient's kidney disease and other medical and psychosocial difficulties. Sexual difficulties must be put in the context of the patient's life stage and his or her adjustment to the demands associated with the particular life stage. The clinician must determine not only if the patient has sexual difficulties, but also if he or she is aware of and concerned about these sexual problems. Most patients do not share their sexual experiences openly with their healthcare provider. It might take multiple attempts and rephrasing of questions to adequately understand the presence or absence of sexual dysfunction. It is important to assess the level of satisfaction with current sexual activities. The frequency of intercourse needs to be determined. Changes in the frequency of intercourse will facilitate the identification of specific symptoms of sexual dysfunction, such as problems with sexual arousal, lack of interest in sexual activity, problems with lubrication, dyspareunia, difficulties getting or maintaining an erection, problems with ejaculation (premature or delayed), difficulties with sexual pleasure, intimacy, and orgasm. In addition, it is important to evaluate patients for the presence of psychosocial problems that may be contributing to sexual dysfunction, such as depression, marital problems, the quality of interaction with spouses and significant others, and family history of psychiatric illnesses. An evaluation of the status of current intimate relationships and the level of discord with these relationships need to be addressed. Additional psychosocial factors to be explored include an assessment of current stressors (loss of job or home, problems of other family members, etc.). It is not uncommon for patients and/or partners to be unavailable for intimacy in the face of these stressors.

A thorough medical history and examination is essential, including an assessment for the presence of vascular disease (especially peripheral vascular disease), autonomic dysfunction, findings of hypogonadism, and a detailed review of current medications. The presence of medical problems that can contribute to, or be responsible for, sexual dysfunction need to be carefully considered. Anaemia and erythropoietin deficiency must be evaluated. A detailed history of menstrual patterns should be obtained in women and a history of erectile function obtained in males. Consideration should be given to laboratory assessment of hormone levels (testosterone, oestrogen, FSH, LH, TSH, PTH, and prolactin levels) and zinc levels based on the specific complaints of each patient.

## 10.6 The treatment of sexual dysfunction

Developing treatment strategies for the sexual dysfunction of a patient with kidney disease presents challenges for the clinician since the causes of sexual dysfunction are frequently multifactorial and it is often difficult to distinguish the primary factor(s) responsible for the sexual dysfunction. It is important to remember that designing therapeutic approaches for each patient is dependent on the systematic evaluation of both the functional and psychosocial problem(s) presented by each patient and the assessment of the cause(s) of the sexual dysfunction.

For both male and female patients, it is important to address the psychosocial factors that may be contributing to the sexual dysfunction. Given the complexity of sexual dysfunction, it is important for the caregivers in the dialysis facilities to engage the patients in a therapeutic alliance. This involves not just the physicians and social workers, but the nurses, technicians, and dieticians as well. An ongoing dialogue between the patient and the clinical team needs to be established. Chronic illness affects relationships, libido, and sexual functioning. Family, marital, or individual counselling in conjunction with medication often needs to be offered. Furthermore, recent studies have suggested that depression is associated with increased morbidity and mortality in patients maintained on dialysis.[31,32] Depression in dialysis patients can be screened for with simple screening instruments (such as the Beck Depression Inventory (BDI)) and then treated with psychotropic medications.[33]

Since medications can affect sexual functioning and patients with kidney disease are often prescribed many medications, these need to be carefully reviewed. Haemoglobin levels should be increased using recombinant erythropoietin, as needed. Zinc levels should be checked, although the use of zinc replacements has been of questionable value, as noted above. Parathyroid abnormalities should be treated. If other endocrine hormonal abnormalities are present, consideration should be given to hormone replacement with oestrogen (with or without progesterone) in females and testosterone in males. Recent studies have also emphasized the importance of testosterone therapy for female libido. Oestrogen replacement alone may not be effective in restoring sexual desire in hypogonadal women, but a combination of oestrogen and testosterone may be more useful. However, the potential side-effects of androgen therapy in women must be kept in mind. Prolactin levels, if elevated, can be reduced with dopaminergic agonists, such as bromocriptine, parlodel, or lisuride.

In male patients, it is important to distinguish between problems with libido and problems with erectile function. ED may be related to problems with autonomic dysfunction and/or vascular disease, as discussed above. Thus, it is important from a therapeutic standpoint to provide an adequate dose of dialysis for patients with ESRD to minimize the deleterious effects of the uraemic environment on nerve function and to create an environment that minimizes the risks of progressive vascular disease. Treatment goals for the latter would include ensuring adequate blood pressure control, lipid control, and phosphate control.

Sildenafil has been used to treat the ED of male patients with ESRD. The response rates to sildenafil have varied in different studies, as discussed above. One reason for the varying response rates to sildenafil may have to do with the use of sildenafil in isolation without consideration being given to the other factors that may contribute to sexual dysfunction. Thus, patients with erectile dysfunction as the primary cause of sexual dysfunction may have a high response rate, while those patients with a multifactorial aetiology of sexual dysfunction may have a lower response rate if the other contributing causes of dysfunction have not been addressed. In male patients with erectile dysfunction who do not respond to sildenafil therapy, treatment options would include intracavernosal injection of alprostadil and/or the use of vacuum/constriction devices.

## Case study

A 52-year-old male accountant with membranous nephropathy has had a gradual decline in his renal function over the past 8 years, with his plasma creatinine increasing from 1.8 mg/dl at the time of his renal biopsy in 1994 to 7.0 mg/dl. He was initially treated with prednisolone and chlorambucil and then switched to ciclosporin in 1995 for 2 years. He has remained with significant proteinuria, greater than 5 g/24 h, despite the various medications, including angiotensin converting enzyme inhibitors and the immunosuppressive drugs. The ciclosporin was stopped in 1997. He has had problems with blood pressure control since 1995 and is currently being treated with 40 mg/day of lisinopril, 10 mg of amlodipine, 50 mg of atenolol, 20 mg atorvastatin, and 80 mg of furosemide.

On his most recent visits, discussions were started concerning the various dialytic and/or transplant options that would become necessary in the near future. The patient expressed concern about his work schedule and his family obligations; he is married, has three children aged 12 to 16, and helps provide support for his ageing parents.

Physical examination on his last visit included a blood pressure of 150/85, an S-4 gallop, trace lower extremity oedema, and a left carotid bruit.

Laboratory data included a haemoglobin of 10 g/l, haematocrit of 30.2, blood urea nitrogen (BUN) of 80 mg/dl, serum creatinine of 6.2 mg/dl, intact parathyroid hormone level of 526 pg/ml, calcium level of 9.6 mg/dl, a phosphorus level of 5.8 mg/dl, and a cholesterol level of 204 mg/dl.

During his last visit, the patient expresses concern over a decreased libido and frequency of intercourse. He reports that he last had intercourse about 3 months ago. He has not discussed this with his wife. He says that he has had difficulty getting and maintaining an erection for the last 2 years but that this problem has worsened in the last 6 months. He has not approached his wife about sexual activity—partly because he says that he is not interested but also because he is concerned about his sexual performance. He generally reports feeling fatigued after work and at weekends.

This case demonstrates the complexity of management of sexual dysfunction. He needs to start on dialysis, he is anaemic, and also has hyperparathyroidism. He is also on beta-blockers. There will also be numerous psychosocial issues in someone approaching dialysis.

## References

1. Finkelstein, S.H., Finkelstein, F.O. (2002). Evaluation of sexual dysfunction in dialysis patients. In: *Dialysis Therapy*, 3rd ed. pp. 368–73. A.R. Nissenson, R.N. Fine. Philadelphia, PA: Hanley and Belfus.

2. Palmer, B.F. (1999). Sexual dysfunction in uremia. *J. Am. Soc. Nephrol.,* **10**: 1381–8.

3. Ayub, W., Fletcher, S. (2000). End-stage renal disease and erectile dysfunction. Is there any hope? *Nephrol. Dial. Transpl.,* **15**: 1525–8.

4. Steele, T.E., Wuerth, D., Finkelstein, S., *et al.* (1996). Sexual experience of the chronic peritoneal dialysis patient. *J. Am. Soc. Nephrol.,* **7**: 1165–8.

5. Schmidt, A., Luger, A., Horl, W.H. (2002). Sexual hormone abnormalities in male patients with renal failure. *Nephrol. Dial. Transpl.,* **17**: 368–71.

6. Guevara, A., Vidt, D., Hallberg, M.C., *et al.* (1969). Serum gonadotropin and testosterone levels in uraemic males undergoing intermittent dialysis. *Metabolism,* **18**: 1062–6.

7. Stewart-Bentley, M., Gans, D., Horton, R. (1974). Regulation of gonadal function in uraemia. *Metabolism* **23**: 1065–72.

8. Tourkantonis, A., Spiliopoulos, A., Pharmakiotis, A., Settas, L. (1981). Haemodialysis and hypothalamo–pituitary—testicular axis. *Nephron* **27**: 271–2.

9. Mitchell, R., Bauerfeld, C., Schaefer, F., Scharer, K., Robertson, W.R. (1994). Less acidic forms of luteinizing hormone are associated with lower testosterone secretion in men on haemodialysis treatment. *Clin. Endocrinol.*, **41**: 65–73.

10. Snyder, P.J., Peachey, H., Berlin, J.A., *et al.* (2000). Effects of testosterone replacement in hypogonadal men. *J. Clin. Endocrinol. Metab.*, **85**: 2670–7.

11. Holdsworth, S., Atkins, R.C., de Kretser, D.M. (1977). The pituitary–testicular axis in men with chronic renal failure. *New Engl. J. Med.*, **296**: 1245–9.

12. Sievertsen, G.D., Lim, V.S., Nakawatase, C., Frohman, L.A. (1980). Metabolic clearance and secretion rates of human prolactin in normal subjects and in patients with chronic renal failure. *J. Clin. Endocrinol. Metab.*, **50**: 846–52.

13. Chen, J., Mabjeesh, N.J., Greenstein, A., Nadu, A., Matzkin, H. (2001). Clinical efficacy of sildenafil in patients on chronic dialysis. *J. Urol.*, **165**: 819–21.

14. Finkelstein, F.O., Wattnick, S., Finkelstein, S.H., Wuerth, D. (2002). The treatment of depression in patients maintained on dialysis. *J. Psychosom. Res.*, **53**: 957–60.

15. Juergensen, P.H., Botev, R., Wuerth, D., *et al.* (2001). Erectile dysfunction in chronic peritoneal dialysis patients: incidence and treatment with sildenafil. *Perit. Dial. Int.*, **21**: 355–9.

16. Ibels, L.S., Alfrey, A.C., Huffer, W.E. *et al.* (1979). Arterial calcification and pathology in uraemic patients undergoing dialysis. *Am. J. Med.*, **66**: 790–6.

17. Goldstein I., Lue, T.F., Padma-Nathan H, *et al.* (1998). Oral Sildenafil in treatment of erectile dysfunction *NEGL. J. Med.*, **338**: 1397–1403.

18. Turk, S., Karalezli, G., Tonbul, H.Z., *et al.* (2001). Erectile dysfunction and the effects of sildenafil treatment in patients on haemodialysis and continuous ambulatory peritoneal dialysis. *Nephrol. Dial. Transpl.*, **16**: 1818–22.

19. Zetin, M., Stone, R.A. (1980). Effects of zinc in chronic haemodialysis. *Clin. Nephrol.*, **13**: 20–5.

20. Antoniou, L.D., Shalhoub, R.J., Sudhakar, T., Smith, J.C. Jr. (1977). Reversal of uraemic impotence by zinc. *The Lancet*, **2**: 895–8.

21. Brook, A.C., Johnston, D.G., Ward, M.K. *et al.* (1980). Absence of a therapeutic effect of zinc in the sexual dysfunction of haemodialysed patients. *The Lancet*, **2**: 618–20.

22. Joven, J., Villabona, C., Rubies-Prat, J., Espinel, E., Galard, R. (1985). Hormonal profile and serum zinc levels in uraemic men with gonadal dysfunction undergoing haemodialysis. *Clin. Chim. Acta.*, **148**: 239–45.

23. Lim, V.S. (1987). Reproductive function in patients with renal insufficiency. *Am. J. Kidney Dis.*, **9**: 363–7.

24. Campese, V.M. (1990). Autonomic nervous system dysfunction in uraemia. *Nephrol. Dial. Transpl.*, **5**(Suppl 1): 98–101.

25. Vita, G., Bellinghieri, G., Trusso, A., *et al.* (1999). Uraemic autonomic neuropathy studied by spectral analysis of heart rate. *Kidney Int.*, **56**: 232–7.

26. Lawrence, I.G., Price, D.E., Howlett, T.A., *et al.* (1997). Erythropoietin and sexual dysfunction. *Nephrol. Dial. Transpl.*, **12**: 741–7.

27. Schaefer, F., van Kaick, B., Veldhuis, J.D., *et al.* (1994). Changes in the kinetics and biopotency of luteinizing hormone in hemodialyzed men during treatment with recombinant human erythropoietin. *J. Am. Soc. Nephrol.*, **5**: 1208–15.

28. Beusterien, K.M., Nissenson, A.R., Port, F.K., *et al.* (1996). The effects of recombinant human erythropoietin on functional health and well-being in chronic dialysis patients. *J. Am. Soc. Nephrol.*, **7**: 763–73.

29. Schaefer, R.M., Kokot, F., Wernze, H., Geiger, H., Heidland, A. (1989). Improved sexual function in haemodialysis patients on recombinant erythropoietin: a possible role for prolactin. *Clin. Nephrol.*, **31**: 1–5.

30. Steele, T.E., Finkelstein, S.H., Finkelstein, F.O. (1976). Marital discord, sexual problems, and depression. *J. Nerv. Ment. Dis.,* **162**: 225.

31. Kimmel, P.L. (2001). Psychosocial factors in dialysis patients. *Kidney Int.,* **59**: 1599–613.

32. Lopes, A.A., Bragg, J., Young, E., Goodkin, D., Mapes, D., Combe, C., *et al.* (2002). Depression as a predictor of mortality and hospitalization among hemodialysis patients in the United States and Europe. *Kidney Int.,* **62**: 199–207.

33. Wuerth, D.B., Finkelstein, S.H., Ciarcia, J., Peterson, R., Finkelstein, F.O. (2001). Identification and treatment of depression in patients maintained on chronic peritoneal dialysis. *Am. J. Kidney Dis.,* **37**: 1011–17.

# Chapter 11

# Spiritual care of the renal patient

Chris Davies and Ira Byock

## 11.1 Introduction

The term 'spiritual' is one which can mean different things to different people. In 1992 the UK Department of Health produced a circular entitled 'Meeting the spiritual needs of patients and staff'.[1] This document, whilst clear, assumes that the reader will understand what spiritual needs actually are, yet little clarification is forthcoming within it. Despite the growing secularization of society on both sides of the Atlantic, healthcare professionals are still being asked to ensure that the spiritual and religious needs of their patients are fully taken into account at all times. The aim of this chapter is to explore the terms 'spiritual' and 'religious' and to see how they may have bearing upon the supportive care of the renal patient.

Spirituality is more an art than a science. Each human life is unique and precious. As a consequence, there can be no single definition of spirituality; rather there are innumerable expressions of it. It is indeed akin to an art class working on a portrait. Each student will create a painting that will be unique. So it is with spirituality and religion. There may be a common theme but the way an individual experiences that theme will depend upon their life's experience and system of beliefs. Attempts are being made to describe and quantify spiritual care within a quasiscientific model. Some of the research carried out will be of interest to those working in the field of spiritual caregiving. However, what follows seeks to understand spirituality as an art rather than a science in order to enable clinicians to include a patient's spiritual and religious needs into their overall care plan.

With this in mind this chapter aims to address the subject in two distinct yet complementary ways. Ira Byock comes to it as an American physician. Chris Davies explores it from the viewpoint of an Anglican priest steeped in the culture of the UK. As with two people painting the portrait of someone sitting before them there will be not only some distinctive insights but also some overlap.

It is to be hoped that readers will take from either or both approaches insights and experiences that will help develop an approach to the spiritual and religious care of their patients that in no way compromises their own integrity as human beings.

## 11.2 Portrait one: spiritual care from the perspective of a UK hospital chaplain

Modern best practice in healthcare demands that a patient is given the opportunity to exercise an 'informed choice' at every possible point in their treatment.

When speaking with nurses about such matters I invariably begin by asking them to consider how they should ask a patient whether they might have any spiritual or religious needs whilst in hospital. The question ought to be routinely asked on admission but is often omitted. It is clear that how the question is asked is as important as asking it in the first place. A nurse who is an ardent member of a faith community may ask it in a way that can only elicit a 'yes response'; i.e. 'You would like to see the chaplain wouldn't you?' Whereas a nurse who is an atheist may ask in a way that will produce a 'no response'; i.e. 'You don't need to see the chaplain do you?' Both extremes are inconsistent with offering the patient balanced information in order for them to make an informed choice. As with the nurse, who is admitting a patient, the doctor's views on spirituality and religion will also affect how comfortable a patient will feel about disclosing such needs. Unlike asking a phlebotomist to carry out a procedure, a doctor will not always be able to call in the chaplain or other spiritual caregiver to deal with matters raised at the bedside. I am not arguing for all clinicians to have a faith, far from it! I am, however, asking that clinicians, whatever their personal beliefs, take the spiritual needs of their patients seriously and allow for them to be addressed.

## 11.2.1 What is meant by spirituality?

In recent years there has been an explosion of books addressing spirituality in the context of healthcare. It is clear from such written material that there is no one clear definition of spirituality and if we see this subject as an art form, then this is to be expected. There are likely to be as many definitions of spirituality as there are human beings!

I understand spirituality to be about making sense of myself in relation to the world around me. It is about looking for meaning: who I am in relation to my past, my present, and my future and what the reference points are on my life journey. In the context of disease I would add questions such as: 'Why is this happening to me?', 'What have I done to bring this upon myself?', 'So what has my life been all about and what has been the point of it all?', 'Who will be affected by my pain and death and why should they be?' Speck[2] notes that 'spiritual' relates to a concern with ultimate issues and is often seen as a search for meaning. This definition echoes Frankl[3] who has said, 'Man is not destroyed by suffering, he is destroyed by suffering without meaning'.

Religious needs on the other hand relate to how an individual seeks to find such meaning within a framework that gives expression to his or her life as a whole. This may be as one of an organized faith community or not. The essential aspect is that it is a framework that others are part of and share in whether they are physically present or not. There is, therefore, a significant difference between spiritual and religious needs.

Perhaps an analogy might help. I liken the difference between spiritual and religious needs to that of a four-stroke petrol engine. Such an engine powers a motor car and requires an electric spark in order to do so. This spark is produced by a spark plug. However, different makes of car have different types of spark plugs. The spark plugs perform an identical function but are usually brand specific. Humanity can be likened to such a car. Our spiritual nature is an integral part and can be compared with the engine. Our religious nature will depend upon our personal histories and will be different accordingly, as are the spark plugs in the various makes of cars. It is important that healthcare professionals, including chaplains, acknowledge such differences and seek to ensure that a patient's spiritual needs are addressed by appropriate means be they religious in the traditional sense or otherwise. Chaplains are 'spiritual mechanics'. They carry a ' virtual tool bag' in which will be found the resources for a wide range of religious needs.

## 11.2.2 Assessing the spiritual and religious needs

'Am I going to die doctor?' is a question often asked by patients. This is a clear, straightforward question, or so it seems. Yet what is being asked maybe something completely different. The patient, rather than wishing to know the prognosis, may in fact want to be told that they are going to get better. Words convey a variety of meanings and it is only by 'listening to the whole person' that we communicate effectively. Listening is about using all our senses in harmony. Quietly asking for clarification of a patient's questions is essential to good care. Taking note of their countenance, their surroundings, and their network of relationships all play a part in seeking to help address their spiritual and religious needs.

## Case study

It was 3 p.m. one Sunday afternoon, I had been busy with bedside prayers for most of the day and was very tired. The renal unit called me to attend one of their patients who had been missed off of my visiting list. The patient was a young blind woman with end-stage renal failure. I introduced myself and said that I had brought her Holy Communion to which she replied, 'no thank you'. I was perplexed by her reply and wondered why she had refused. She was sitting beside her bed and appeared quite agitated by my presence. I gently asked her if I had upset her in any way and she said, 'no I hadn't'.

As I sat with her and apologised for not coming during the morning her agitation lessened. I said to her that I felt that she appeared upset by my arrival and wondered why. After a long pause she explained to me that ever since her childhood she would only go to church on a Sunday morning. She had expected me to come that morning and when I failed to arrive then she thought no more of it. However, to turn up unexpectedly on a Sunday afternoon had terrified her. She could not see my face but felt that I was rather anxious, which of course I was, for I had failed to see her earlier. Arriving as I did made her feel that there was some sort of emergency and that I wasn't just bringing her Holy Communion but had come because the staff had called me to attend as she was near to death. I had come, so she thought, to give her the 'last rites' and she did not want that at all. This was the starting point of a series of visits during which she began to talk of her fear of death.

It may be that the patient is unaware of some deep profound worry that has been thrown into focus by their disease. They may be unclear and unable to articulate what is troubling them. Listening to the whole person and not to just their words can enable the clinician to begin to help the patient face what is upsetting them. Sometimes it is unwise to offer the services of a chaplain immediately. It may be that only after several difficult conversations it becomes appropriate to suggest that perhaps someone like a chaplain might be able to help.

The most important factor in all of this is time and reflective listening.

Assessing spiritual needs can be a slow process. This is not so when it comes to religious needs. Members of major faith communities will usually know what they need. It may be a place to pray, or the attendance of their minister for prayers and support. We all do well to remember that meeting the religious needs of a patient may not meet their spiritual needs at all. Assumptions can be made all too easily.

## Case study

On one occasion a local minister called to commend one of his congregation to me. He was a recently retired professional man who was now actively involved in his church's outreach work. He had come in for tests and a tumour had been found in his kidney. He was awaiting its removal and further tests. I found him in a four-bedded unit with three other very talkative male patients. We sat on his bed and spoke for some considerable time about his new work with his church, of what was happening now, and how things might or might not go after surgery. As I drew our conversation to a close I suggested that we prayed together. He immediately withdrew from me saying, 'no thank you I would rather not if you don't mind'. I respected his wishes shook hands waved goodbye to the other three patients and went on my way perplexed. Why did this committed Christian refuse to pray with me at such a difficult time in his life? Some weeks later I met him after an out patient appointment and asked how he was getting on. Before replying he said how sorry he was for rejecting my invitation to pray with him. He went on to explain that it had been such a terrible shock to discover the tumour so soon after starting out on a ministry that he had really wanted from his youth. To have prayed openly with me in that unit would have meant that he would then have had to bring his message to the other three patients. At that moment his own inner turmoil was such that he just needed time to come to terms with what was going on in his life without having the pressure of wanting to tell others about his faith. In this instance I had made wrong assumptions and this led me to focusing on what I perceived to be the patient's religious needs to the exclusion of his spiritual ones.

Care must be taken to ensure that both are addressed in a balanced and sensitive way. Hindsight is a wonderful gift, what would have been more helpful might well have been to have taken the patient into a quiet room off the ward where he could have shared both his spiritual and religious needs away from the ever watchful eyes and ears of other patients.

## 11.2.3 Questions, questions, and even more questions

When a patient is seeking to make sense of what is happening to them they will ask themselves and may ask others a host of questions. Questions often begin with an adverb such as 'how' or 'where', or 'when'. The most powerful of them all is 'why'. It is all too easy for those working in a healthcare setting to proffer an immediate answer to a patient's questions. Yet for many of the 'why' questions there is no ready answer. We may be able to answer why a patient's dialysis is no longer effective, i.e. vascular access is no longer possible and why it has come to this point. But why with this particular patient at this particular point in their life is not a question that we can even begin to answer. It is here that we must be prepared to say that we just do not know. For some faith groups sense is made of such an awful position by stating that it is the will of God. For many of our patients the struggle to make sense of what is happening to them is not satisfied by such a faith position. Their agony can only be helped by the listener staying with the patient's questioning and not running away from the pain that is engendered. Helping a patient by just being there as they seek to find words to articulate their innermost distress is fundamental to spiritual care at every level.

Many patients talk of their fear not of death but of dying. It is often a fear of a painful and undignified death. The great advances in palliative care over recent decades have gone a long way to ensure that no patient need die in physical pain any longer. However, it is not for us to decide for a patient that they should be pain free at the expense of all else.

## Case study

A 72-year-old widow dying slowly of end-stage renal failure had one son now living in Australia. She had not seen him for 26 years. He was flying across to see his mother but would not arrive until the following day. The staff felt that she would benefit from analgesia and sedation. However, her wish was to see and speak with her son. Care and expertise needed to be used in order that her wishes could be observed. It meant that until she and her son could have some time together her physical pain could not be as effectively controlled as the team would have wished. As a result of listening to her needs and respecting them she was able to be with her son in a way that meant so much to them both.

### 11.2.4 Peace and reconciliation

As a patient struggles with his disease and the prospect of death it is often the case that part of his or her spiritual struggle is with events that have taken place in the past that have never been resolved. The patient may not know how to put things right, or believe that it is too late to make amends. Memories can come flooding back that feel unbearable. A patient's agitated state may be as much to do with the past as with their present circumstances and imminent death. Helping patients talk through their painful past is an important part of their spiritual care. It may be that they are torn apart by something they did, they said, or even thought which was hurtful to someone else. The person concerned may no longer be available for them to see and they are at a loss to know what to do. Feelings of guilt can become so great that the patient does not know how to cope. In such cases, those from within a religious background may be helped by a recognized ritual such as sacramental confession. For those without such a framework just verbalizing what is troubling them to someone who is non-judgmental can in itself be all that is required. The reverse may also be the case, i.e. the patient is the one who has been wronged and has never come to terms with what took place. Here bitterness, anger, and depression may be mistakenly attributed to the patient's disease pathway rather than to an event or events that took place many years before. By telling their story slowly and perhaps over and over again the patient may begin to come to terms with all that had happened. The listener should be slow to reassure and to justify what took place, rather he or she needs to be present with the telling of the story, however painful and upsetting that might be. Acceptance and forgiveness can come about but they are both slow and painful processes.

Making present the past, in the presence of another and facing it head on can be a truly healing experience. To be at peace with oneself as death beckons has always been seen as most desirable. For some this will never be so, yet it is possible to facilitate it. Clinicians as well as chaplains may find opportunities with their patients to offer the support and encouragement needed for them to face the painful past in order that they may be more at peace with the present so as to accept the future with courage.

### 11.2.5 Meeting a patient's spiritual needs is a two-way process

Very often renal patients have been associated with a renal unit for months or years. Their disease may have taken a long time to run its course. Doctors, nurses, and associated healthcare professionals will usually get to know much about such patient's families and friends and history. They can almost become part of the furniture! Staff may become very attached to such patients, which can be a positive experience but also a source of stress. Being with another person as they seek to come to terms with what is happening to them as a result of their disease has a cost to doctors and nurses. How we are with thoughts about our own mortality can help or hinder our involvement. The patient may remind us of a member of our own family who has gone through a similar illness. This may be extremely painful for us and we may avoid any references to death and dying because of this. The patient may also remind us of someone close to us now and this can be traumatic. 'It could be my wife or my child in that bed.' Again such painful projections can lead the clinician to avoid any mention of issues relating to the patient's spiritual needs. My own father died after many months of illness in an intensive care unit (ITU). Treatment was withdrawn as my mother and I sat by his bed. He died peacefully and with dignity. However, when I was next called to ITU to be with a family in a similar situation I found it extremely painful and difficult to be there with them fully. The emotional and spiritual cost to clinicians can be large. It is vital, therefore, that appropriate support networks, including the provision of spiritual care to the team, and a system of clinical supervision are readily available. This is not only necessary for the well-being of the clinician but will also ensure that a patient's spiritual needs are not overlooked because of any unresolved issues raised for team members.

It is also important to note that any supportive care of the patient will also include their closest family members and carers. They too will be struggling to make sense of what is happening to their loved one. It may well be that clinicians spend as much if not more time with family and friends than with the patient grappling with issues related to spiritual needs. Again it is here that referral to a spiritual caregiver may be the most appropriate form of action. To care for and support the patient will always include support of their family and friends. All in all the support of a renal patient as they move towards the end of their life is a complex web, involving staff, relatives, and friends. It is support that will take many forms and will vary from patient to patient.

### 11.2.6 Final brush strokes

I have tried to 'paint' my picture of the spiritual and religious needs of a renal patient that should be part and parcel of the supportive care offered by clinicians. As with all portraits it will be clear which of those aspects are particularly important to me as a hospital chaplain. It would be presumptuous of me to tell patients what to believe and how to address their spiritual agonies. However, it is a great privilege to be invited into a patient's life at such a personal and deep level. By actively listening to their searching questions, I hope, that should they ask me how I make sense of my life in relation to God and the universe, I might be able to share with them a sense of hope and peace that gives them courage to face all that lies before them.

## 11.3 Portrait two: spiritual and religious issues from the perspective of a US clinician

### Case study

KF is a 79-year-old man with longstanding insulin-dependent diabetes, renal insufficiency, and peripheral vascular disease. He has been maintained on haemodialysis for the past 3 years and has needed bilateral below-knee amputations. Bouts of severe depression in the past have usually responded to antidepressant medication. Vascular access has become progressively more difficult and within the past 4 months, two vascular grafts have become unusable, despite multiple procedures.

He recently moved into the home of his daughter and her family as 3 months previously his wife of 27 years died suddenly of a stroke, plunging him into grief and depression. He now feels an increasing burden on his daughter and her family. He has a strong Christian faith, but has been unable to attend church regularly because his health problems have led to difficulties in access. During a routine visit

**Case study** *(continued)*

with the dialysis social worker, KF asked about the option of discontinuing dialysis. He asked her whether it was allowed, and how it was different from suicide. After consulting with his nephrologist, the social worker and a peer counsellor[4] began meeting him over a period of weeks and listened to his concerns. He had many questions concerning what would happen and how he would be cared for if he were to stop dialysis. He was particularly concerned about his daughter and her family. Hospice referral was made to respond to his questions. The hospice medical director spoke to his doctor and recommended a modest adjustment in his dose of antidepressant medication. The hospice chaplain contacted his congregation and encouraged the minister to visit.

The minister visited the very next day and was apologetic that he had not known of KF's recent misfortunes. They prayed together. This visit affirmed his sense of worth and the minister arranged for him to be visited by members of the congregation's caring committee. Transportation was arranged and he was able again to attend services each Sunday.

On a follow-up visit, the hospice chaplain asked KF, 'What is most important to you in your life now?' He readily responded that God, his children, and his grandchildren are what give his life meaning. Working with the chaplain he was able to identify specific tasks he wanted to accomplish. He had in mind gifts of memorabilia and a photo album of his and their grandmother's early life he wanted to assemble for his family, especially his grandchildren. The church's caring committee members helped and he found the projects enjoyable and meaningful. Through informal life review, KF developed a sense of how much he had contributed to others—his family, friends and community—and gradually came to accept their love and support. His depression lifted and he again engaged in life, exhibiting a renewed sense of self-worth. He assumed the responsibility of after-school childcare for his two grandchildren.

Through this process he came to feel that nothing was left unsaid, and to accept his new life, with all its difficulties. Although discontinuation of dialysis remains a consideration and may become necessary if vascular access is lost, KF now has a sense of worth and value in his current life.

## 11.3.1 Interior realms: responding to mystery, seeking meaning and connection

Spirituality is an inherent aspect of the human condition. Our ability to reflect upon ourselves, our lives, and our relationships to others and to the world embeds the human experience with spiritual dimensions. This is not a philosophical assertion as much as it is an anthropologic fact. In the devoutly secular culture of American medicine, the existence of spirituality as a fundamental feature of humankind cannot be emphasized too strongly. A person may choose to characterize him- or herself as 'religious' or 'spiritual'. An individual's cultural heritage and upbringing, as well as his or her unique preferences and perspectives, influence that person's specific beliefs and the level of interest and intensity of feeling invested in the spiritual aspects of life. Labels such as 'religious', 'spiritual', 'non-religious', 'atheist', or 'existentialist' may convey information, at times clinically useful, about the individual's interest and particular beliefs. However, any person with the capacity for self-awareness and reflection must be assumed to have aspects of his or her life experience that can properly be termed, spiritual.

The realms of the interior and transcendent commonly swell in proportion to other aspects of life for persons living with progressive illness, and they can be sources of solace or suffering. It is, therefore, especially important for clinicians who care for patients with life-limiting conditions to develop a vocabulary and some familiarity with spiritual domains of patients' experiences.

Definitions and terms are critical to discussing spirituality. Often the words spirituality and religion are used interchangeably. Here the term spirituality is used to refer to experiences, thoughts, and emotions that arise in response to mystery, pertain to a source of meaning, or a sense of connection to something larger than oneself, and which extends into an open-ended future. The drive to seek meaning and a connection as a response to the at times awe-inspiring and at times terrifying mystery of life is rooted in the depths of the human psyche. There is value in considering meaning and connection to be distinct; however, these constructs are frequently intertwined. A person's connection to God or to country, for instance, may also provide him or her with a predominant source of meaning.

Religion refers to a combination of beliefs, values, eschatology, knowledge, techniques, rituals, customs, and practices which foster a sense of connection and meaning and a way of dealing with the mystery of existence. Religion may be thought of as a way human beings have reached out to one another, in community and across generations, in confronting primal issues of life and death. Particular religions often involve specific beliefs related to a supreme being, but some, including Taoism, Shintosim, and Buddhism, do not include a belief in a deity. Therefore, someone may describe themself as religious but not believe in a God.

People who have a deep religious faith often find it affords a well of strength and source of comfort in dealing with injury, illness, disability, caregiving, death, and grief. In some circumstances, however, religion can be at the root of a person's suffering causing an individual to feel that his or her illness or misfortunes are caused by some moral failing or the lack of sufficient faith. Any such dilemmas need to be addressed with a patient with due care and sensitivity.

## 11.3.2 Spiritual care is integral to supportive and palliative care

Spiritual care is an integral part of whole-person supportive and palliative care for patients with end-stage renal disease. When a person is confronted with the new diagnosis of a life-limiting illness or when a serious complication of long-standing illness raises the possibility of death, questions of spiritual content often acquire special relevance and urgency.

'Why is this happening to me? Why now? What caused this illness or injury? Is there some deeper meaning to this misfortune? What is my life worth now that I cannot do the things I used to? What has my life meant to myself, to others? Will I be remembered, and if so, how will I be remembered? What will happen after I die? Does "life"—my existence and self-awareness—really end, or will I awake in an afterlife? How does God view my life and me? What does God want from me in this situation?'

Some of these questions carry obvious religious assumptions and invite further inquiry and response within the context of a person's religious orientation. Others among these questions when stated in written form sound distinctly philosophical. However, for a person living with the symptoms, functional limitations, and emotional and social consequences of serious illness, these questions arise from the physical reality and mundane events of daily life.

## 11.3.3 Meaning

Although the concept of meaning is central to the definition of spirituality offered here, and has profound importance for clinicians engaged in spiritual assessment and care, the word 'meaning' may never cross a patient's lips. People universally have a sense of meaning, or suffer from the lack of meaning, but they may not think in such terms. Many people do ponder meaning of and in their lives; however, meaning or its absence is predominantly felt. Far from being a merely philosophical construct, a person facing the end of life may have a visceral sense of meaning that is related to tangible entities, events, and people in his or her life. A father of three grown children, who are all successful with young children of their own, need only look around the room at a family gathering to feel a sense of meaning about his life. That sense of satisfaction may be eroded when he considers his failures in business, the loss of his children's inheritance in bad investments, or perhaps through gambling. The myriad of influences that shape an individual's life and sense of meaning are diverse and unique. Yet this uniqueness does not exclude elemental commonalties. Cassell's construct of personhood encompasses an individual's physical body and emotional temperament, as well as his or her past, cultural heritage, habits and aversions, family, hopes and fears, and sense of the transcendent.[5] This multidimensional concept of personhood suggests predictable aspects of life in which both contributors to and detractors from meaning may reside. Accomplishments, failures, the people we have loved and lost, as well as those we have hated, all have roles in shaping a person's sense of themselves and their sense of meaning.

## 11.3.4 Therapeutic implications of the drive to make meaning

An inventory of contributions and barriers to meaning suggests a basic therapeutic strategy. If meaning is central to spiritual well-being, it follows that helping people to identify meaning in their lives is essential to achieving that process. A meaning-based interview can identify sources of satisfaction and pride as well as areas of regret and shame. Most often this takes the form of life review. The word meaning may or may not be used at all. The most direct question, 'What gives your life meaning?' may evoke a long and cogent reflection on life from one person and shrugged shoulders from another. 'What is most important to you in life?' may be more likely to yield a response.

  Many people will readily identify the things in their lives they are most proud of and, along the way, mention things they wish they had done differently. In providing spiritual care to patients with life-threatening conditions, it is important to listen sensitively and avoid probing to uncover old wounds that have not been mentioned. Life review is not insight therapy. People need not sift through an inventory of failures to reach some predetermined spiritual goal. Within a developmental approach, our goal is to help people to achieve a sense of meaning. They can be helped to grieve, forgive and let go of the sad, tragic, painful, and shameful regrets of the past. I often reflect to patients that none of us is perfect. We are just human. When feelings of regret or shame or lack of worth are contributing to a person's suffering, I may ask the person to have some mercy. 'If you were reading this story as a biographical novel, how would you feel toward the main character? Can you please bring yourself a little mercy?'

## 11.3.5 Listening: the principal skill of spiritual care

Listening is the fundamental skill necessary for effective spiritual care. As a physician, I inevitably bring my own taxonomy and conceptual way of thinking about spiritual experience to the clinical encounter. However, it is important for me to learn how the patient thinks and talks about issues of mystery, meaning, and connection so that I may discuss these matters in his or her own terms. Here again, labels people choose in describing their perspectives and beliefs can help, but it is prudent to assume that not every Catholic, Jew, or Buddhist thinks like every other, or has adopted the world view of their religious heritage. It is wise to explore how each patient's religion or philosophical stance is uniquely experienced and understood by them.

## 11.3.6 Connection

Humans share an inherent drive to feel connected. While relatively few people believe in immortality *per se*, it is nearly universal to seek a connection to some thing or to people who will remember us after we have gone. The sense of connection to something larger than oneself that will endure into an open-ended future is the basis for transcendence. For many people the sense of connection to God is vibrant and in itself is a response to the mystery.

This sense of connection to a supreme being has been described as a feeling that, 'mother is at home'. It is a confident sense of being loved, of being cared for.

It is not necessary to have a belief in God to have a passionate sense of connection. Dr Ned Cassem (personal communication, 2002) asks, 'Is there anyone or anything you would be willing to die for?' An individual's answer to this question may point toward a secular source of felt connection that transcends the boundaries of the person's finite life.

For many people, their family and the community of their friends and acquaintances provides a sense of connection that will endure beyond their life and death. When someone tells stories from her past, the process contributes to a sense of meaning about her life. In recording or otherwise preserving her life stories, she is creating an heirloom for her children, grandchildren, and generations yet to come. For people who are physically debilitated and feeling a burden to others, the preserving and conveying of their personal history can be a tangible way of continuing to contribute to their family and community. In this way the connection to others is strengthened in a manner that not even death can destroy.

Not uncommonly, patients tell me that they are comforted by knowing that they will be buried on a plot of earth that has been in their family for generations; or that their ashes will be scattered from a peak or at a high mountain lake that has special importance for them. This sense of connection to nature and the understanding that their physical self will go back into the earth has value, dare I say meaning, for them.

The fundamental way in which clinicians can contribute to a patient's sense of connection is to remain involved. Many times in the past, when cure is no longer possible, patients have described feeling abandoned by their doctors. An often quoted American phrase is one that holds that 'ninety-five percent of life is "showing up"'. It is certainly true in the realm of care for patients nearing the end of life. As clinicians, being present at the bedside or at the home of an ill and possibly dying person provides tangible evidence that we care; that the person still matters to us.

## 11.3.7 The developmental approach to spiritual experience with progressive, incurable illness

The uniqueness and individuality of each person is not diminished by recognizing that there are elemental commonalties within the human experience of living with the knowledge of the approach of death. By building on the methodologies and knowledge base of childhood development and developmental psychology, the conceptual framework and terminology of human development can be used as a valuable clinical tool for approaching the personal experience of life-threatening illness and injury. The developmental approach encompasses spiritual dimensions of experience and offers a robust framework for assessment and individualized, patient-centred intervention, and a well-established foundation for clinical research. Since the concept of life-long human development is commonly taught in primary and secondary schools, it also provides a familiar vocabulary for clinical training.

If human development is life-long, it follows that people may grow, or suffer developmental delays, during the latter stages of life, just as they might at its beginning. A schema of relevant developmental landmarks and task-work enables practical and clinically meaningful assessment of individual patients in a manner that informs therapeutic intervention (Box 11.1).[6]

An important advantage of a developmental approach is that it is not confined, as is the problem-based approach to medical care. Although all too common, suffering is only one pole of human experience associated with nearness to death. Personal experience associated with illness and dying extends from suffering on the one hand to a heightened sense of well-being on the other. Suffering in the context of end-stage illness may involve pain and other physical distress, but often extends to the realms of spirit. Suffering has been described as a sense of impending disintegration[5] based on a felt loss of meaning and purpose in life. In the resulting isolation that accompanies the gradual destruction of one's sense of value and purpose and in the resulting isolation that follows its loss, all suffering is spiritual. Pain is just pain if one knows it will end, and if it doesn't threaten the integrity of one's self and one's place in family and community. Recognizing the myriad potential sources of suffering experienced by our patients, and encountering so much suffering in the course of our busy clinical practices, can at times make it seem that suffering is inevitable, and the best we can do is make it a little less intolerable. Sometimes that is true; however, our clinical models of human experience are challenged to accommodate the empiric evidence that some individuals experience preserved or even heightened quality of life in the face of death.

We may be helped to understand our patient's experiences through the words of others such as Dr Roger Bone, an eminent American pulmonologist, who wrote during the months in which he was living with progressive, incurable renal cancer:[8]

> Death has opened my eyes to life—literally. Since learning that I have a terminal illness, I believe that my mind has expanded and its appetite has become insatiable. I want to know and experience everything. . . . No life is without gift, even when it may seem giftless to others. Contemplation and introspection in the context of nature have brought me to a point of enlightenment I would probably not have had under other circumstances. Cancer has allowed me a measure of insight.

## Box 11.1 Developmental landmarks and task-work for life closure

### Sense of completion with worldly affairs

◆ Transfer of fiscal, legal, and formal social responsibilities.

### Sense of completion of relationships with community

◆ Closure of multiple social relationships (employment, commerce, organizational, congregational).

◆ Components include: expressions of regret, expressions of forgiveness, acceptance of gratitude and appreciation.

◆ Leave taking; the saying of goodbyes.

### Sense of meaning about one's individual life

◆ Life review.

◆ The telling of 'one's stories'.

◆ Transmission of knowledge and wisdom.

### Experienced love of self

◆ Self-acknowledgement.

◆ Self-forgiveness.

**Box 11.1 Developmental landmarks and task-work for life closure** *(continued)*

## Experienced love of others

♦ Acceptance of worthiness

## Sense of completion in relationships with family and friends

♦ Reconciliation, fullness of communication and closure in each of one's important relationships.

♦ Component tasks include: expressions of regret, expressions of forgiveness and acceptance, expressions of gratitude and appreciation, acceptance of gratitude and appreciation, expressions of affection.

♦ Leave-taking; the saying of goodbyes.

## Acceptance of the finality of life—of one's existence as an individual

♦ Acknowledgement of the totality of personal loss represented by one's dying and experience of personal pain of existential loss.

♦ Expression of the depth of personal tragedy that dying represents.

♦ Decathexis (emotional withdrawal) from worldly affairs and cathexis (emotional connection) with an enduring construct.

♦ Acceptance of dependency.

## Sense of a new self (person hood) beyond personal loss

♦ Developing self-awareness in the present.

## Sense of meaning about life in general

♦ Achieving a sense of awe.

♦ Recognition of a transcendent realm.

♦ Developing/achieving a sense of comfort with chaos.

## Surrender to the transcendent, to the unknown—'letting go'

♦ In accomplishing this last landmark, the doer and 'task-work' are one. Ultimately, little remains of the ego except the volition to surrender.

Marie de Hennezel observed:[9]

> Life has taught me three things: The first is that I cannot escape my own death or the deaths of the people I love. The second is that no human being can be reduced to what we see, or think we see. Any person is infinitely larger, and deeper, than our narrow judgements can discern. And third: he or she can never be considered to have uttered the final word on anything, is always developing, always has the power of self-fulfilment, and a capacity for self-transformation through all the crises and trials of life.

Understanding how some individuals who are approaching death are able to transition from experiencing a sense of meaninglessness and impending annihilation to a sense of wholeness and 'well-ness' has profound practical implications for psychosocial and spiritual assessments and interventions. If a sense of impending disintegration and the loss of meaning underlie suffering, it is not surprising that a sense of well-being involves the preserved or enhanced sense of integrity and meaning. We can aid people in developing a sense of meaning about their life and life in general. For instance, clinicians and trained volunteers can work with patients on life review and the recording of stories. We can help people explore things that they feel would be left undone if they were to die suddenly. It is often important to people to complete relationships with others who have been important to them in the past. At times this involves resolving past differences. Care providers can help patients make contact with significant others and assist with correspondence, phone calls, or travel arrangements.

As spheres of a person's life become less relevant to their changed situations, they can be completed and released. We can assist people to complete these tasks. In this manner, a person need not disintegrate, but may instead be thought of as becoming less 'corporeal' and progressively more 'ethereal' over time. The metaphor of a person dissolving out of life well describes the peaceful, transcendent deaths palliative care professionals and others sometimes witness.

Families suffering the recent or impending loss of a loved one also have needs and opportunities in spiritual realms. In approaching the death of a beloved friend or relative, people may struggle amidst sadness to find some meaning in the tragedy. Belief systems may help people cope with tragedy and death and religious teachings often provide guidance to those who grieve.

People naturally look for ways to develop a lasting sense of connection to the person. Religious traditions offer prayers, holidays, and memorial customs as ways of establishing and maintaining a sense of connection. Common informal customs include collecting photos, stories, heirlooms, and ashes of the deceased.

In each age and culture our innate human drive to make meaning and seek connection finds relevant expression. One strategy is in some way to deliberately invest the tragedy with meaning. An example of a secular practice that has become fairly common for making meaning from a seemingly senseless death is for the family and friends to establish a scholarship fund or annual event to benefit others in a manner that reflects the deceased's values. In modern America, I have observed in my own practice several family members thoughtfully design and undergo tattoos that memorialize loved ones they've lost. And finally, in a typically American fashion, one company has recently begun offering to manufacture individual cubic zirconium, or manmade diamonds, from carbon of the person's ashes. Those who wish, and can afford to, can wear a bit of their loved one on their finger, from a pendant or as earrings.

## 11.3.8 Final brush strokes

The specific work that a person feels a need for, or interest in doing, as they confront life's end will vary. The end-of-life developmental landmarks and the task-work that underlies them are intended to represent predictable personal challenges as well as important opportunities for people as they die. The general developmental approach can provide a valuable map to clinicians through the inherently difficult landscape of the dying experience and end-of-life care.

Importantly, within this model one need not sanitize nor glorify the experience of life's end to think of a person as having achieved a degree of wellness in their dying. Personal development is rarely easy. The touchstone of dying well is that the experience has value and is meaningful for the person and their family.

## 11.4 Conclusion

Two distinct yet complementary portraits of the spiritual and religious care of the renal patient have been offered in this chapter. Much of what has been written will apply to patients whatever their illness or disease.

It is to be hoped that readers will be encouraged to develop their own portrait of spirituality and religion that will enable them to address the needs of their patients and patients' families as carefully as possible.

The two portraits both highlight the search for meaning as central to any understanding of a person's spirituality. Equally significant is the need to assess a patient's spiritual needs in the context of their home environment, culture, and religious faith (if they have one). The importance of significant others to the patient will also be crucial to the support offered by healthcare professionals.

It is important to note that at times, however hard we try to meet such needs, a patient may die without resolving some if not all of the issues encompassed by the terms 'spiritual' and 'religious'. That does not detract from the importance of making sure that we are aware that, for many people, spiritual and religious experience is a fundamental part of their daily life. It is essential that as healthcare professionals we seek to care for the whole person and not just the disease; that we find ways of asking and then assessing a patient's spiritual and religious needs and opportunities, and that we use the services of spiritual caregivers such as chaplains who are a vital part of the multidisciplinary team to assist in this aspect of care.

As a patient travels along the renal disease trajectory from diagnosis to death clinicians can monitor their spiritual needs and experience at every point. Careful listening to what is going on at that moment for the patient, both what is said and what is not said, will enable the clinician to make an assessment of the appropriate support that should be offered. Whether that support is received and made use of will, in the last analysis, be up to the patient. That is only right and fitting.

As with all aspects of palliative care, and indeed all of medicine, those involved need the support of others. This is especially true when it comes to being with patients who are grappling with the deep and painful questions encompassed by the terms 'spiritual' and 'religious'. It is important that whatever one's own orientation to such matters there should be no hesitation in calling on the services of chaplains and spiritual caregivers to support not only the patient and their relatives and friends but also the professional caregiver.

## Ethical analysis

In any ethical analysis, attention to the patient's values and preferences is central. The recent medical literature documents that patients' spiritual values are more important to them than previously appreciated. In the United States, research shows that 95% of patients believe in God. Focus group research of patients and families indicates that at the end of life patients and families have broader—psychosocial and spiritual—concerns than physicians' often narrow tendency to focus on physical matters. The

**Ethical analysis** *(continued)*

authors of this chapter do well to stress that physicians should take the spiritual needs of their patients seriously and ensure that they are addressed. In this regard, the case of the 72-year-old widow whose son was flying in from Australia is instructive. The physicians were concerned about treating the widow's pain, but the widow was more concerned about being mentally alert for the visit from her son, whom she had not seen in 26 years. Physicians need to understand that patients' values may differ from physicians', and physicians should not underestimate the significance of achieving a patient's spiritual goals in providing treatment to them.

Similarly, the case of KF demonstrates how important having meaning in one's life is to one's overall well-being. KF was on the verge of discontinuing dialysis when interventions by the hospice chaplain and KF's minister helped him to see how continuing to live after his wife's sudden death could have meaning and value for himself and his family. Asking questions is key to helping patients understand the meaning of their lives. The hospice chaplain asked, 'What is most important to you in your life now?' Other helpful questions include 'What might be left undone if you were to die today?' and 'What legacy do you want to leave to your family?'[10] As was accomplished in the case of KF, the goal of a spiritual intervention is to see the patient as a person and help the patient appreciate his/her worth. The 'Patient as person history' presented in the Introduction is also helpful toward this end.

# References

1. NHS Management Executive (1992). *Meeting the Spiritual Needs of Patients and Staff: Good Practice Guide.* London: Department of Health.
2. Speck, P. (1998). *Being There.,* London: SPCK Publishers.
3. Frankl, V.E. (1987 edition) Man's search for Meaning. London: Hodder and Stoughton.
4. Kapron, K., Perry, E., Bowman, T., Swartz, R.D. (1997). Peer resource consulting: redesigning a new future. *Adv. Renal Replacement Ther.,* **4**(3): 267–74.
5. Cassel, E.J. (1982). The nature of suffering and the goals of medicine. *New Engl. J. Med.,* **306**(11): 639–45.
6. Byock, I.R. (1997). *Dying Well: the Prospect for Growth at the End of Life.* New York: Riverhead.
7. Byock, I.R. (1996). The nature of suffering and the nature of opportunity at the end of life. *Clin. Geriatric Med.,* **12**(2): 237–52.
8. Bone, R.C. (1996). A piece of my mind. Maumee: my Walden Pond. *J. Am. Med. Assoc.,* **276**(24): 1931.
9. de Hennezel, M. (1997). *Intimate Death: How the Dying Teach Us How to Live.* New York: Knopf.
10. Lo, B., Quill, T., Tulsky, J. (1999). Discussing palliative care with patients. *Ann. Intern. Med.,* **14**: 27–34.

Chapter 12

# Support of the home dialysis patient

Alastair Hutchison and Helen Hirst

## 12.1 Introduction

The development of the Scribner dialysis shunt in the early 1960s made intermittent haemodialysis treatment possible, in both North America and Europe, for people who would otherwise have died. Despite specifically identified funding, dialysis was only available in a few centres so that only people who were considered 'socially worthy' by hospital select committees were given this scarce and expensive treatment.[1] Consequently during the 1960s the haemodialysis population consisted mainly of white, married, well-educated men, who were less than 50 years of age.[2–5] However, as the spaces within dialysis centres were filled, it became common for patients and their spouses (or other family members) to be trained to perform haemodialysis at home, thereby allowing many more patients access to treatment.[6] The number of dialysis patients in the United States increased from around 300 in 1965, to nearly 3000 by 1969 of whom more than 1000 were dialysing at home.[7]

Even in these early years it rapidly became apparent that patients and their carers experienced a variety of psychological stresses associated with home haemodialysis, and that it demanded a degree of technical expertise and psychological resilience beyond that of any other treatment available then or now. Some patients were reported to resist all efforts to train them, and others took many more months than expected.[1] Once a patient was established at home it became clear that carer-assistants experienced as much, or possibly more, anxiety, in particular relating to the possibility of their spouse dying during dialysis.[8] The investigating psychiatrists highlighted the fact that home haemodialysis necessitated a spouse carrying out a treatment that is both life-saving and potentially lethal on their partner. During the 1970s there was a dramatic increase in home haemodialysis patients with an increasing number of female patients whose employed husbands were not available as carer-assistants. Furthermore, in the United States Medicare legislation included some economic disincentives to home treatment and consequently the percentage of patients dialysing themselves declined from 40% in 1972 to 13% in 1979. Nevertheless health professionals, most notably nurses, social workers, and psychologists, began to design studies to examine the impact of home dialysis on patients and their families using conceptualizations derived from systems theory.[9] In turn clinicians described interventions that focused on helping family assistants adapt to their situations through support groups and improved communication with their spouse. Gradually an understanding of the support required by a home dialysis patient and his or her family began to evolve.

The development of continuous ambulatory peritoneal dialysis (CAPD) in the late 1970s radically altered the nature of home dialysis and made it available to many patients who would previously not have been considered, including a greater proportion of women. CAPD had minimal capital costs compared with home haemodialysis and the training period of 1 to 2 weeks was vastly shorter than the 3 to 4 months required for haemodialysis. In addition no carer-assistant was thought to be required if the patient was otherwise able-bodied. However, in time it became evident that older patients and those with significant additional co-morbidity did require the help of a carer, and that generally this was a female member of the family—wives, daughters, and even adult sisters.

Full rehabilitation of home dialysis patients (return to gainful employment, full-time studies, or homemaking) has been shown to be difficult, but equally possible amongst haemodialysis and CAPD patients. Rubin *et al.*[10] found no significant differences between dialysis modalities in this respect, whilst acknowledging that the majority of patients were not rehabilitated.

In order to understand the support required for a home dialysis patient, whether on CAPD or haemodialysis, healthcare professionals require a significant understanding of the family relationships involved, as well as an awareness of stereotypical role expectations which can vary from one family to another, and are influenced by a variety of cultural and ethnic factors.[11] It has been emphasized that many health professionals reinforce the belief that women are responsible for family care-giving so that a wife may be expected to take on the role of dialysis assistant where a husband would not. Similarly it was noted that a husband assisting his wife to dialyse was invariably offered in-home cleaning services, care services, and community resources, whereas a wife assisting her husband often did not receive or ask for such help.

The collective findings of a variety of studies leave no doubt that home dialysis has always been a complex and stressful experience for patients and their families.[1] Over the past 25 years the dialysis population has become increasingly elderly and suffers from multiple complex and debilitating medical problems as outlined in the case study at the end of this chapter. Long-term survival is not a serious consideration for many patients taken on to home dialysis programmes despite selection of patients. Nevertheless, advanced care planning in patients with chronic kidney disease remains woefully inadequate considering that the average annual mortality for all dialysis patients is around 25%.[12] The modification of the 'Sheffield model' for renal palliative care implicitly acknowledges that life expectancy is significantly shortened by end-stage renal disease, and that increasing support therapies will be required in time, for all patients (see Fig. 12.1 and Table 12.1). This model emphasizes the importance of advance planning and provides a useful template for healthcare professionals to apply to home dialysis patients, accepting that dialysis is not a curative treatment and that the nature of the required support changes with time. Although certain features of supporting a home dialysis patient are

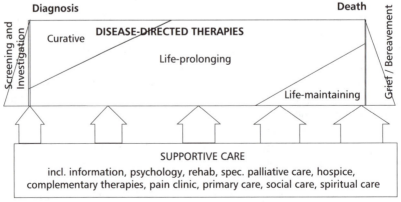

**Fig. 12.1** The Sheffield model of palliative care.

**Table 12.1** Comprehensive supportive care as described by the Sheffield model

| |
|---|
| Primary care team |
| Physiotherapy and occupational therapy |
| Psychology |
| Rehabilitation |
| Dietetics |
| Social Work |
| Chaplaincy |
| Pain Clinic |
| Complementary therapies |
| Information services |
| Palliative care |

unique to the home environment, many of the other chapters within this book will be of direct relevance. For example the symptoms of renal disease, sexual problems, psychological and psychiatric considerations, and the use of advance directives are no different for the home patient than for the 'in-centre' patient.

## 12.2 Selection of home dialysis patients

It is self-evident that not all patients are suitable for home dialysis, either because they are unable or unwilling to dialyse themselves, or because their home circumstances are unsuitable. However, in the UK, the National Institute for Clinical Excellence (NICE) (on behalf of the government) has recently published guidance for healthcare professionals on the location in which haemodialysis is carried out.[13] Although use of home haemodialysis has declined compared to its peak in the early 1970s, NICE recommends that 'all suitable patients should be offered the choice between home haemodialysis or haemodialysis in a hospital'. The guidance[13] alludes to selection of suitable patients, stating that patients suitable for home haemodialysis will be those who:

- have the ability and motivation to learn to carry out the process and the commitment to maintain treatment;
- are stable on dialysis;
- are free of complications and significant concomitant disease that would render home haemodialysis unsuitable or unsafe;
- have good functioning vascular access;
- have a carer who has (or carers who have) also made an informed decision to assist with the haemodialysis unless the individual is able to manage on his or her own;
- have suitable space and facilities or an area that could be adapted within their home environment.

The guidance also states that patients and their carers 'will require initial training and an accessible and responsive support service'. It does not identify how to assess ability, motivation, commitment, stability on dialysis, ability to make an informed decision, or what constitutes an accessible and responsive support service. Nevertheless it is clear that support and training for the patient and their family should ideally begin in this 'pre-dialysis' phase in order that a firm bond of trust is built. Conversely, failure to address a patient's perceived problems at this stage, or, for example, failure to plan and create dialysis access appropriately, will result in a loss of confidence that may not be recoverable later. Under such circumstances, establishing a patient on home dialysis may become almost impossible.

## 12.2.1 Pre-dialysis education

A prospective home dialysis patient needs to have sufficient knowledge, skill, and ability to carry out their treatment regimen without direct supervision from healthcare personnel. Therefore patient education is an important component in the management of end-stage renal disease (ESRD).[14] The suitability or otherwise of a patient for home dialysis may first become apparent during the process of pre-dialysis education (Table 12.2).

A review of the literature shows that a number of different models have been used for patient education[15–18] but most include information on dialysis techniques and modalities, the impact on patients' and families' lives, plus information about the local renal unit and available resources. Commonly cited goals include informed choice of treatment options, decreased anxiety for patients and their families, and enhanced self-care strategies. Klang *et al.*[19] evaluated the effects of a pre-dialysis patient education programme on functioning and well-being in 28 uraemic patients and compared them with an age- and sex-matched group of patients who had not been through the programme. She found participating patients to have better mood, fewer mobility problems, fewer functional disabilities, and lower levels of anxiety compared with controls. These differences disappeared after 6 months on dialysis, but it is not clear whether this was because the control group improved or the 'educated' group slipped back. However, the initial 6 months of home dialysis are perhaps the most important, as the patient and carers learn to adapt to a radically new home environment, so that the benefits listed above could only be helpful.

## 12.2.2 Training for home dialysis and the patient's role in treatment

Although technological advances have simplified many aspects of dialysis over the past 30 years, the statement of Lancaster in 1979 concerning home dialysis remains true in the 21st century: 'No other chronic illness in today's society requires as many diet restrictions, as many medications, or as large a volume of technical knowledge as is required for the patient with end-stage renal disease'.[20] However, self-care moves the patient away from traditional medical paternalism, fostering dependence and the sick role, and offers a positive approach to adaptation to a

**Table 12.2** Process of establishing home dialysis

| |
|---|
| Pre-dialysis education programme |
| Training for patient and helper |
| Input from nursing staff, dietician, social worker, clinician, dialysis technician |
| Conversion of suitable area in home for dialysis and storage |
| Transition to home dialysis with community renal nurse (CRN) assistance |
| Independent home dialysis with visits from CRN |

chronic illness. It involves patient control over treatment and a choice of therapies.[21] Its medium- and long-term aim is to place the patient back in their own environment and to make them independent, to the fullest extent possible, of the hospital environment and the sick role. In so doing it makes the patient and their carer the 'experts' and equips them to prevent, or deal with, the majority of likely complications. The restoration of confidence to a previously devastated life can be almost miraculous to witness, but it requires a highly organized and skilful team to do so.

Methods employed in training patients for home dialysis are outside the scope of this chapter, but it is vital to realize the importance of the bond of trust and friendship that should develop between trainer and trainee. All of us remember our teachers, both good and bad, from our past education and realize the impact that the relationship can have on eventual 'grades'. So it is with the home dialysis trainee. A good trainer will inspire confidence and trust, and the trainee's perception of the entire support structure of the renal unit will be influenced by this early experience. In this way, the process of involving the patient and carer in the multidisciplinary 'renal team' will begin and, perhaps for the first time, they will start to feel that they are gaining control of the illness rather than vice versa.

The length of the training period varies according to the chosen mode of dialysis, the patient's aptitude, and the frequency of training sessions, and will include continued teaching on diet and fluid management. A predetermined expectation of length of training is unhelpful since it encourages both trainer and trainee to think in terms of 'slow' and 'fast' learners. If the selection process is essentially sound, and the trainer is a good one, very few patients should fail to 'graduate'. Nevertheless, a significant integration of manual dexterity and cognition is required by the patient and carer for home dialysis to be feasible.[21]

Once the initial training period is completed, further training will be required in the patient's home, initially under the close supervision of the community renal nurse (CRN). He or she will continue the training process and lead the patient to real independence as a home dialyser.

## 12.3 An accessible and responsive support service

'Accessible' and 'responsive' are key aspects of a home dialysis support service. It is essential that from the first day at home the patient feels secure in the knowledge that if a complication arises the full resources of the local renal unit are readily available, and can deal with it promptly and efficiently. If at any stage (but particularly in the first few weeks and months) this appears not to be the case, the patient's confidence will rapidly diminish and home dialysis will become progressively more problematic.

The two most immediate sources of support for the newly established home dialysis patient are the CRN and the telephone 'help-line' to the local renal unit (Table 12.3). Ideally the CRN will have already been involved with the patient at earlier stages of education and training, and must have several years of dialysis nursing behind them to exude an air of calmness, confidence, and 'seen it all before'! In the United States, Medicare regulations require follow-up visits to home dialysis patients, yet they require a large amount of personnel time. Theoretically the cost of these visits in both time and money may be offset, at least in part, by the savings from complications and in-patient episodes avoided as a result of recommendations made, and changes implemented during a home visit.[22] Many dialysis patients refer to 'their' CRN as their 'lifeline', and mean it quite literally. The CRN will usually act as a focal point for the majority of the patients' and carers' problems, and is ideally placed to refer on to other members of the multidisciplinary support team such as the dietician, social worker, counsellor, or physiotherapist (Table 12.3).

**Table 12.3** Renal unit support for the home dialysis patient

| |
|---|
| Planned home visits from CRN |
| Telephone help-line giving 24/7 access to technical, nursing, and medical advice |
| Planned hospital clinic visits and blood testing |
| Drop-in clinic for unplanned medical examination and assessment |
| Monitoring of water quality for haemodialysis patients |
| Appropriate ease of access to: |
|    renal medical and nursing staff |
|    dietician |
|    social worker |
|    psychologist/counsellor |
|    home dialysis administrator |
|    physiotherapist and occupational therapist |
|    chaplaincy and spiritual care |
| Inpatient bed and medical or surgical management of complications |

Obviously the CRN cannot be available 24/7, and therefore a telephone help-line is required for problems that arise at other times. Many home haemodialysis patients will choose to dialyse at times outside the usual working day, and therefore adequate back-up must always be available. This is not as easy as it might seem at first sight. The telephone number must be invariable—an anxious patient in the middle of a dialysis does not want to have to consult a rota to decide which number to call. This means that for most renal units the phone line will be to ward area which is always open, rather than to a dialysis area which may close down overnight. When the phone rings it must be immediately obvious to the staff that the call is from a home patient, so that it is not left to ring for several minutes as can often happen on a busy ward. Whoever answers the phone must be capable of dealing swiftly with a distressed patient or carer in the midst of a dialysis crisis—the last thing the caller wants to hear is 'could you hold on for a moment, all the nurses are busy just now', even though this may be true!

The outcome of a phone call may be that the patient needs to come up to the renal unit for a medical assessment, and therefore an 'open access' or 'drop-in' clinic facility is required. Peritoneal dialysis (PD) patients should be encouraged to utilize this facility immediately they develop 'cloudy bags' or think they may have peritonitis for any other reason. Patients will often use this facility for all manner of minor ailments rather than going to their GP or primary care physician, but it provides an ideal setting for on-going education about dialysis and chronic kidney disease. It requires appropriate nurse staffing and ready access to patient notes, a renal physician, and the possibility of surgical review if required.

The availability of a psychologist or counsellor with experience of chronic disease is imperative, and can be useful to both patients and staff. The counsellor perhaps straddles the boundary between the multidisciplinary renal team and the other sources of support that patients may utilize outside the renal unit's physical provisions.

## 12.3.1 Psychosocial and social support

The demands and coping skills required of people with chronic kidney disease and their families are enormous.[21,23] The home dialysis patient must overcome, or at least cope with, a large

**Table 12.4** Crisis points in chronic kidney disease

| |
|---|
| First diagnosis of chronic kidney disease |
| Hospitalization |
| Access surgery |
| Initiation of dialysis |
| 6 months after initiation of dialysis |
| Changes in restrictions or dialysis schedules |
| Modality change |
| Complications |
| Significant change in health status |

number of internal and external stressors if the process of dialysis itself is to be acceptable within the home environment. Various coping strategies will manifest themselves initially and may be helpful or otherwise. Reactions such as fear, anxiety, depression, denial, anger, and emotional dependency must be recognized and carefully worked on in a partnership between the patient and carer, and the healthcare team with the psychologist/counsellor taking a lead role. The counsellor also has an important role in educating other members of the multidisciplinary team whose reactions to patient denial or anger may otherwise be unhelpful.

'Crisis points' in chronic kidney disease have been identified by Steffen[24] and it is important that these are recognized in all dialysis patients, but particularly those dialysing at home (Table 12.4). A crisis occurs when the patient's state of equilibrium is disrupted and the usual coping mechanisms are ineffective. The patient adopts new strategies in an attempt to restore equilibrium and these result in either healthy or unhealthy adaptation. The crisis may therefore eventually be a very positive experience for the patient who finds that they can adapt, but an awareness of the crisis points amongst the healthcare team allows unhealthy adaptation to be picked up as early as possible and appropriate support to be provided.

## 12.3.2  Patient peer support

National and local peer support groups such as the Kidney Patients' Association, provide invaluable aid to many home dialysis patients who may otherwise be relatively isolated from fellow sufferers (Table 12.5). Information on peer support groups should be made available

**Table 12.5** Other sources of support for the home dialysis patient

| |
|---|
| Family and friends |
| Primary care physician/GP |
| Spiritual care |
| Palliative care teams |
| Patient organisations |
| Internet advice |
| Nursing homes and rehabilitation facilities |
| Employer |

during the training period, but it should be recognized that some patients would rather have nothing to do with them because it 'places' them within a lifestyle group from which they are striving to escape. Nevertheless, for many home patients, communication with someone who has 'been there' provides enormous encouragement, and also an opportunity to help others. Meeting patients with successful renal transplants can also provide significant hope for the future and a sense of purpose. Purvis quotes a patient as saying 'Having been on treatment for a long time, the group has helped me remove the isolation attached to life on home dialysis'.[25]

In many renal units, formal peer support groups exist and meet together regularly, some coordinated by a psychologist.[26] Many units such as our own have a tradition of an annual holiday for CAPD patients organized by two or more CRNs. The favourite destination for these groups from Manchester is Majorca in the Mediterranean. For some patients this can be a very bonding time, and it is sometimes the first international holiday they have ever had. Travel abroad produces a great sense of achievement in both patient and carer and gives them a feeling of freedom, or of having broken the shackles that were clamped on them when they started dialysis. Many then go on to organize their own family holidays in subsequent years.

Another approach to peer support is to pair experienced, coping patients with new dialysis patients to assist adjustment during the early months.[27]

### 12.3.3 Family support

The importance of a supportive family environment cannot be overestimated, and may be more important for the more elderly patient. Carey et al.[28] used the Beavers–Timberlawn Family Evaluation Scale to rate the supportive nature of families of 294 CAPD patients, with ratings from 1 (representing a chaotic family structure) to 9 (representing an orderly 'egalitarian' structure). Patients over the age of 60 years in families with low scores were four times more likely to transfer to in-centre haemodialysis as a result of peritonitis or psychosocial factors than were patients from families with high scores. As a result almost 70% of patients more than 60 years of age with low scores transferred within a year of starting home dialysis. The authors emphasize the importance of considering psychosocial factors in selection of patients suitable for home dialysis, and in particular those at the older end of the age spectrum.

Family members often assist with haemodialysis and may assume the total burden associated with dialysis therapy.[29] Since the 1960s both clinicians and researchers have reported that home haemodialysis is as stressful, if not more stressful, for the carer than for the patient.[1] Family involvement in home care significantly influences the outcome of home haemodialysis patients, just as the patient's health and functioning influence the family. Haemodialysis patients assisted by paid care workers experienced significantly greater morbidity and greater financial burden than patients cared for by family members.[30]

Family carers of CAPD patients are similarly affected, and often assume some, if not all, of the responsibility for providing care.[31] This is particularly common in certain patient groups such as infants, children, the frail elderly, and otherwise disabled patients such as those who have undergone lower limb amputation.

### 12.3.4 Financial support

In most Western countries financial support for dialysis patients is provided in varying ways by the state. Private health insurance usually ceases in whole or in part to contribute to the costs associated with home dialysis at around the time the patient first commences dialysis.

In the UK, the National Health Service pays all the bills, although dialysis facilities overall do not match demand. This has resulted in greater dependence on home dialysis, and in particular CAPD. All associated costs are paid by the local renal unit, to the dialysis equipment manufacturer.

In the United States, dialysis patients may voluntarily choose to become a home patient, but the final decision is based on whether the patient meets Medicare guidelines. Medicare will pay 80% of the cost of home dialysis for all patients who are eligible for Medicare. The remaining 20% is usually paid either by the patient's private insurance company or by Medicaid and in many states other programmes will assist patients who have neither insurance nor Medicaid eligibility. The cost of home dialysis for each approved dialysis centre is determined by Medicare. Home dialysis patients can choose between two payment options, method I and method II. Under method I the patient's dialysis unit provides all the facilities required for home dialysis either directly or under arrangements with other providers, and Medicare pays the unit directly. Under method II the patient chooses to deal directly with a single supplier to obtain all dialysis equipment and supplies, but a local dialysis unit must agree to provide backup dialysis and support services in the event of problems arising.

### 12.3.5 Monitoring and audit of home dialysis support

Regular monitoring or audit of home dialysis can provide early signs that support is not as good as it should be, and may point to inadequacies in the service. A monthly or quarterly review of parameters such as number of in-centre haemodialysis sessions, in-patient days, drop-in clinic visits, telephone help-line calls, peritonitis and catheter exit site infections in PD patients, unplanned home visits by CRNs or technical staff can quickly identify deficiencies in support to home patients. An increase in in-centre haemodialysis sessions may suggest inadequate home support, whereas an increase in unplanned home visits or peritonitis may suggest inadequate training.

## 12.4 The long-term home dialysis patient

A patient who has managed their own dialysis for a number of years can present particular challenges for the healthcare team. In our own programme we have a number of home haemodialysis patients who have looked after themselves for over 20 years, and who therefore have more experience of their treatment than many quite senior staff members. Such patients will immediately recognize a junior nurse or doctor's inexperience, whilst the nurse or doctor may frequently fail to recognize the patient's vast wealth of experience! Under these circumstances conflicts may occur, particularly when the staff member's instinct is to be cautious and perhaps recommend admission when the patient was simply seeking advice or reassurance. They may specifically avoid junior members of the team at clinic visits because they recognize that they know more about dialysis and its complications than a recently qualified nurse or doctor. It is important that home patients of this type have access to the most senior staff available on a given day, and that all staff recognize that enquiries from them are unlikely to be frivolous or clinically unimportant.

Inevitably long-term patients eventually enter a phase of decline and will by this stage have seen many of their dialysis colleagues fall victim to complications of one sort or another. They will therefore be well aware of their own limitations and mortality so that the transition to greater dependency requires enormous skill and sensitivity. Although the multidisciplinary team remains essential to provide the range of care required at this time as much as any other, it is likely that the patient and their carer will look to one or two particularly trusted members to advise and guide them through this period.

## 12.4.1 End-of-life care for the home dialysis patient

Patients who have maintained the independence afforded by home dialysis rarely wish to relinquish it as they near the end of their life. Ninety per cent of the respondents to a Gallup survey commissioned in the United States by the National Hospice Organization in 1996,[32] expressed a desire to die at home. In contrast to this, as modern medicine developed increased technology to treat illness, death moved out of the home and into institutions, so that now fewer than 20% of people in the United States die within their own homes.[33] The majority of deaths are predictable and could be managed at home, as is the case for many dialysis patients—not just those utilizing home treatments. However, formal education in 'end-of-life care' is lacking in most medical schools but other organizations have taken a lead. The American Medical Association conceived the Education for Physicians on End-of-life Care (EPEC) Project—EPEC is intended to help physicians take care of their portion of the responsibility to develop good end-of-life care, and is particularly appropriate to any physician looking after home dialysis patients. Topics include:

◆ negotiating goals of care and treatment priorities;
◆ advance care planning;
◆ medical futility;
◆ requests for physician-assisted suicide;
◆ requests to withhold or withdraw life-sustaining therapy.

If the Sheffield model is applied to care of the home dialysis patient then appropriate supportive care will have been deployed from the earliest signs of kidney disease, so that when a patient enters the end-of-life period described by the EPEC Project there should be no difficulty in initiating the change in the nature and intensity of support required to enable the home dialysis patient to die peacefully at home. Planning end-of-life care for a home-based patient should in fact be easier than planning similar care for a hospital-based patient who is less likely to have the network of support services already in place.

Planning the end-of-life care of a home dialysis patient incorporates all the aspects discussed in the other chapters of this book. However, the role of the CRN in end-of-life care of a home dialysis patient cannot be over-emphasized. He or she will probably be the member of the multidisciplinary team who will know the patient, the carer, and the home circumstances best. It will probably be the CRN with whom the question of discontinuation of dialysis will first be discussed, and of whom questions about mode of death will be asked. If the patient becomes frail, visits to the hospital clinic and repeated measurement of laboratory parameters become unnecessary. The emphasis on dialysis as a life-prolonging treatment shifts towards it being a means of controlling symptoms. If the patient has acquired a life-threatening condition in addition to chronic kidney failure, such as an incurable cancer, then the dialysis patient may be in the 'fortunate' position of being able to decide at what point to discontinue dialysis and plan the timing of their death. Many questions arise in the patient's and carer's mind at this time and may require a home visit by the dialysis physician. EPEC type training at this stage is invaluable to both the patient and physician.

## Case study

Mary is a 66-year-old female with a primary diagnosis of Type I diabetes mellitus from the age of 24 years. She has co-morbidities of hypertension, retinopathy, neuropathy, and depression. She required temporary haemodialysis while on holiday in the United States at the age of 63 years and she commenced CAPD 7 months later. She lives at home with her husband; one son died due to diabetic coma and the other son is alive with two sons of his own. Mary's mobility is poor and limited.

Mary was first introduced to the renal team in the low-clearance clinic having been referred by her diabetes consultant at a local district hospital. She attended with her husband. A full history and examination was followed by meetings with the pre-dialysis nurse and renal dietician. Mary was noted to be very quiet and her husband did most of the talking and questioning. In view of the known poor prognosis for patients with diabetic nephropathy and extensive co-morbidity, palliative care was discussed along with dialysis options. A 3-week follow-up appointment was made.

She did not have any uraemic symptoms at this time but was noted to be anaemic and erythropoietin was commenced. At the follow-up visit the pre-dialysis nurse spent more time with Mary and her husband to discuss issues around her impaired vision and osteoarthritis in both knees. She had decided that she wanted dialysis treatment, and because she did not like hospitals wanted a treatment that would reduce hospital admissions or attendances. CAPD was discussed and Mary felt that with help from her husband she would be able to do it. A home visit with the community renal nurse was arranged. This was an opportunity for the CRN to meet Mary and her husband in their own home.

At the third visit to the low-clearance clinic Mary was referred for insertion of a Tenckhoff catheter as her results were worsening. The pre-dialysis nurse continued to provide education and support during this stage, liaising closely with the CRN. Subsequently Mary's training took place in hospital but she attended as a daily outpatient. Once home on treatment the CRN initially visited frequently to provide a high level of support for both Mary and her husband.

For the first 18 months at home Mary managed reasonably well. She and her husband experienced many emotions and difficulties during this period and it became clear that in particular she was having difficulty coping with her other disabilities rather than the dialysis. The CRN involved the renal social worker to examine ways of alleviating some of the difficulties. Increased opportunities for communication allowed time for Mary and her husband to discuss their problems, and enabled the team to analyse strategies to overcome and support them appropriately to good effect.

However, 6 months later Mary had become less communicative and displayed evidence of depression. She was reviewed by the nephrologist and commenced on an antidepressant. The CRN increased the frequency of visits to provide support for both Mary and her husband. It became evident that Mary's husband was doing increasingly more as her level of independence deteriorated, and he required increased support from the social worker in order to organize various aspects of Mary's care, including carers to sit in the house whilst he was able to get out for short periods. Mary's GP became involved at this stage and a 1-week hospital admission was organized to allow Mary's husband a respite and to reassess Mary's condition. There was little evidence of any new medical issues but Mary was unable to manage most of her daily living needs and required lots of help from nurses. Once at home again Mary continued to deteriorate. The CRN arranged a home visit by the nephrologist to discuss with Mary and her husband how best to mange her from this point. Her bed was now downstairs and her husband was doing all her dialysis. She had become increasingly immobile and had significant pain from her arthritis. Mary expressed clearly that her quality of life was now so poor that she could no longer battle against all her difficulties. A referral was made to the palliative care team who liaised closely with the GP, district nurses and CRN. Although dialysis was not stopped the number of PD exchanges was reduced. Mary's husband needed a lot of support and the family were at the bedside constantly. Mary died peacefully at home, approximately 30 months after starting dialysis.

## References

1. Brunier, G.M., Mckeever, P.T. (1993). The impact of home dialysis on the family: literature review. *ANNA J.,* **20**(6): 653–9.

2. Brunner, F.P., Gurland, H.J., Harlen, H., Scharer, K., Parsons, F.M. (1972). Combined report on regular dialysis and transplantation in Europe, II, 1971. *Proceedings of the European Dialysis and Transplant Association,* **9**: 3–34.

3. Katz, A.M. (1970). Patients in chronic haemodialysis in the United States: a preliminary survey. *Soc. Sci. Med.,* **3**: 669–77.

4. Morrin, P.A.F. (1966). A survey of chronic renal failure in Southeastern Ontario. *Can. Med. Assoc. J.,* **94**: 1353–6.

5. Price, J.D.E., Ashby, K.M., Reeve, C.E. (1978). Results of 12 years treatment of chronic renal failure by dialysis and transplantation. *Can. Med. Assoc. J.,* **118**: 263–6.

6. Shambaugh, P.W., Kanter, S.S. (1969). Spouses under stress: group meetings with spouses of patients on haemodialysis. *Am. J. Psychiat.,* **125**(7): 928–36.

7. Evans, R.W., Blagg, C.R., Bryan, F.A. (1981). Implications for healthcare policy: a social and demographic profile of haemodialysis patients in the United States. *J. Am. Med. Assoc.,* **245**(5): 487–91.

8. Shambaugh, P.W., Hampers, C.L., Bailey, G.L., Snyder, D., Merrill, J.P. (1967). Hemodialysis in the home: emotional impact on the spouse. *Trans. Am. Soc. Artif. Intern. Organs.,* **13**: 41–5.

9. Osmond, M.W. (1987). Radical-critical theories. In: *Handbook of Marriage and the Family,* ed. M.B. Sussman and S.K. Steinmetz, pp. 103–24. New York: Longman.

10. Rubin, J., Case, G., Bower, J. (1990). Comparison of rehabilitation in patients undergoing home dialysis. Continuous ambulatory or cyclic peritoneal dialysis vs home haemodialysis. *Arch. Intern. Med.,* **150**(7): 1429–31.

11. Anderson, J.M., Elfert, H. (1989). Managing chronic illness in the family: women as caretakers. *J. Adv. Nursing,* **14**: 735–43.

12. United States Renal Data Service (2000). *Annual Data Report 2000.* http://www.usrds.org/adr_2000.htm

13. Adam, J., Akehurst, R.L., Angris, S., *et al.* for the National Institute for Clinical Excellence (2002). *Guidance on Home Compared with Hospital Haemodialysis for Patients with End-stage Renal Failure.* London: National Institute for Clinical Excellence.

14. Falvo, D.R. (1995). Educational evaluation: what are the outcomes? *Adv. Ren. Replace. Ther.,* **2**(3): 227–33.

15. Nitz, J., Shayman, D. (1986). A model for patient education. *ANNA J.,* **13**(5): 253–5.

16. Ahlmen, J., Carlsson, L., Schonborg, C. (1993). Well-informed patients with end-stage renal disease prefer peritoneal dialysis to hemodialysis. *Periton. Dial. Int.,* **13**(Suppl. 2): S196–S198.

17. Binik, Y.M., Devins, G.M., Barre, P.E., Guttmann, R.D., Hollomby, D.J., Mandin, H., *et al.* (1993). Live and learn: patient education delays the need to initiate renal replacement therapy in end-stage renal disease. *J. Nerv. Ment. Dis.,* **181**(6): 371–6.

18. Hayslip, D.M., Suttle, C.D. (1995). Pre-ESRD patient education: a review of the literature. *Adv. Ren. Replace. Ther.,* **2**(3): 217–26.

19. Klang, B., Bjorvell, H., Berglund, J., Sundstedt, C., Clyne, N. (1998). Predialysis patient education: effects on functioning and well-being in uraemic patients. *J. Adv. Nursing,* **28**(1): 36–44.

20. Lancaster, L.E. (1984). *The Patient with End-stage Renal Disease,* 2nd edn., New York: John Wiley.

21. Summerton, H. (1995). End-stage renal failure: the challenge to the nurse. *Nursing Times,* **91**: 27–9.

22. Ponferrada, L., Prowant, B.F., Schmidt, L.M., Burrows, L.M., Satalowich, R.J., Bartelt, C. (1993). Home visit effectiveness for peritoneal dialysis patients. *ANNA J.,* **20**(3): 333–7.

23. Gathercole, W.K. (1987). Psychosocial aspects of end stage renal disease. *Nursing,* **17**: 633–6.

24. Steffen, C. (1989). Psychosocial issues at critical times in the course of dialysis. *9th Annual Conference on Peritoneal Dialysis* (presentation). University of Missouri, Columbia.

25. Purvis, P.J. (1991). A support group for patients with renal insufficiency on maintenance dialysis. *EDTNA-ERCA J.,* **17**(3): 25–7.

26. Cerruti, G., Cotto, M., Rivetti, M., Servetti, L., Baracco, M., Ferrero, R. (1993). Patients' group experiences. *Periton. Dial. Int.,* **13**(Suppl. 2): S199–S201.

27. Prater, J. (1985). An exploration of coping behaviors within a dialysis caseload. *Dial. Transplant.,* **14**(9): 504–10.

28. Carey, H., Finkelstein, S., Santacroce, S., Brennan, N., Raffone, D., Rifkin, J., *et al.* (1990). The impact of psychosocial factors and age on CAPD dropout. In: *Peritoneal Dialysis in the Geriatric Patient. A Supplement to Advances in Peritoneal Dialysis,* ed. A.R. Nissenson, **6**: 26–28.

29. Wicks, M.N., Milstead, E.J., Hathaway, D.K., Cetingok, M. (1997). Subjective burden and quality of life in family caregivers of patients with end stage renal disease. *ANNA J.,* **24**(5): 527–38.

30. Walker, P.J., Diaz-Buxo, J.A., Chandler, J.T., Farmer, C.D., Farres, M., Cox, P., *et al.* (1981). Home care: paid home dialysis aides: the experience of a single program. *Contemp. Dial.,* **2**(4): 50–4.

31. Srivastava, R.H. (1988). Coping strategies used by spouses of CAPD patients. *ANNA J.,* **15**: 174–9.

32. The Gallup Organization (1996). *Knowledge and attitudes related to hospice care. Survey conducted for the National Hospice Organisation.* Princeton, NJ: The Gallup Organization.

33. Emanuel, L.L., von Gunten, C.F., Ferris, F.D. (1999). *The Education for Physicians on End-of-life Care (EPEC) Curriculum.* Princeton, NJ: The Robert Wood Johnson Foundation.

Chapter 13

# Initiation and withdrawal of dialysis

Lionel U. Mailloux

## 13.1 Introduction

As patients and their families realize they can exercise their rights, more are becoming involved in decision-making about all aspects of their medical care, e.g. dialysis, cancer chemotherapy, or surgical procedures. This is having a direct impact on the practising nephrologist. The ready availability of dialysis leads to a feeling of obligation by nephrologists to offer renal replacement therapy to all patients with the common biochemical indications for dialysis.[1–3]

In fact, some nephrologists feel that most, if not all, patients requiring renal replacement therapy should receive dialysis; refusal may be seen to represent a failure on the physician's part to provide total care. However, as patients become more educated and involved with decision-making, conservative management (i.e. not starting dialysis) and withdrawal from dialysis are assuming greater prominence. How this happens varies in different countries depending on local healthcare cultures and medical law. The main body of this chapter reflects American practice with a commentary at the end by Edwnia Brown highlighting the differences in practice in the UK.

Dialysis withdrawal is now one of the most common causes of death in patients with end-stage renal disease (ESRD); more than 20% of dialysis patients in the United States discontinue dialysis before death.[3] In the United States the revised Center for Medicare and Medicaid Services (CMS) Health Care Finance Administration (HCFA) form 2746, a form required for all ESRD patients who die, no longer identifies withdrawal as a specific cause of death; it is therefore not known whether withdrawal is the absolute cause of death.[3] Patients, families, and the healthcare team should work together on advance directives to achieve the goals of life with quality and death with dignity consistent with the patient's wishes. These issues can, however, become a source of conflict between physicians, patients, and their families.[4,5] A new clinical practice guideline to facilitate ethical facets of dialysis consultations 'Shared decision-making in dialysis: the new RPA/ASN guideline on appropriate initiation and withdrawal of treatment'[6] provides excellent guidance describing all aspects of these conflicts, and is discussed in the introduction to this book. In the ensuing case studies we look at the following areas:

- shared decision-making
- informed consent or refusal
- estimating prognosis
- conflict resolution
- advance directives
- withholding or withdrawing dialysis

- special patient groups
- time-limited trials
- palliative care.

## Case study 1: Mrs L

Mrs L was a 90-year-old woman who had had very slowly progressive renal insufficiency for several years superimposed upon peripheral vascular disease, degenerative joint disease, and hypertension. She had also had recent trauma with a dislocated right shoulder and at the same time developed poor bladder control; ultimately she required dialysis. Although she lived semi-independently, she required assistance for activities of daily living and was tired and lethargic. A further fall caused a fracture of her right hip, requiring surgical fixation, following which she went to a rehabilitation facility from where she was discharged to her daughter's home where she needed increased assistance to mobilize. While at her daughter's she talked of her concern that she had now become a 'real burden' to her family. One of her neighbours was on dialysis and tried to convince her to think positively about it. Numerous cardiac medications added to the burden of her disease. Physical examination at that time revealed a frail lady, clearly chronically ill, who needed one assistant and a walker to ambulate. She had obvious wasting but was alert, oriented, and fully responsive. Pertinent lab data revealed a depressed serum albumin.

### Case comment

This lady felt unable to perform peritoneal dialysis and did not want to burden her family, she was also extremely negative about the possibility of initiating haemodialysis, therefore no planning was made for either, including no provision for vascular access. In addition she showed clinical evidence of protein calorie malnutrition. Her children were in full agreement with her decision, because she was competent. She had no healthcare proxy or advance directive but had clearly expressed her views which were supported by her family. Her grandchildren were quite upset that she was not willing to start dialysis, however they respected her wishes. The nephrologists concurred with the decision-making process, made over a period of months as she deteriorated. She passed away peacefully at home in her own bed 3 weeks later. There was considerable relief in the family with closure of the clinical situation.

This case demonstrates several of the principles noted above, i.e. shared decision-making, conflict resolution, and informed refusal to initiate an extraordinary therapy. The patient, with the support of children, consciously decided to forego dialysis, a decision which was accepted despite the fact that she did not have an advanced directive. She was uraemic, but competent to make her own decisions and her family supported her.

## Case study 2: patient HA

Mr HA was 76 at the time of his death. He had been on dialysis for more than 6 years when he elected to withdraw. His end-stage renal disease was caused by adult polycystic kidney disease with significant underlying coronary artery disease, hypertension, peripheral vascular disease (S/P bilateral lower extremity amputations), and severe pulmonary hypertension with right-heart failure. One of his children had begun dialysis in 2001 and another child had advanced chronic kidney disease awaiting a renal transplant. The patient himself had chronic pain requiring narcotic analgesia. In mid 2001 he began to express concern about his inability to care for himself. He used expressions such as 'my son has to carry me', 'I can't breathe', 'I need oxygen at all times', and 'my wife doesn't have a single free minute except when I'm in the hospital'. He needed six hospitalizations in 2001 and five in 2002. He was, however, well

## Case study 2: patient HA *(continued)*

dialysed, often receiving additional ultrafiltration or dialysis. At this time, because of his increasing dependence and his need for constant oxygen therapy, he started to talk about his wish to stop dialysis. Initially his family had great difficulty discussing the idea of withdrawal from dialysis, feeling that one did everything medically until death occurred. They were referred to their pastor for a discussion in which the nephrologists participated. His wife and daughter had been appointed healthcare proxies and were aware of his concerns. Six months after opening the conversation about withdrawal, a decision to withdraw was made. It was accomplished after a quick trip to their summer home for a last visit (the journey 250 miles away nearly killed the patient). The daughter on dialysis also had to arrange for a trip east from California; she stayed for 3 months receiving dialysis in the same ambulatory unit as her father. He died in the hospital within 18 h of admission when he developed agonal breathing, 5 days after withdrawing. His family was at his bedside.

## Case comment

This patient was absolutely miserable on dialysis as his peripheral vascular disease and pulmonary hypertension progressed further. He did have an advance directive, in which he had expressed his wish not to be a 'total burden', but his entire family needed to be involved in the decision-making process. They eventually 'bought into' the process and everyone was at peace with the decision. This case also illustrates some of the above principles: shared decision-making, informed consent or refusal, estimating prognosis, conflict resolution, and having advance directives in place.

## Case study 3: Mrs GA

Mrs GA was 68, legally blind with Type 2 diabetes mellitus, hypertension, underlying coronary artery disease and who had undergone a two-vessel coronary artery bypass graft years earlier (S/P myocardial infarction, angina pectoris, and arrhythmias.) During the previous 6 months, she had been hospitalized twice for a myocardial infarction and cerebrovascular accident with minimal residual weakness on the left side. It was noted that she had chronic kidney disease. Three months later, a full evaluation for anaemia revealed the presence of multiple myeloma with bony lesions. The patient was hospitalized on several occasions for pain control, congestive heart failure, and eventual initiation of chemotherapy after developing severe hypercalcaemia. Her renal function deteriorated and she developed progressive uraemia. She had expressed the wish to withhold dialysis. Despite an advance directive, her two children felt that she should initiate dialysis in the hope of controlling the myeloma. She therefore consented to a 'trial' of dialysis. Additional therapy included thalidomide, narcotics, oral hypoglycaemic agents, antiangina medication, antihypertensive medication, and erythropoietin. At that time she had generalized pain and discomfort throughout her body, she had experienced episodes of bleeding, examination revealed a debilitated lady with markers of chronic ill-health and numerous bruises and ecchymoses. In addition she had decompensated congestive heart failure. She remained significantly anaemic and thrombocytopaenic (haemaglobin always $< 8.8$ g/dl) despite escalating doses of erythropoietin with appropriate iron replacement. Dialysis was initiated as an inpatient. There was no recovery of renal function; bone pain persisted, and she developed gastrointestinal symptoms which became worse. By week 9, the patient met her whole family, held private discussions with the oncologists and nephrologists, and decided to withdraw from dialysis at the end of week 10. She died at home with her children and grandchildren 16 days later.

> **Case study 3: Mrs GA** *(continued)*
>
> **Case comment**
>
> This lady's advanced directive had clearly stated that she wished no extraordinary measures should she be critically or terminally ill. She had also expressed the desire to withhold dialysis, but after full discussion with her oncologist, nephrologists, and family, she elected to set a time trial on dialysis because her healthcare team had convinced her that there was a possibility of some recovery. A review was subsequently undertaken, as agreed, at which time her family acquiesced with her wishes.

### 13.1.1 Discussion

National and regional data show that withdrawal from dialysis is the second commonest cause of death in Canada (after cardiovascular disease) in patients with end-stage renal disease and the third most common cause in the United States (after cardiovascular and infectious diseases), when it was tracked by the United States Renal Data System (USRDS).[3,6–8] Withdrawal means the discontinuation of maintenance dialysis, while withholding dialysis is defined as the foregoing of dialysis in a patient in whom it has yet to be initiated. The terms may be used interchangeably in patients with acute or chronic renal failure. The expected outcome from choosing either of these options is death within a variable period of time (usually 7 to 14 days after withdrawal and up to 90 days when not initiating dialysis).

## 13.2 Foregoing initiation of dialysis

Although less well publicized, foregoing the initiation of dialysis probably occurs more frequently in the United States than does withdrawal. In a survey of American nephrologists, nearly 90% reported withholding dialysis at least once in the previous year and over 30% reported withholding it at least six times.[9] In a prospective Canadian study, about 25% of patients with advanced chronic kidney disease (CKD) referred for initiation of haemodialysis were not offered it.[10] These patients had very poor functional capacity, severe cardiovascular disease (50% with diffuse atherosclerosis and renovascular disease), diabetes mellitus, or neurological disease. Only two of the 23 patients survived for 6 months, confirming the terminal prognosis in 91% of the patients. Primary care physicians can also withhold dialysis by not referring the patients to nephrologists for evaluation of their progressive CKD. One study among physicians in West Virginia, for example, found that 20 of 76 primary care providers (26%) had effectively withheld dialysis from at least one patient through non-referral to a nephrologist.[11] The most common reasons given by the physicians were end-stage heart, liver, or lung disease, old age, or that the patient chose not to be referred.

Many nephrologists feel it is appropriate to withhold dialysis in the following specific clinical settings:[8,10–14]

- Patients with severe and irreversible dementia.
- Patients who are permanently unconscious (as in a persistent vegetative state).
- Patients with end-stage lung, liver, cancer, or heart disease, who are confined to bed or chair or in a hospice and who need assistance with activities of daily living.
- Patients with severe mental disability who are unable to cooperate with the procedure of dialysis itself, are unable to interact with the environment or other people, or are persistently combative with family or staff.

- Patients with severe, continued, and unrelenting pain in whom dialysis may prolong life for a short period of time but will also prolong suffering.

- Hospitalized patients (especially the elderly) with multiple organ system failure that persists after 3 days of intensive therapy. The mortality rate of such patients is very high.

Reliable data for the factors associated with withholding dialysis are not available. Reasons for dialysis withdrawal noted in the USRDS death notification form in order of declining percentage in 1991 to 1992 included:[3]

- failure to thrive (42%)

- medical complications (35%)

- access failure (4%).

## 13.3 Withdrawal from dialysis

Several factors are known to be associated with withdrawal from dialysis including advanced age, diabetes mellitus, extensive atherosclerotic disease, White race, low Karnofsky scores, female gender, higher physical discomfort index, and higher educational level.[15–17] The withdrawal rate rises with age, representing a significant part of the high mortality rate in the elderly ESRD patient population. For example, in one review of USRDS data, dialysis was discontinued in about 6% of patients under 65 years of age, but in 14% of those over 65 years of age.[17] In one of the original reports about discontinuation of dialysis, death followed withdrawal of dialysis occured in 56% of deaths in those over the age of 85.[18]

Certain co-morbid conditions are also frequently present near the time of withdrawal, including diabetic gastropathy, neuropathy, the need for surgery, overall burden of dialysis, neoplastic disease, neurological deterioration, extremely poor quality of life, and increasing pain.[8,18–20] Dialysis is occasionally begun as a therapeutic trial in an attempt to improve an extremely poor quality of life; it is subsequently discontinued if no improvement occurs.

### 13.3.1 Factors for consideration when withholding or withdrawing dialysis

There has to be an appropriate sequential clinical approach to the withholding or withdrawing of dialysis, which involves some or all of the following important elements:

- Assessment of the patient's decision-making capacity.

- Assessment of possible reversible factors.

- Detailed and effective communication with the patient.

- Full family involvement, with appointment of a surrogate if wished.

- Interdisciplinary dialysis team involvement.

- The presence of an advanced directive, either through a living will or healthcare proxy.

- A trial period of dialysis if appropriate.

- Commitment to support the patient's decision whether it is to continue dialysis, withdraw, or to forego initiation.

#### 13.3.1.1 Assessment of the patient's decision-making capacity

The withholding of or withdrawal from dialysis may be suggested by the patient, the patient's family, the nephrologist, or other members of the healthcare team. Before proceeding with such a decision the physician should satisfy him or herself that the patient (or appropriate surrogate) is competent and fully comprehends that the consequence of the decision includes death, usually within 1 to 2 weeks in the case of withdrawal.

### 13.3.1.2 Assessment of reversible factors

Patient or family requests to withdraw from or withhold dialysis should be explored by the health-care team as there may be reversible or acute issues which precipitate the initial contemplation of withdrawal. Potentially remediable factors may include painful needle insertions, frequent hypotensive episodes, intradialytic muscle cramps, uncontrolled pain, and depression. The nephrologist, with other members of the healthcare team, should address and modify these factors where possible, with an agreement to review the situation at an appropriate time to assess benefit or otherwise.

### 13.3.1.3 Detailed and effective communication with the patient

Effective communication about foregoing dialysis or the possibility of withdrawal starts at the first nephrology consultation and should continue as appropriate throughout the patient's care. This will help the nephrologist determine the patient's true wishes. It is particularly important to ensure that requests for withdrawal are not either a reflection of untreated depression or a cry for help for unrecognized distress. Using the full resources of the multidisciplinary team will aid recognition of remediable family or communication issues. A full and open communication, maintained at all times will contribute to the patient being able to reveal his or her true needs.

### 13.3.1.4 Involvement of patient's family and appointment of a surrogate

The nephrologist must ensure that the patient and his or her family or significant others are aware of a decision to forego or withdraw from dialysis and the consequences of such a decision; this includes the designated surrogate, if appointed. The patient, in most cases, is likely to be helped by the support of these people as he or she comes to a decision. Where there is conflict between the patient's wishes and those of his family, professionals from the nephrology team or separate from that team may be helpful for an individual to clarify his or her own wishes.

### 13.3.1.5 Interdisciplinary dialysis team involvement

The decision to forego or withhold dialysis is both complex and of enormous consequence. All members of the healthcare team, social workers, physicians, clergy, and dialysis nurses can contribute to the decision-making along with the patient and family and thus provide support to the patient and family and to the nephrologist.[19]

### 13.3.1.6 Importance of having an advance directive (living wills or healthcare proxies)

If the patient has limited capacity; the presence of an advance directive, detailing his or her desires concerning their future care in the event they become incompetent or critically ill on life support, or the prior identification of a surrogate agent (healthcare proxy) simplifies the decision-making process. There are data suggesting that in ESRD patients advance directives may contribute to 'good and peaceful deaths'.[21]

### 13.3.1.7 Trial period of dialysis

A trial of dialysis may last 30 to 90 days during which the patient is closely monitored, and at a predefined point a discussion is held with the patient and family to assess its success or failure. A decision is then made to continue or withdraw treatment. This may be particularly useful in a patient who is depressed, in whom fear over the dialysis technique is contributing to a decision to withhold dialysis. Many such patients often remain on dialysis once their trial period is over.

### 13.3.1.8 Commitment to support the patient and family whatever the decision made

Once the discussions are completed, the competent patient who chooses to withdraw from long-term dialysis, or those who choose not to initiate dialysis, should be supported in this decision by the healthcare team whatever their own views might be. Likewise, this is true for the occasional patient who the nephrologist feels is not a good dialysis candidate, but who nevertheless chooses to continue or initiate dialysis treatments.[22]

### 13.3.1.9 Support to patient and family following withdrawal of dialysis

Patients typically survive 1 to 2 weeks after discontinuing long-term dialysis. Most patients express great relief with the lifting of a heavy burden, become very comfortable, and are at peace with their decision. At this point, major healthcare attention should be directed toward the total comfort of the patient, including pain control if that was a precipitating factor. Care in the place of the patient's choice should be offered if possible; this will include care within the hospital familiar to them, their own home, or hospice care. Palliative care support can be provided whatever the setting. Comfort care includes the prevention where possible of foreseeable problems so intravenous fluids, tube, or parenteral nutrition become inappropriate since they may precipitate fluid overload and pulmonary oedema which are most uncomfortable. Fluid and sodium intake can be liberated to include what the patient wishes. As Kjellstrand has stated, 'if a patient has willingly begun dialysis with a fully open communications policy (atmosphere), then this same patient should be able to withdraw, exercising his or her own best judgement'.[23] The expertise of the nephrology team should remain available to the patient and family to guide the care of the dying patient by supporting the patient's priorities and discussing, in advance, the effects of the dying process with the patient and family.[24] Non-palliative medications should be withdrawn and optimal pain control instituted.

## 13.4 UK practice (by Edwina Brown)

The different healthcare culture and patient expectations in the UK, as well as a different emphasis, means that the approach to the problems discussed are at times dissimilar. Referral patterns differ and very few patients will have advance directives. The sick elderly are often cared for in the community by primary care physicians and will initially be referred to physicians for the elderly. Historically, few such patients, especially if no longer independent, have been referred to nephrologists, although this is changing.

Potential dialysis patients are assessed by pre-dialysis teams consisting of nurses, social workers, counsellors, and medical staff. It is not uncommon for some patients not to want dialysis for the reasons already discussed. Supportive care or a trial of dialysis, and dialysis withdrawal are discussed with frail patients. The decision not to dialyse is the patient's alone if he/she is mentally competent. If the patient is not mentally competent, then the healthcare team, not the relatives, makes the decision on behalf of the patient; in UK law, no relative can make health-related decisions for mentally incompetent patients. Families are involved in discussions so they can provide support for the patient and contribute to the decision-making process. As they do not make the eventual decision, they are not made to feel responsible for 'letting a relative die'.

Other aspects of dying also need to be discussed with patients—do they want to be resuscitated (a decision that can be made without also withdrawing from dialysis) and where do they want to die. The decision about resuscitation follows the same principles discussed above, i.e. it is made by the patient, if mentally competent, and if not, it is made by the doctor in charge (usually after discussion with the rest of the healthcare team and an informative discussion with the family). Often the patient and family would prefer death to take place at home; in this case, the general practitioner needs to be involved and community care organized.

The following case history of a patient with severe autism illustrates the approach used to come to the decision that dialysis was not appropriate.

## Case study 4: Miss SS

SS is a 43-year-old woman living in a special care home because of severe autism. She had been brought up as a child by her parents but had move to a residential home in her 20s. She was first found to have renal failure when she was admitted to another hospital with severe vaginal bleeding. At presentation, haemoglobin was 4.4 g/100 ml and plasma creatinine was 650 $\mu$mol/l. She was given a blood transfusion and had an ultrasound which demonstrated uterine fibroids and two small kidneys. SS hated needles and needed sedation for blood tests so no more were done after the immediate management. On discharge, she was referred to a nephrologist to consider further management. On that first visit, she refused to have a blood test which was only done subsequently when a nurse visited her at the care home and she had been given diazepam. Plasma creatinine had fallen to 350 $\mu$mol/l. A diagnosis of acute on chronic renal failure was made. Immediate chronic dialysis was fortunately not needed. The chance that SS's renal function would deteriorate again and the fact that it was felt that she would be unsuitable for this mode of treatment was discussed with her carers. Initially, they were antagonistic as they felt that SS was being discriminated against. The counsellor and pre-dialysis nurse made several visits to the residential home and the carers visited the dialysis unit, thus gaining an understanding of what dialysis would entail for SS. This enabled all to be in agreement with the decision made by the medical team. Currently she attends the renal clinic every 3 months; sometimes she is willing to have blood tests. These show that renal function is slowly deteriorating, as expected.

## Ethical analysis

The working group who drafted the Renal Physicians Association/American Society of Nephrology (RPA/ASN) guideline and its 27 reviewers reached a consensus: just because we can perform dialysis does not mean that we should. This consensus recognized that there are cases in which it is ethically permissible to stop dialysis or not to start it. The RPA/ASN guideline recommended that it is appropriate to withhold or withdraw dialysis in the following circumstances: when the patient either verbally or though an advance directive refuses it; when the patient's legal agent refuses it for a patient who has lost decision-making capacity; and when because of profound permanent neurological impairment the patient has lost the potential for human relationship (Recommendation 6). The decisions not to start dialysis in the cases of Mrs L and SS, and the decisions to stop it in the cases of HA and GA, are solidly supported by this recommendation. In the case of Mrs L, her nephrologists concurred with her decision not to start dialysis. They estimated her prognosis to be poor (Recommendation 3) because she had all four of the worst prognostic indicators described in the RPA/ASN guideline—advanced age, poor nutritional status, poor func-

**Ethical analysis** *(continued)*

tional status, and multiple severe co-morbidities. In the case of SS, who hated needles and needed seda-tion to have blood drawn, the decision to withhold dialysis is supported by the RPA/ASN guideline (Recommendation 7). The case of Mrs GA is regrettable because she really did not want dialysis, and her outcome with dialysis was predictably very poor. Both the healthcare team and the family were unrealis-tic. In the future, dialysis of such unfortunate patients may be avoided as nephrologists acquire knowl-edge with increased dissemination of the RPA/ASN guideline and more research on prognosis in ESRD. As all four cases illustrate, nephrologists and renal care teams will need to improve their skills in com-municating with and supporting families so that dialysis of patients for whom the burdens substantially outweigh the benefits will not be undertaken.

# References

1. Levinsky, N.G. (1993). The organization of medical care: lessons from the Medicare end-stage renal disease program. *New Engl. J. Med.,* **329**: 1395.

2. Klahr, S. (1990). Rationing of health care and the ESRD program. *Am. J. Kidney Dis.,* **16**: 392.

3. US Renal Data System (USRDS) (2002). *Annual Data Report: Atlas of End-Stage Renal Disease in the United States.* Bethesda, MD: National Institutes of Health, National Institute of Diabetes and Digestive and Kidney Diseases. [Also 1995, 1999, 2001 editions.]

4. Moss, A.H. (1998). 'At least we do not feel guilty': managing conflict with families over dialysis discontinuation. *Am. J. Kidney Dis.,* **31**: 868.

5. Holley, J.L. (2002). A single-center review of the death notification form: discontinuing dialysis before death is not a surrogate for withdrawal from dialysis. *Am. J. Kidney Dis.,* **40**: 525–30.

6. Moss AH for the Renal Physicians Association and American Society of Nephrology Working Group (2001). A new clinical practice guideline to assist with dialysis-related ethics consultations. Shared decision-making in dialysis: the new RPA/ASN guideline on appropriate initiation and withdrawal of treatment. *Am. J. Kidney Dis.,* **37**: 1081.

7. Canadian Organ Replacement Register (1995). *1993 Annual Report.* Don Mills, Ontario: Canadian Institute for Health Information.

8. Mailloux, L.U., Bellucci, A.G., Napolitano, B., *et al.* (1993). Death by withdrawal from dialysis: a 20 year clinical experience. *J. Am. Soc. Nephrol.,* **3**: 1631–7.

9. Singer, P.A. (1992). Nephrologists' experience with and attitudes towards decisions to forego dialysis. *J. Am. Soc. Nephrol.,* **2**: 1235.

10. Hirsch, D.J., West, M.L., Cohen, A.D., *et al.* (1994). Experience with not offering dialysis to patients with a poor prognosis. *Am. J. Kidney Dis.,* **23**: 463.

11. Sekkarie, M.A., Moss, A.H. (1998). Withholding and withdrawing dialysis: the role of physician specialty and education and patient functional status. *Am. J. Kidney Dis.,* **31**: 464.

12. Moss, A.H. (1995). To use dialysis appropriately: the emerging consensus on patient selection guide-lines. *Adv. Renal Replace. Ther.,* **2**: 175.

13. Moss, A.H., Stocking, C.B., Sachs, G.A., *et al.* (1993). Variation in attitudes of dialysis unit medical directors towards decisions to withhold. *J. Am. Soc. Nephrol.,* **4**: 229.

14. Eiser, A.R., Seiden, D.J. (1997). Discontinuing dialysis in persistent vegetative state: the roles of autonomy, community, and professional moral agency. *Am. J. Kidney Dis.,* **30**: 291.

15. Leggat, J.E., Bloembergen, W.E., Levine, G., *et al.* (1997). An analysis of risk factors for withdrawal from dialysis before death. *J. Am. Soc. Nephrol.,* **8**: 1755.

16. Bloembergen, W.E., Port, F.K., Mauger, E.A., *et al.* (1995). A comparison of mortality between patients treated with hemodialysis and peritoneal dialysis. *J. Am. Soc. Nephrol.,* **6**: 177.

17. Nelson, C.B., Port, F.K., Wolfe, R.A., *et al.* (1994). The association of diabetic status, age and race to withdrawal from dialysis. *J. Am. Soc. Nephrol.,* **4**: 1608.

18. Neu, S., Kjellstrand, C.M. (1986). Stopping long-term dialysis. An empirical study of withdrawal of life-supporting treatment. *New Engl. J. Med.,* **314**: 14.

19. Cohen, L.M., McCue, J.D., Germain, M., *et al.* (1995). Dialysis discontinuation: a 'good' death? *Arch. Intern. Med.,* **155**: 42.

20. Tobe, S.W., Senn, J.S. (1996). End-stage renal disease group. Foregoing renal dialysis: a case study and review of ethical issues. *Am. J. Kidney Dis.,* **28**: 147.

21. Holley, J.L., Nespor, S., Rault, R. (1993). The effect of providing chronic hemodialysis patients written material on advance directives. *Am. J. Kidney Dis.,* **22**: 413.

22. Holley, J.L., Nespor, S., Rault, R. (1993). Chronic in-center hemodialysis patients' attitudes, knowledge towards advance directives. *J. Am. Soc. Nephrol.,* **3**: 1405.

23. Kjellstrand, C.M. (1988). Giving life–giving death. Ethical problems of high-technology medicine. *Acta Med. Scand. Suppl.,* **725**: 1–88.

24. Hines, S.C., Glover, J.J., Holley, J.L., *et al.* (1999). Dialysis patients' preferences for family-based advanced care planning. *Ann. Intern. Med.,* **130**: 825.

# Chapter 14

# A multidisciplinary approach to end-of-life care

Erica Perry, Julie Gumban Roberts, and George Kelly

## 14.1 Introduction

Quality personal relationships between renal patients, their families, and the renal team are fundamental to effective, meaningful end-of-life care. It is family-like relationships that invite listening and trust, and relationships that open doors to discussing frightening possibilities. Relationships empower choice, and also see staff through difficult times and return them enriched and more open to the next challenge.

This chapter will look first at the impact of relationships on the functioning of the renal team; then at how we are trained and what happens to how we function over the course of time. Lastly it will look at the significance of our relationships with our patients and families in end-of-life care, and at opportunities to integrate palliative work as fellow travellers along the biopsychosocial journey that we all take together.

## Case study

Michael, a 20-year-old with multiple complications from continuous ambulatory peritoneal dialysis, a failed living-related transplant, and subsequent haemodialysis access was transferred to University Hospital as a last resort. He had multiple admissions for abdominal pain, pancreatitis, recurrent seizures, and jejunal feeding tube placement. He required intensive pain control and antidepressive therapy.

Prior to his illness, Michael had been a successful high school student, academically and in sports, and was beloved among his student body. A college career with a scholarship was awaiting him when his acute multisystem illness struck. His mother, stepfather, sister, and surviving grandparents were deeply involved and supportive.

Shortly after transfer, Michael withdrew into a fetal position on dialysis, communicating rarely. His condition continued to deteriorate despite excellent dialysis delivery and stable 'core indicators'. The transplant team was concerned about his stability for surgery, even though a living donor (stepfather) was ready to donate. Nurses found it increasingly difficult to fend off requests for pain medication at dialysis, and were extremely uncomfortable witnessing this young man's slow 'crawl' toward death. The dietitian also was devastated to see her patient wasting away. Occasionally, the nephrologist was able to talk sports and history with Michael, and the peer mentor, a volunteer patient committed to empowering patients on dialysis, would play cards with him. In one of these non-medical moments, Michael shared that, although he was not ready to die, he also was not afraid to do so.

The team had become so upset in caring for this young man that the social worker arranged a family meeting including his mother, stepfather, grandmother (widowed), concerned team members and Michael. His mother was able to share her anguish over Michael's suffering, her guilt regarding

**Case study** *(continued)*

previous medical decisions, and her horror at the thought of losing him. The grandmother, on the other hand, spoke directly to Michael about his close relationship with his grandfather who had died peacefully after refusing extensive radiation treatment. When discussion turned to possible transplant surgery, Michael suddenly was able to say he wanted it all to stop. When asked what he wanted to do, he chose to stop dialysis and go home and die. Later, the family shared that they did not know that withdrawal from treatment was an option until the social worker brought it up in the family meeting.

The following few days were filled with friends and love. The nephrologist, peer mentor, and social worker visited him at home and found a Michael who was funny and at peace among family and friends. He was honoured at the Friday night football game and, on a pickup tailgate; he cruised in his wheelchair around the field to a standing ovation. That weekend, Michael died peacefully at home.

## 14.2 The multidisciplinary nephrology team

In the United States nephrology is unique among medical fields in that a multidisciplinary team is mandated by Medicare to collaborate and provide comprehensive care to the patient with end-stage renal disease[1] and his of her family. Both medical literature and the Centers for Medicare and Medicaid Services have agreed that dialysis patients require a wide variety of support to successfully adapt to a life dependent upon technology.[2] Further, they agree that a multidisciplinary team consisting of nephrologist, nephrology nurse, renal dietitian, and renal social worker can best address these needs. Though this group of professionals is mandated to care for the renal patient and family from the onset of kidney failure to death, little is written about the impact of their personal interaction and relationship, especially in end-of-life care. Although the importance of the multidisciplinary team is emphasized in studies of patients' quality of life and mortality, the implication is that staff are an interchangeable, faceless lot and that the protocols, interventions, and core indicators are the major contributors to the improved outcome. The value of the interpersonal relationships in the 'renal team' is less well researched than the 'harder' medical measures. Yet we feel that these relationships contribute significantly to a patient's quality of life.

### 14.2.1 Challenges in developing a collaborative relationship on the team

Many phenomena complicate team collaboration besides lack of time and conflicting schedules. Professionals with such dissimilar training can be likened to diverse tribes, each with its own language and culture. It takes perseverance, shared life experience, and listening skills to appreciate the blessings that this wide array of orientation and agenda can provide. These professional differences are illustrated by the variety of answers each renal team member would give to the question: who sets treatment goals? Physicians and dietitians are trained to generate treatment prescriptions. Nurses are trained to implement treatment protocols. Social workers are trained to encourage the client to generate his or her own goals; three points of view each fundamental to a notion of care.[3] Each point of view is needed in the care of the renal patient at different times in the patient's biopsychosocial journey. Working together with awareness of each other's contribution, the group of professionals can be a team 'for all seasons'.

In the same way, each profession learns different beliefs, standards, and ethics that sometimes handicap them from utilizing themselves to the fullest extent possible in developing relationships with patients and their families. Social workers are trained to avoid transference and boundary confusion, such as not allowing a patient to buy them a cup of coffee. Nurses are trained to attend to formularies and not to cry in front of their patients. Dietitians are trained to focus on the dietary compliance and lab values of patients and not to consider eating as a major quality-of-life indicator. Physicians are often trained in paternalism and to take a militaristic stance in the fight against death. In the past they have been shaped to be ultimately responsible and often view themselves as 'lone rangers'. In a synergistic team, these pre-established ways of operating can be transcended when needed, and roles can be shared as the team works out of their collaborative commitment to each other and to renal patients and families.[4]

There is some overlap between professional roles (i.e. dietitians and physicians, nurses and social workers[5]) which can create occasional 'turf wars', especially when resources are threatened and staff experience stress, e.g. during the growth of managed care and capitation of renal programmes. In the US healthcare system, as 'for-profit' dialysis companies mushroom, pressure has been exerted to change some professional roles for the purposes of expediency. For example, expanded roles of admission coordinator and insurance watchdog have been delegated to renal social workers in many for-profit companies. This additional role significantly shifts time spent away from a role as counsellor/coach,[6] crucial to fostering support throughout the course of treating a dialysis patient. This supportive role can facilitate palliative and gentle end-of-life care.

## 14.3 Theoretical, operational contexts: acute versus chronic

Most medical professionals are shaped in their formal education by an acute care model of service delivery. In this model, patients have little say and look to the medical staff to assess, diagnose, and create a treatment plan that will hopefully 'fix what ails' them. In some ways, dialysis appears to require this kind of orientation. It is certainly one of the most technological arenas of medicine and has a high mortality rate. Kidney Disease Outcomes Quality Initiative (KDOQI)[7] guidelines focus on 'numbers', as the technology of dialysis itself forces the renal team to attend to the mathematics of the treatment regimen.

Compounding this technological orientation, nurses, medical social workers, dietitians, and physicians are trained to a large degree in a model that is disease/pathology oriented. In this mode, staff set the treatments goals and are in control, and it is not necessary to communicate with the patient beyond the domains of brain and body.

Experienced renal teams realize that people on dialysis can live for many years and will never be cured. Further, they see that attending to purely medical issues will not necessarily ensure an acceptable quality of life for the patient nor will it ultimately satisfy the team. A growing body of literature underscores the need to focus on the biopsychosocial needs of patients if they are to integrate the severe treatment regimen and still experience quality in their lives.[8–11] Kimmel's work emphasizes the importance of psychosocial factors like depression, social support, and perception of the effects of the illness on differing survival rates of the dialysis patient.[10,11] Clearly, both quality and quantity of life depend on our willingness to attend to the whole patient in the context of family and in how he or she sees their world.

### 14.3.1 Differences between chronic and acute illness

In order to shift the context of the renal team, we have to appreciate the differences between chronic and acute illness. For instance, chronic and acute illnesses are perceived in different ways in our culture. There are no greetings cards saying 'wishing you the best in your life with chronic illness'. Instead, they say either 'get better quickly' or send 'sympathy' to the relatives.

The very word 'handicap' (literally translated from cap in hand, meaning begging for alms) reminds us of the invisible stigma of chronic illness. There is denial and negativity in the 'chronic illness narrative', the filter through which a patient views having a chronic illness, that our culture itself generates. When patients enter the 'dialysis community', they step into our society's real ambivalence about their worth and value.

In the acute care model, the patient may see his or her physician and nurse only once or twice with very little personal detail revealed about the medical professional's or patient's life. Once on dialysis, staff will accompany the patient from the beginning of kidney failure to its conclusion often over decades. Patients and staff will share major events in their lives along the way, such as weddings, births, graduations, and significant losses.

Finally, the goals of treatment are different. In his book *The Illness Narratives: Suffering, Healing, and the Human Condition* Kleinman makes eloquent distinctions between acute and chronic care:[9] 'Whereas acute care aims to restore one's freedom from illness, the goal of chronic care is to sustain meaning in a life lived with—and in spite of—illness. The primary obligation of chronic care medicine, then, is not keeping [a patient] from being affected by illness—that is impossible—but rather to assist the person in keeping the transformative power of illness under control, to integrate the patient's new wants and needs into a coherent and satisfying life.'

### 14.3.2 Medical decision-making in the context of chronic illness

> I need to be included as a member of the team. This is my life, and I have every right to be part of the decision-making process. I have a voice and it needs to be heard.

The patient and family are the 'hub' around which the team revolves in a chronic illness model. Treatment decision-making needs to be as consensual as possible, and this process will evolve as relationships grow with staff, and as the patient and family learn and experience more and more on the dialysis journey. In this chronic context, the word compliance, which has been defined as coercing one agenda on another, will not work. Patient-determined compliance or active self-management more closely approximates the actual situation.[12] Clearly, patients have the upper hand in what they are willing and not willing to do. If the team can adopt this practical point of view, patients will be in the best position to learn about medical decision-making and the consequences of their informed choices.

### 14.3.3 Relationships in the chronic model

> Share a little of yourself with me and I'll share twice as much with you. I need to know it's OK to be open and have human frailty.

Though medical professionals are formally trained in an acute care model, life experience often leads them to a shift in paradigm and they find themselves fellow travellers with patients and families on the road of chronic illness.[13] One physician describes how patients with whom he engages in end-of-life discussions imprint their own identity, as that of a family member.[14] Another remarks that 'a doctor's job would be so much more interesting and satisfying if he would occasionally let himself plunge into the patient, if he could lose his own fear of falling'.[15]

In fact, some renal teams are beginning to adopt a 'medical family' identity with their patients and families.[13] Many patients already view renal teams in this way.[16] In a recent article, Swartz describes his team's work with patients with chronic renal failure (CRF). The renal team see their 'patients frequently and recurrently, get to know them more closely, and assist with or take responsibility for aspects of patients' lives that even some family members do not

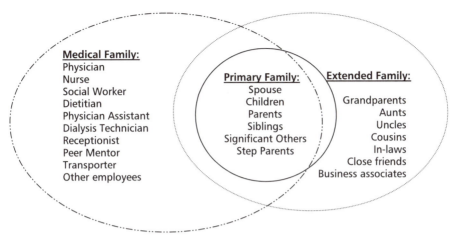

**Fig. 14.1** The medical family.

address'. The intensity of this relationship has prompted some team members to say that they feel 'almost like family'. In effect, the relationship may well be familial in nature, sharing obligations, dependency, and emotional attachments that exist in many family interactions. He suggests using the term 'medical family' to describe these interactions, 'implying a relationship that encompasses all parties participating in and affected by a patient's chronic illness and its management'. Fig. 14.1 offers a theoretical model that describes the relationship of the medical family to the traditional primary and the extended family.[13]

The medical family includes some, though not necessarily all, of those mentioned above and may include other persons who are not part of the patient's traditional family. These individuals become a community of support with the patient.

### 14.3.4 Relationship research

Though professional publications often portray staff as anonymous entities, the renal team grows and evolves as human beings along with their patients on the journey of chronic illness. Research is currently being conducted for patients on the phenomenon of the impact of relationships and the dialysis milieu on patients and, reciprocally, on staff.[17] Early findings show that when staff report more shared feelings with patients (intimacy), they have less work stress, less job burnout, and more job satisfaction and meaning. Similar results were obtained looking at the relationship between patients' well-being and their 'intimacy' with staff. Thus, more open interpersonal relationships in the dialysis unit correlate consistently with both patient and staff well-being. These and other future studies that look at the influence of relationships and the dialysis milieu have the potential to significantly enhance patient outcomes and staff satisfaction.

### 14.3.5 Challenges and new approaches

Many authors point to how difficult it is for physicians (and other medical staff) to 'plunge' into the lives of their patients. Jung calls empathy the merging of the viewer and the viewed. Harries sees it as 'a feeling of being at home with the object contemplated', as with a friend.[18] Howard Spiro in his insightful article[19] talks about how empathy is bred out of medical students and replaced by equanimity and detachment. He suggests that physicians move beyond the detached 'I want to help you', with their patients, families, and team and allow themselves to feel the empathic 'I might be you'.

To foster the development of relationships, the building of trust, and consensual decision-making, Elisabeth Kubler-Ross suggests a model in which we see patients as having four 'parts': physical, emotional, intellectual, and spiritual.[20] By attending only to the physical and intellectual aspects of patients we create a hierarchy since staff are physically well and more medically knowledgeable than the patient. In the chronic care setting, patients take their place on the team where their emotional orientation (illness narrative) and spiritual values are incorporated into their care and they can assist in facing and giving meaning to life's ups and downs and to strengthen their ability to create quality in thier own lives.[21]

Various value-assessment tools are available to help the team develop the practice of attending to the total person, but it is important to remember that they are aids and not 'answers'. Delbanco[15] acknowledges the growing distance between physician and patient and offers an excellent patient review that includes seven dimensions of care.

Ann Fadiman in her book *The Spirit Catches You and You Fall Down*,[22] posed eight questions aimed at drawing out patients' and families' personal view of their illness narrative using the Hmong culture from south-east Asia as an interesting example. For instance, when the physician tapped the explanatory model of Hmong medicine by asking, 'What do you think has caused the problem?' The reply was 'soul loss'. Fadiman suggests that the notion of compliance loses any meaning when one looks at cross-cultural medicine and that negotiation and involvement of someone from that particular culture would be more effective. Antonovsky[23] describes spirituality as a positive, pervasive way of seeing the world that renders illness more manageable and comprehensible. Furthermore, there is some evidence that spirituality is associated with lower levels of anxiety and psychological distress[24] (see Chapter 11).

### 14.3.6 Peer mentoring: creating a caring community in dialysis units

> By empowering us, you foster well-being and the desire to take an active part in care and decision-making. This in turn generates acceptance and a positive outlook. This positive outlook shines through and helps others as we role model that there is life beyond dialysis.

We see the value of support groups in the lives of alcoholics, people who want to lose weight, in breast cancer, AIDS, and in other arenas of chronic conditions. This kind of support is also very effective in dialysis settings. Peer mentors provide support to patients and families and a role model that life with chronic illness may be inconvenient, but that it does not have to be hopelessly intrusive. Kimmel's research underscores the importance of social support and role modelling to successful living with chronic kidney failure, and to achieving a better quality and quantity of life for renal patients.[10]

On every dialysis unit there are patients who are committed to contributing to others who are also managing a life with chronic illness. These individuals have time for volunteer work. They may not have enough energy to return to work, but they want to make a difference and most renal teams know who these individuals are. Very naturally, new patients are introduced to them by staff to view their fistula or to share an empowering experience. This informal support by veteran renal patients referred to as peer mentoring has been formalized and expanded in many American states.[25] The US National Kidney Foundation has adopted the programme nationally. It provides 16 hours of training to dialysis and transplant patients and family members consisting of empathic listening, problem solving, value clarification, assertiveness, sexuality, and end-of-life issues. Patients fine-tune their own listening skills and become more self-aware regarding how they have integrated life with dialysis.

New levels of relationship and support enter the dialysis setting when the peer mentor is added to the team. The powerful interventions of the peer mentor will be illustrated as we explore the biopsychosocial journey with patients and families later in the chapter.

## 14.4 Adding a palliative approach to the chronic care model

Recognizing the prevalence of death in nephrology, a palliative approach is beginning to filter through into the operational context of the renal team.[26] Despite a high mortality rate[27], renal staff are not formally educated, trained, or mandated to address death and dying with their patients and families.

We have seen, in addition to the benefits to patients, that there is tremendous personal growth and satisfaction, with reduced burnout, for staff who develop palliative care skills and incorporate a palliative approach to their work.

### 14.4.1 Relationship and advance directives (see Chapter 4)

The inherent value of advance directives (ADs) is that they provide a vehicle for the development or relationships and trust. In terms of comfort level, social workers were by far the most comfortable discussing ADs and did so with 60% of their patients. Nephrologists were more uncomfortable and talked with 38% of their patients about ADs. Nurses were quite uncomfortable and discussed ADs with 25% of their patients. In this study, the renal team looked to the social worker and the nephrologist to take the lead in discussion of ADs with patients.[28,29,30]

### 14.4.2 Integrating discussion of advance directives into the renal team

There are ways to incorporate the whole team in the process of introduction, discussion, and execution of ADs that take into account professional concerns. For instance, nurses can give the patient the initial AD question and answer fact sheets and the AD document; they do not need to spell out its legalities but can refer the patient to the social worker for discussion. The social worker can bring in the nephrologist when discussion is required. In any family meeting about end-of-life decision-making, the dietitian is often extremely helpful as quality-of-life issues are sorted out which often include dietary questions and eating difficulties as the end of life approaches.

In the ordinary course of interaction with staff, patients tend to bond with at least one particular staff member. It may be, as in the case study, that they have a mutual interest in sports, and, through this shared human interest, trust is created. This provides a foundation for the trust that is necessary in end-of-life discussion. If every renal team member took some part in naturalizing the end-of-life discussion, credibility and trust might be established more effectively ahead of time in this existential, often fearful, domain.

Certainly initial introduction to ADs can be frightening to patients and families. In fact, in one study,[31] 60% of the patients acknowledged initial anxiety when staff brought the subject up. Several months later, when the subject was raised, this percentage of anxiety decreased to 23%, and after a year was only at 3%. The Robert Wood Johnson Foundation recently awarded a grant to the National Kidney Foundation of Michigan, Inc., to assess the impact of discussion of ADs initiated by a peer mentor. The hope is that less anxiety about death would be triggered via this format of presentation. A Michigan pilot study for this grant, indeed, did show a significant increase in completion of ADs and a decrease in patient discomfort when peer mentors portrayed completing an AD as a means to preserve control rather than as an indicator of imminent death. Patients view peers as more experienced and successful in integrating chronic illness into their lives. If peers do not show discomfort in discussing their own AD, patients tend to adopt this attitude.

This chapter contends that relationships between patients, family, and staff are crucial to end-of-life discussion and that they evolve over time. There are predictable milestones on the journey of chronic kidney disease (CKD) with opportunity for the development of relationships as well as end-of-life discussions. This relationship can begin with visits to the clinic where the peer mentor can meet clients and discuss the different types of modalities available to them. Discussions about haemodialysis, peritoneal dialysis, transplant, and even no treatment can alleviate some of the fears that the patient may be experiencing. The peer once again serves as a role model showing that end-stage renal disease with its various treatments is by no means the end of life as they knew it. Patients can also be invited to patient education meetings where modalities are discussed by nurse educators as well as peers. Visits to the dialysis unit can also help to calm fears of the unknown. When a patient meets with a peer who they identify with, and see that the peer is having the treatment in question (home dialysis, transplant, etc.), they often quickly agree to sign on to this treatment even when they were reluctant or sceptical when it was explained by the nurse or physician.

The remainder of this chapter is dedicated to this journey

EMPOWER ME

Equip me with the tools I will need as I enter
the arena of dialysis so that I might
fight the valiant battle.

Be honest! For I can see what you're
not saying.

Listen to me as you would your own
family. I have important things
to say to you.

Help me from the dark shadows of
Despair so that I might see
The path more clearly.

Stand by me from the first day to the
Last and allow me a dignified death.
A good death!

The truth shall be my guide.
EMPOWER ME,
AND YOU WILL ALSO BE EMPOWERED!

George Kelly, peer mentor and kidney/liver transplant patient/consumer

## 14.5 Stages of the biopsychosocial journey: windows for relationship development and end-of-life discussion

The truth is the most important thing that you can share with me. I don't want to go through this experience thinking one thing and have another happen. The truth will help to prepare me for a road filled with potholes and wild turns. . . .

## 14.5.1  At initial diagnosis of chronic kidney disease

My world is falling apart. What did I do to deserve this? I can't handle this! How am I going to tell my family?

### 14.5.1.1  Patient and family experience

A sense of unreality often accompanies early diagnosis of CKD. One part of the patient senses the life-shaking change ahead; another part keeps this fear at bay, carrying on as long as possible with the comforting normality of routine. Denial is often serviceable until the patient is forced to step into the unknown dimension of total kidney failure and of life and death.

### 14.5.1.2  Relationship with the team

The renal team can serve as a 'guide' in this early phase and provide support to both the renal patient and their family. Establishing trust at this juncture supports both the patient and the team when end-of-life issues become the predominant focus later on. A trusting relationship can be nurtured by the offer of telephone contact by a peer mentor, someone who has been there and who would be happy to answer any questions.

### 14.5.1.3  End-of-life discussion opportunities

Many new dialysis patients have beliefs within their illness narrative that initiating treatment is the 'beginning of the end'. Depending on age and medical circumstances, this might, in fact, be the case, and it affords an important opportunity to engage the patient in discussions about quality of life and the real options that are available.[30]

## 14.5.2  Just before dialysis begins

I need to know what this thing called dialysis really is. I want to know what it's going to do to me. Will this cure me? If this doesn't work, where can I go from here? AM I GOING TO DIE?

### 14.5.2.1  Patient and family experience

Prior to beginning dialysis, patients will face many physical, social, and emotional changes. It is a difficult time to be making important healthcare decisions and many patients are clinically depressed.[33,34]

### 14.5.2.2  Relationship with the team

Prior to the initiation of dialysis, the patient needs non-threatening education. Nephrologist referrals to CKD education programmes have been found to delay the progression of the disease, decrease acute hospitalizations, and increase compliance.[35] Peer mentors should be included in these groups and can have new patients feel their fistulas and listen to why they chose one dialysis modality over another. Patients are more likely to choose home dialysis if they identify with a peer using this modality. Also, individuals and families who are seen by a renal social worker before initiating dialysis have been shown to have a decreased incidence of depression and will demonstrate increased compliance with treatment when dialysis begins, as well as increased quality of life and positive adaptation to dialysis.[32,34,35]

### 14.5.2.3  End-of-life discussion opportunities

Patient and family pre-dialysis education programmes that include peer mentors shift patients' understanding about life on dialysis. The pre-dialysis programme is an opportunity in a group setting for the peer to raise advance directives, why they themselves completed them, and what their family's response was to them; this neutralizes and naturalizes end-of-life discussion.[37]

## 14.5.3 Starting dialysis

I'm scared as hell to walk through that door. This is surreal. If I turn around and leave, will I die?

### 14.5.3.1 Patient and family experience

Individuals newly experiencing dialysis have many fears, including pain related to needle sticks, dependence on dialysis for survival, body image changes, sexuality changes, financial issues, and the fear of decreased independence, to name a few.[32] Although many renal patients appear to cope well with being a 'novice' to dialysis, 28% were found to experience difficulties in adapting to kidney failure.[35] In the first 3 months after initiating chronic dialysis, 52% of individuals self-reported anxiety and 43% displayed symptoms of depression.[34] Since depression is a factor associated with increased mortality,[34] this should be a red flag for staff. The depressed patient will demonstrate decreased self-management with medical treatment both before and during the initiation of dialysis.[32,36]

Spouses, family members, and significant others[38] face changes in lifestyle when a loved one is diagnosed with CKD and begins life on dialysis. Stress experienced from dialysis may increase tensions within the marriage, have an impact on sexuality and perceived intimacy, as well as decrease effective communication.[38]

Please don't forget that there are those of us who have people in our lives that don't meet the conventional family definition. This person is still an integral part of my life. Include him. Don't leave my heart out of my life with chronic illness.

It is vital to identify and recognize those who are important to the patient in the broad definition of 'family'.

### 14.5.3.2 Relationship with the team

The renal social worker helps the newly diagnosed patient with kidney failure adapt to dialysis in many ways. While providing education and support to the individual and family, the social worker also builds a relationship with them. A 1994 study found that 91% of dialysis patients believed that access to a renal social worker enhanced their treatment.[35] Dobroff *et al.*[34] found that social work practice with both 'identified patient' and family was associated with increased compliance and decreased hospitalizations and emergency department visits.[34]

The peer mentor can play a significant role at this early stage. Patients new to dialysis have not yet learned the chronic illness context for relationship with staff, but will share concerns and speak more freely with a peer who has 'been there'. A trained peer mentor will not give medical advice, but will 'coach' the new patient to seek professional staff who can address their concerns, such as the dialysis nurse, dietitian, and social worker, thus ensuring communication early on.

### 14.5.3.3 End-of-life discussion opportunities

Many patients will not experience an increased quality of life when dialysis is initiated, such as a nursing home resident with Alzheimer's disease. Dialogue about when 'enough is enough' and beliefs regarding death and mortality need to be addressed as part of the medical relationship between the patient and the renal team. If this does not happen, a conspiracy of silence is set up that will make end-of-life discussion much more difficult when it is needed later on.[39,40]

## 14.5.4 Maintenance dialysis

Be vigilant and hear what I'm not saying. Notice that I am in a dark foreboding place which takes over my entire being. I need you to help me find my way back.

### 14.5.4.1 Patient and family experience

Once stabilized on dialysis, many patients achieve a measure of predictability in their lives. Fear decreases regarding treatment, and survival is no longer in the forefront of the patient's mind. When the individual reaches physical and emotional homeostasis with dialysis, the next task is to integrate meaning into life with a chronic disease.

During this stage, the patient's support system also contributes to well-being and positive outcomes. Dobroff *et al.*[34] found that patients on dialysis who have good family support are more likely to experience a positive adaptation to chronic dialysis. When families are educated about CKD and chronic dialysis, the overall quality of life improves as the family motivates compliance with treatments and dietary restrictions.[32,34,35]

### 14.5.4.2 Relationship with the team

At this time, it is important that the renal team open up conversation regarding some important quality-of-life issues. Physically, sexual dysfunction is common in both men and women as is sleep disturbance, fatigue, itchiness, restless legs, and thirst. The team needs to naturalize discussions about changes in sexuality, be open to patient and family concerns, and to address returning to work, if the patient has been on medical leave.

This may be a time when the team needs to talk about 'tough love' with the spouse who may be wearing her/himself out caring for the loved one who is correspondingly feeling regressed and more and more of a burden. Peers can help to empower the patient to take control of their disease. They also can address 'compliance' in a way that is not perceived as scolding or blaming.

### 14.5.4.3 End-of-life discussion opportunities

In the course of a patient's dialysis 'career', they will see patients whom they have known and cared about who will suddenly not be there any more. If the renal team is operating from denial, no mention will be made to other patients about these deaths. This 'conspiracy of silence' communicates to patients that something must have gone wrong, somebody was at fault, that death is a tragedy rather than a natural event.

If the renal team is incorporating a palliative approach, it will let the other patients know about the death, and will honour the patient who has died in some way. Some units put a rose on the chair of the patient who died. Others develop remembrance gatherings once a year in which other patients and families of the deceased are invited to remember their loved ones. Peer mentors can play a crucial role in these palliative approaches by sending cards, inviting families to the gatherings, or just sharing with other patients that their friend has died.

## 14.5.5 Deterioration

I'm falling apart. What did we do wrong? My family doesn't want to hear that the end is near. Neither does my healthcare team. Help me make it through this final journey. Be part of the end as you were part of the beginning . . .

### 14.5.5.1 Patient and family experience

As deterioration gains momentum, the patient and family experience multiple kinds of stress. Caregivers can be overburdened, transportation to dialysis may be difficult (and expensive) to arrange, and pain and suffering may be the rule rather than the exception. Though perhaps there was an agreement among family to never consider nursing home placement, this may be the time when, besides stopping dialysis, it is the only realistic discharge plan. The hospital system may no longer greet the deteriorating patient with open arms as it did in the past when conditions could be reversed.

A crisis in health will bring family strengths and pathologies bubbling to the surface. The 'daughter from California' syndrome may cause many breakdowns within the renal team, when the uninvolved adult child requests that a parent receive cardiopulmonary resuscitation and will not accept other family members' wishes that comfort care be initiated.[38] When the renal team is in partnership with the family and aligned with the patient's wishes, breakdowns in end-of-life care can be dealt with and not become the focus of the dying process. Reiss[41] has found that individuals who are dying are more likely to die sooner than expected if their family is involved with medical decision-making and ambivalence about dying is addressed.

Families may differ in views of end-of-life care in relationship to cultural and social factors, such as ethnicity, education, and spirituality. Some cultures may be more accepting that dying is a part of life and are better able to process end-of-life planning.

Many African Americans have a basic mistrust of the healthcare system having long experienced that healthcare has been delivered along racial lines. These patients and families need to know that advanced care planning can be a vehicle for asking for the healthcare that they need and want.[42,43]

### 14.5.5.2 Relationship with the team

Family meetings build the foundation for end-of-life discussion. The relationship with staff establishes conditions that lay the foundation for good outcomes in end-of-life planning. There is also the opportunity for family members to raise possibly delicate or painful issues and for the staff to assess family support systems for future planning and decision-making.[13]

### 14.5.5.3 End-of-life discussion opportunities

Palliative care needs are best met at this stage if they were discussed before the onset of dialysis treatment.[32,40]

Early education meetings naturalize death by having peers share that advance directives are one way of maintaining control of quality living and quality dying. In discussions with staff, patients should have been informed of the 'fourth option', the right to stop dialysis, and be encouraged to discuss their wishes with their families during the stable dialysis years. The stage is now set for the next level of discussion including questions like: 'what death can be like', 'how long it might take', 'what kind of support options do families have?'

If the team, patient and family suspect that the end of life is approaching, it is time to begin to look at the components of a good dying process. These include pain control, finishing 'unfinished business', expressions of love given and received, and an opportunity to participate in a life review. At this time the dying patient may express wishes regarding their body after death and the ceremony they would envision for themselves.[26,29]

## 14.6 Conclusion

Nephrology is in a unique position in the field of chronic illness. With a federally mandated treatment team and a 'captive' group of patients who we will be followed for the duration of their lives on dialysis, we have the opportunity to be leaders in several important ways. First, we can pioneer the integration of the chronic disease model with palliative care. Second, we can naturalize death in a world that has made it exceedingly unnatural. Third, we can rediscover the value of relationships with our patients and families, not only in terms of their outcomes but our own well-being as well.

This chapter concludes with the following inquiries for the renal team:

1. Are we willing to be synergistic in our commitment with each other, our patients, and families?

2. Are we willing to see our patients and families as fellow travellers as opposed to passive recipients of our knowledge and healthcare?

3. Are we willing to see 'good' dying as a legitimate outcome?

4. What is the possibility that we will create end-of-life care that nourishes us rather than depletes us?

## Ethical analysis of the case study

A key part of the process of ethical decision-making is learning the patient's values (see the Introduction to Ethical Case Analysis in the Introduction, p. xvii). Often the best way to learn a patient's values is to take a Patient as Person History (see the Introduction, p. xvii) and learn the narrative of the patient's life. In this case, the renal care team should ask Michael what is most important to him and what gives his life meaning. The team should also learn what Michael would want to avoid in his treatment. Though the case does not explicitly say so, it appears that the social worker understood that Michael had undergone all the pain and suffering he could tolerate and that he needed a way to end his life narrative in a meaningful way. Through the family meeting and the story of Michael's grandfather with whom Michael had a close relationship, an acceptable end to Michael's narrative (he died like his grandfather, refusing further therapy) was found. After satisfying themselves that Michael was making an autonomous, voluntary, informed decision not unduly influenced by depression or encephalopathy (see the ethical case analysis in Chapter 2 for a systematic evaluation of a patient request to stop dialysis), the renal care team should accept his decision to stop dialysis to honour the ethical principle of respect for patient autonomy. Dialysis patients do not always make the decisions the renal care team would make for them. The role of the renal care team is to make certain that their patient's decisions are authentic and informed and then to honour them in a way that promotes their comfort, dignity, and support.

## Acknowledgements

To the enduring spirit of our beloved patients who constantly teach us about living and dying.

To the following reviewers for their wonderful suggestions and editing: Beth Witten, MSW, ACSW, LSCSW, renal social worker of renal social workers; Tracy Shroepfer, MSW researcher; Lea Fischer, MSW hospice social worker; Richard D. Swartz, MD, Director of Acute Dialysis Programs at the University of Michigan Medical Center; and Maurie Ferriter, Program Services Director, NKFM, Inc.

## References

1. Fried, B., Leatt, P., Deber, R., Wilson, E. (1988). Multidisciplinary teams in health care: lessons from oncology and renal teams. *Health Care Management Forum* 1(4): 28–34.

2. Federal Register (3 June 1976) 41(106): 22520.

3. Temkin-Greener, H. (1983). Interprofessional perspectives on teamwork in health care: a case study. *Milbank Memorial Fund Q. (Health Society)*, **61**(4): 641–58.

4. May, W. (1983). *The Physician's Covenant. Images of the Healer in Medical Ethics*. Philadelphia, PA: The Westminster Press.

5. Fried, B.J., Leatt, P. (1986). Role perceptions among occupational groups in an ambulatory care setting. *Hum. Relations*, **39**: 1155–74.

6. Pearson, P. (1983). The interdisciplinary team process or the professional tower of Babel. *Dev. Med. Child Neurol.*, **25**: 390–5.

7. National Kidney Foundation (2002). K/DOQI: clinical practice guidelines for chronic kidney disease: evaluation, classification and stratification. *Am. J. Kidney Dis.*, **39**(2) (Suppl. 1): 51–5246.

8. Burnell, M.S. (1997). The hemodialysis patient: object of diagnosis or part of the treatment team? *Adv. Renal Replacement Ther.*, **4**(2): 145–51.

9. Kleinman, A. (1988). *The Illness Narratives: Suffering, Healing, and the Human Condition*. New York: Basic Books.

10. Kimmel, P., Peterson, R., Weihs, K., Simmens, S., Alleyne, S., Cruz, I., *et al.* (1988). Psychosocial factors, behavioral compliance and survival in urban hemodialysis patients. *Kidney Int.*, **54**: 245–54.

11. Kimmel, P., Peterson, R., Weihs, K., Simmens, S., Alleyne, S., Cruz, I., *et al.* (2000). Multiple measurements of depression predict mortality in a longitudinal study of chronic hemodialysis patients. *Kidney Int.*, **57**: 2093–8.

12. Anderson, R. (1985). Is the problem of compliance all in our heads? *Diabetes Educ.*, **11**: 31–4.

13. Swartz, R.D., Perry, E. (1999). Medical family: a new view of the relationship between chronic dialysis patients and staff arising from discussion about advance directives. *J. Women's Health Gender Based Med.*, **8**(9): 1–7.

14. Quill, T. (1993). Doctor, I want to die. Will you help me? *J. Am. Med. Assoc.*, **270**: 870–3.

15. Delbanco, T. (1993). Enriching the doctor–patient relationship by inviting the patient's perspective. *Ann. Intern. Med.*, **116**(5): 414–18.

16. *Ann Arbor News* 5 June 2002. Eulogy of Ilene Brunson '. . . The family wishes to express a special thank you to the University of Michigan Dialysis Center for including Ilene in their family . . .'

17. Swartz, R.D., Perry, E., Swartz, J., Brown, S., Vinokur, A. (2001). Impact of the interpersonal milieu on clinical outcome, mental health and well being in the chronic dialysis unit [abstract]. *Am. Soc. Nephrol.* Annual Meeting 2001. San Francisco.

18. Harries, K. (1973). Empathy. *Dictionary of the History of Ideas II*, ed. P.P. Wiener. New York: Scribner's.

19. Spiro, H. (1992). What is empathy and can it be taught? *Ann. Intern. Med.* **116**: 843–6.

20. Kubler-Ross, E. (1991). *Life, Death, and Transition Intensive, Headwaters, Virginia*. Workshop.

21. Sermabeikian, P. (1994). Our clients, ourselves: the spiritual perspective and social work practice. *Social Work*, **39**(2): 178–83.

22. Fadiman, A. (1997). *The Spirit Catches You and You Fall Down*. Farrar Straus & Giroux. New York.

23. Antonovsky, A. (1987). *Unraveling the Mystery of Health: How People Manage Stress and Stay Well*. San Francisco, CA: Jossey-Bass.

24. Kaczorowski, J.M. (1989). Spiritual well-being and anxiety in adults diagnosed with cancer. *Hospice J.*, **5**: 105–16.

25. Kapron, K., Perry, E., Bowman, T., Swartz, R. (1997). Peer resource consulting: redesigning a new future. *Adv. Renal Replacement Ther.*, **4**(3): 267–74.

26. Cohen, LM., Poppel, D.M., Cohn. G.M., Rieter, G.S. (2001). A very good death: measuring quality of dying in end stage renal disease. *J. Palliative Med.*, **4**(2): 167–72.

27. United States Renal Data Service (USRDS) (1996). *1996 Annual Data Report*, publication 96–3176. Bethesda, MD: The National Institutes of Health, National Institute of Diabetes and Digestive and Kidney Diseases.

28. Holley, J.L., Hines, S.C., Glover, J.J., Babrow, A.S., Badzek, L.A., Moss, A.H. (1999). Failure of advance care planning to elicit patients' preferences for withdrawal from dialysis. *Am. J. Kidney Dis.*, **33**: 688–93.

29. Swartz, R., Perry, E. (1993). Advanced directives are associated with good deaths in chronic dialysis patients. *J. Am. Soc. Nephrol.*, **3**(9): 1623–30.

30. Perry, E., Swartz, R., Smith-Wheelock, L., Westbrook, J., Buck, C. (1996). Why is it difficult for staff to discuss advance directives with chronic dialysis patients? *J. Am. Soc. Nephrol.*, **7**(10): 2160–8.

31. Perry, E., Buck, C., Newsome, J., Berger, C., Messana, J., Swartz, R. (1995). Dialysis staff influence patients in formulating their advanced directives. *Am. J. Kidney Dis.*, **26**(1): 226–8.

32. Kimmel, P.L. (2000). Psychosocial factors in adult end stage renal disease patients treated with hemodialysis: correlates and outcomes. *Am. J. Kidney Dis.*, **35**(4): S132–S140.

33. Callahan, M.B. (1998). The role of the nephrology social worker in optimizing treatment outcomes for end stage renal disease patients. *Dial. Transplant.*, **27**(10): 630–7, 641–2, 674.

34. Dobroff, J., Dolinko, A., Lichtiger, E., Uribarri, J., Epstein, I. (2000). The complexity of social work practice with dialysis patients: risk and resiliency factors, interventions, and health related outcomes. *J. Nephrol. Social Work*, **20**: 21–36.

35. Funk Schrag, W. (2001). The K/DOQI chronic kidney disease guidelines: defining the role of the social worker in pre-dialysis education. *J. Nephrol. Social Work*, **2**: 9–12.

36. McClellan, W., Stanwyck, D.J., Anson, C.A. (1993). Social support and subsequent mortality among patients with end stage renal disease. *J. Am. Soc. Nephrol.*, **4**(4): 1028–34.

37. Rothchild, E. (1994). Family dynamics in end of life treatment decisions. *General Hospit. Psychiat.*, **16**(4): 251–8.

38. Daneker, B., Kimmel, P., Ranich, T., Peterson, R. (2001). Depression and marital dissatisfaction in patients with end stage renal disease and in their spouses. *Am. J. Kidney Dis.*, **38**(4): 839–46.

39. Davison, S. (2001). Quality end-of-life care in dialysis units. *Semin. Dial.*, **15**(1): 41–4.

40. Quill, T. (2000). Initiating end-of-life discussions with seriously ill patients: addressing the 'elephant in the room'. *J. Am. Med. Assoc.*, **284**(19): 2502–7.

41. Reiss, D. (1990). Patient, family, and staff responses to end-stage renal disease. *Am. J. Kidney Dis.*, **15**(3): 194–200.

42. Byrd, M., Clayton, L. (1991). The 'slave health deficit': racism and health outcomes. *Health PAC Bull.*, **25**: 236.

43. Byrd, M. (1990). Race, biology, and health care: reassessing a relationship. *J. Healthcare Poor Underserved* Winter: 278.

# Chapter 15

# End of life

Jeremy Levy

## 15.1 Introduction

Dialysis saves lives. However, dialysis does not provide normal life expectancy, and patients die on dialysis with chronic renal failure (CRF) and end-stage renal disease (ESRD) contributing to their death. Patients with renal failure live significantly shorter lives than the general population, and life expectancy on dialysis is vastly less than for age-matched controls. Furthermore, death on dialysis or with ESRD tends to be even more medicalized than death in general in the 21st century.

There are few published data for death rates and causes of death for patients with renal impairment of various degrees prior to dialysis, but it is likely that cardiovascular disease is the leading cause of death at all stages of chronic kidney disease. In one of the few studies examining mortality in pre-dialysis patients, Holland and Lam studied contributory factors in the deaths of 37 patients out of a cohort of 362 patients prior to their need for dialysis.[1] Death was significantly associated with increasing age, diastolic hypertension, a history of myocardial infarction, heart failure and angina, a lower haematocrit and baseline creatinine >300 μmol/l. By multivariate analysis only female sex, a history of angina, and increasing age were independent predictors of death.

There are many more data available for patients with ESRD. In the United States, for example, a 49-year-old man on dialysis will only live an average 7 years, compared with 30 years in the general population. There is marked variation though in mortality rates between different countries (see later). The United State Renal Data Service (USRDS) provides the most detailed data for mortality in ESRD, and shows that overall for all patients with ESRD, death rates are higher for Whites than African Americans (193 versus 157 per 1000 patient years), slightly higher for women than men (206 versus 187 per 1000 patient years), and not surprisingly significantly higher for patients with diabetes than hypertension, glomerulonephritis, or other causes of ESRD (236, 209, 90 and 130 per 1000 patient years respectively). All of these death rates are higher for dialysis patients than transplant recipients, in whom death rates approach (but do not reach) those of the general population.[2] The overall death rates for transplant recipients was 35 per 1000 patient years compared with 234 for all dialysis patients. The Australian ANZDATA registry reported death rates of 157 and 192 per 1000 patient years for dialysis patients in Australia and New Zealand respectively, and 32 and 25 for transplant recipients.[3]

Cause of death for patients with ESRD has not changed significantly over the last 20 years. American data show that cardiac disease in general is the major cause, and more specifically, cardiac arrest. This is twice as common as septicaemia, followed by acute myocardial infarction and cerebrovascular disease.[2] Other cardiac causes follow, including arrhythmia and cardiomyopathy. Some of these terms are open to variable interpretation, and not used in other registry data sets, but the overall picture emerges of cardiac and vascular disease as the major cause of death in ESRD. Malignant disease is one-sixth less common than cardiac disease, but relatively more important in transplant recipients. Cause of death does not vary substantially between patients receiving peritoneal or haemodialysis. The Australasian registry has very similar results (although the classification of death varies somewhat), with 46% of dialysis patients dying from cardiac causes overall (including both acute myocardial infarction and cardiac arrest), 12% from infections (mostly septicaemia), and 10% from vascular disease (mostly cerebrovascular).[3] However, in the ANZDATA registry a large proportion of patients (21%) are identified as dying from refusal for further therapy or therapy being ceased—causes not explicitly coded in USRDS data.[3] In Brazil the epidemiology of death is also broadly similar, although with more infections: 30% of patients die from cardiovascular causes, 20% from infections, and 13% from cerebrovascular disease.[4] In the Lazio region of Italy 50% of patients are identified as dying from a cardiac cause, 15% from vascular disease, and 4% from infections.[5] Single-centre studies have shown some variations in mortality. For example, Mailloux followed 532 patients with ESRD over 16 years, of whom 222 died.[6] In this cohort infections were the commonest cause of death (36%) followed by dialysis withdrawal (21%) and then cardiac disease, sudden death, and vascular causes. Infections and cardiac causes were more common in patients dying during the first 4 years on dialysis, while infections and withdrawal more common beyond 4 years.

Although the causes of death are roughly similar between countries, the overall death rate of dialysis patients is consistently higher in the United States than in other countries. Several explanations have been proposed for this including increased co-morbidities in patients dialysed in America, an increased number of diabetic patients, older age at start of dialysis, and inadequate dialysis. Certainly more patients are accepted onto dialysis programmes in America than in the rest of the world, and this reflects a greater referral rate to nephrologists by other physicians in the US, and by a greater reluctance to withhold dialysis.[7] Inadequate dialysis as an explanation for the shorter survival of patients in the US could have been historically due to attempts to reduce the number of hours patients spent on haemodialysis in the 1970s and early 1980s, when attempts were made to shorten the number of hours on dialysis by using newer high-efficiency and high-flux dialysers. Data reporting higher death rates in the 1980s led to attempts to increase the dose of dialysis delivered by increasing times on dialysis once again, and 1-year mortality in new haemodialysis patients fell from 280 per 1000 patient years in 1988 to 150 by 1997. The experience in Tassin in France, where patients receive 24 h of dialysis per week and have exceptional survival and low morbidity, has also led to much investigation into the major factors determining outcome on dialysis.[8]

## 15.2 Risk factors for increased mortality in ESRD

Most patients with ESRD have several co-morbidities which potentially increase their risk of an early death. Pre-existing coronary artery disease not surprisingly increases the risk of dying in ESRD, since cardiac causes account for most deaths on dialysis. However, the risk factors for heart disease in renal failure are not necessarily the same as for the general population. Hypercholesterolaemia, for example, is not associated with increased cardiovascular events in ESRD, and there is good evidence that atherosclerosis is not the key underlying pathophysiological cause of vascular disease. Despite this, some studies have shown that markers for vascular damage (such as carotid artery intima–medial thickness) are associated with cardiovascular death in dialysis patients.[9] Hypertension certainly predisposes to left ventricular hypertrophy, and this may be much more important in renal patients since sudden cardiac death is commoner than acute myocardial infarction as a cause of death, and hypertensive ventricular hypertrophy may be more associated with ventricular abnormalities than coronary ischaemia. Over 80% of patients starting dialysis are hypertensive, and have had hypertension for many years, usually poorly controlled.

Many patients starting dialysis are now diabetic and hence have a host of metabolic derangements leading to premature vascular disease (in this case including atherosclerosis). Diabetic patients may also have pre-existing peripheral arterial disease, myocardial disease, and hypertension. Dyslipidaemia is common, although usually hypertriglyceridaemia rather than hypercholesterolaemia.

Hyperphosphataemia and an elevated calcium phosphate product are increasingly recognized as important causes of vascular calcification, certainly in ESRD and probably earlier in chronic renal insufficiency, and this may be more significant than previously identified.[10] Coronary artery calcification may be the major substrate for cardiac arrhythmias, sudden death, and myocardial ischaemia. Patients with systemic collagen vascular diseases such as systemic lupus erythematosus (SLE) and vasculitis are also at increased risk of premature vascular disease, even without significant renal failure.

Which factors are most important in predisposing to an early death remain unclear. Foley et al.'s analysis suggested that age, diabetes, cardiac failure, ischaemic heart disease, cancer, coma, sepsis, and liver failure were independent prognostic indicators of an early death (in less than 6 months after starting dialysis).[11] The underlying cause of renal disease has some impact on survival, but usually through systemic effects. Hence diabetic patients have the worst survival on dialysis, followed by patients with hypertension as primary diagnosis, and finally those with primary glomerulonephritis or polycystic kidney disease. Age has a controversial impact on survival.[12] In one study from the UK of patients over the age of 70 undergoing dialysis, only age over 80 years was associated with an increased relative risk of death (relative risk 2.79), as was the presence of peripheral vascular disease (relative risk 2.83).[13] There was no excess risk associated with diabetes, ischaemic heart disease, cerebrovascular disease, or sex, and overall survival was very similar to patients aged 60 years. In contrast Letourneau et al. from Montreal examined the outcome of 67 dialysis patients over 75 years of age compared with 66 aged 50–60 years.[14] The younger patients had been referred earlier. Survival rates at 1 and 3 years were 93% and 74% for the younger patients and 80% and 45% for the older patients ($p = 0.002$). More than 50% of the patients aged over 75 years had died within 2 years, and had a mean survival of 31 months. The younger patients had a mean survival of 44 months. Joly et al. studied their octogenarians reaching ESRD in France, and collected 144 patients with a creatinine clearance of less than 10 ml/min aged over 80 years.[15] Thirty-seven decided on conservative care only and 107 started dialysis. The only factors associated with a poor survival in the dialysed patients were a low Karnofsky performance score, late referral for dialysis, and low body mass index. It should be remembered that various measures of quality of life do not suggest a differential effect of dialysis in elderly patients compared with their younger dialysees, or elderly controls, especially for mental rather than physical quality of life.

Data on the impact of race on survival, mostly from the US, have proved intriguing.[16] African Americans consistently have a significantly lower mortality rate on dialysis than Whites; at 5, 10, and 15 years survival is almost 50% higher in Black patients.[2] Furthermore, this is despite lower apparent delivered dialysis doses in African Americans in general, higher co-morbidities, higher rates of diabetes, and lower socioeconomic status. Pei et al. reported a similar effect (better survival on dialysis) in patients from South and Southeast Asia.[17] Nutrition is another crucial determinant of survival on dialysis, and nutritional status at the start of dialysis has a great impact on short- and long-term survival. Patients with poor nutrition (however measured) have significantly shorter life expectancy on dialysis. Perhaps as a corollary, serum albumin alone is a strong predictor of survival on dialysis, although of course a low albumin is possibly more importantly a reflection of a generalized inflammatory state than simply a marker of malnutrition. Socioeconomic factors are also very important and act independently in predicting patient mortality. Patients' support networks, family structures, perception of illness, social isolation, and depression, interacting with compliance, have a similar impact on mortality at 1 and 5 years as more purely medical risk factors and co-morbid diseases. Finally some studies have suggested that time accrued on dialysis itself increases mortality rates, with a 6% increased risk of death for every additional year on dialysis, all else being equal.[18] This has not been replicated in all centres, when account is taken of modifiable factors such as high phosphates, low haemoglobin, and dose of dialysis delivered to patients.[19] Under these circumstances length of time itself does not increase the risk of death on dialysis.

One recent study from the Lister dialysis unit in the UK examined factors affecting survival in a single centre between 1992 and 1996. During this period 292 patients with ESRD started dialysis. The four major determinants of survival were age, co-morbidities, Karnofsky performance score, and whether the presentation for dialysis was planned or unplanned.[20] Age less than 50 years was associated with a significantly better outcome (85% 5-year survival) compared with those who were older (30% 5-year survival). Five-year survival for patients with no co-morbidities, moderate, or severe co-morbidities were 70%, 30%, and 0% respectively. The Karnofsky score was also strongly associated with survival; 65% of patients with normal activity scores survived for 5 years compared with 20% of those with poor functioning. An unplanned admission reduced survival by 25% at all times up to 5 years. In this study diabetes did not predict a poorer outcome. Using a combination of the four individual predictors it was possible to identify patients with an appalling or excellent prognosis. In contrast, Walters *et al.* from Leicester, UK, were unable to identify patients with a poor prognosis using co-morbidity and age alone.[21]

Pre-dialysis nephrological care has emerged more recently as yet another important factor determining outcome on dialysis, although definitions of late and timely referral vary. Patients referred to a nephrologist more than 6 months before the need to initiate dialysis survive significantly longer then those referred late. Jungers *et al.* reported death rates of 77% and 59% for patients followed by a renal physician for less than 6 months or more than 3 years.[22] A longer duration of pre-dialysis care led to increased survival. Walters *et al.* found that more than 50% of patients dying within the first year on dialysis in a UK centre had never seen a nephrologist prior to renal replacement therapy,[21] and there was an association with a very high rate of temporary access use (more than 85% patients) and septicaemia. Stack found a strong association between pre-dialysis ESRD care and survival in his cohort of 2264 patients.[23] The relative risk of dying was 1.68 in late referred patients (less than 4 months prior to dialysis) compared with those referred early, both at 1 and 2 years. Essentially identical results were obtained in Leeds.[24] Winkelmayer *et al.* reported 36% excess mortality in patients referred late, but the effect only lasted 3 months.[25] Van Biesen *et al.* found that 30% of all patients were referred less than 1 month before the need to start dialysis, and this led to an increased mortality from 16% to 27%.[26] Late referral has detrimental effects because of the lack of interventions which might slow progression of renal failure, the failure to plan for renal replacement therapy, failure to plan vascular access, and failure to provide psychological support. It leads not only to increased early death rates but also increased hospitalizations and lower quality of life.[27]

## 15.3 Dialysis factors affecting survival

There has been enormous controversy in determining, firstly, whether the mode of dialysis (peritoneal or haemodialysis) has any effect on mortality rates in ESRD, and secondly whether dialysis dose affects outcome. Most studies of mode of dialysis have shown no significant difference in survival between patients receiving peritoneal dialysis (continuous ambulatory peritoneal dialysis (CAPD) or ambulatory peritoneal dialysis (APD)) or any form of haemodialysis. However, all these studies have been confounded to a degree by the differential selection of patients for the different dialysis modalities—there have never been (and never will be) a prospective study allocating patients randomly to either peritoneal or haemodialysis. Data from individual centres have shown both increased and decreased survival for patients on peritoneal versus haemodialysis.[28–31] Several epidemiological studies have suggested that patients on peritoneal dialysis seem to have a significantly lower risk of death in the first 2 years of dialysis only.[32] Longer-term survival does not seem to differ significantly between patients, regardless of initial mode of dialysis. A significant factor affecting these survival data, and usually unaccounted for, is residual renal function. Patients with preserved residual renal function have better outcomes than those without, and renal function is better preserved on peritoneal dialysis. Similarly when looking at survival data in peritoneal dialysis alone, retention of native renal function is fundamentally important.

For patients on haemodialysis there has been much debate about the effect of dialysis dose on survival. Clearly there are issues about measuring 'dialysis dose' but for now I will use this as a generic term. It is certainly clear that patients dialysing at home have lower mortality rates than those dialysing in centres, whether by conventional thrice-weekly haemodialysis, daily, or nocturnal haemodialysis. Survival rates as high as 90% at 5 years and 75% at 15 years have been reported. This survival advantage is maintained even when corrected for age, race, socioeconomic status, and co-morbidities, although the numbers in most studies have been small, and by the nature of home dialysis patients are a selected group. Despite this benefit less than 1% of patients in the United States dialyse at home, 10–12% in the UK and Canada, and 18% in Australia.

Does the specific nature of the haemodialysis programme determine survival? Patients in Tassin, France, survive significantly longer than anywhere else in the world and dialyse for 24 h per week, until recently with low-flux modified cellulose dialysers.[8] A 15-year survival rate of 65% was reported. Most other centres around the world have attempted to replicate these survival rates but using shorter hours, and substituting high-efficiency or high-flux dialysers, haemodiafiltration, or even daily dialysis. All of these interventions are undertaken in the belief that improved small molecule clearance will translate into better survival, which may of course not be true. Too short a time on dialysis undoubtedly leads to poor survival—as shown in the United States during the 1970s and 1980s, where mortality rates doubled when dialysis hours were reduced significantly.

A huge literature has been published trying to assess whether solute removal (as measured by $Kt/V$ or urea reduction ratios) can be associated with survival, and whether there really is an association between more dialysis and lower mortality. A number of retrospective studies have shown that increasing $Kt/V$ led to better survival; however, all these studies were confounded. Despite this various reports suggested that, for example, for every 0.1 increase in $Kt/V$ the relative risk of death due to coronary artery disease was 9% lower, other cardiac disease 12% lower, cerebrovascular disease 14% lower, infection 9% lower, and dialysis withdrawal 9% lower.[33] The recent HEMO study attempted to solve this question once and for all. This was a prospective randomized trial comparing survival in both new and existing haemodialysis patients achieving a single pool $Kt/V$ of 1.25 or 1.65, and using either low- or high-flux dialysis membranes.[34] Overall, and to the surprise of many nephrologists, there was no survival advantage in achieving higher urea clearances or in using high-flux membranes. Clearly the study will become the subject of much analysis and reanalysis, but does not support the universal use of high-flux dialysers to improve patient survival, nor that survival improves with continually increasing solute clearance.

Finally there has been a suggestion that earlier initiation of dialysis leads to better survival and lower death rates. The major problem with such research is 'lead time bias', and identifying the true length of time the patient would have dialysed had they not started early, Traynor *et al.* tried to overcome this by calculating estimated glomerular filtration rate (GFR) in patients with chronic kidney disease, and compared patients starting dialysis with creatinine clearances above and below the median clearance for the whole group (8.3 ml/min).[35] Having adjusted for the earlier start, they found an inverse relationship between survival and earlier start to dialysis, in other words the longest survivors had started with the lowest clearances. Similar results have been reported in other centres. There seems therefore to be no justification for starting early to improve survival.

## 15.4 Specific causes of death

The major cardiac causes of death in general are not atherosclerotic coronary artery disease or cardiac ischaemia, but rather sudden death, often labelled as sudden *cardiac* death, and cardiac arrest. A single study from Japan has looked in more detail at dialysis patients dying suddenly.[36] From 1979–1999 35 of 93 dialysis patients undergoing autopsies had died suddenly. Overall (for all 93) most patients had died from cerebrovascular disease (26%), 19% from a true cardiac event, 17% from infections, 15% from malignancy, and 5% from a dissecting aneurysm. For patients dying suddenly, a cause was identified in most cases: 14% had an aortic dissection, 9% intracerebral haemorrhage, 9% a subdural haematoma, and 6% each an acute myocardial infarction and acute ischaemic stroke. Thus sudden death has mixed causes and cannot be simply ascribed to 'cardiac' causes. Bleyer *et al.* examined the distribution of sudden and cardiac deaths through the week.[37] In peritoneal dialysis there was an equal incidence on all days; however, in haemodialysis they noted a large excess of both sudden and cardiac deaths on Mondays and Tuesdays. Twenty per cent of patients on haemodialysis died on a Monday and 20% on a Tuesday, compared with 14% expected for each day. The authors suggested that these deaths may be caused by metabolic abnormalities or abnormally large electrolyte swings (especially potassium) on the first dialysis of the week after the longer weekend break, or to volume overload.

Cardiac arrest remains a 'difficult' cause of death in haemodialysis patients. It raises many issues of resuscitation, 'do not resuscitate' orders, consent to treatment and non-treatment, and communication, and may take place in the very pubic forum of the busy dialysis unit. A number of studies have looked at the outcome of cardiac arrest in dialysis patients. Moss *et al.* reported in 1992 on the outcomes of 221 patients with cardiac arrest over 8 years.[38] Thirty-four per cent of these patients underwent attempted resuscitation, compared with 21% of 1201 control cardiac arrests within the institution. Attempted resuscitation was therefore more common on the dialysis unit. The outcome, however, was worse, with only 8% of the 74 resuscitated patients actually leaving hospital, compared with 12% of the non-dialysis patients. By 6 months only two of the dialysis patients (3%) were still alive, compared with 23 of the 247 control (9%; $p = 0.044$). Finally, of those patients who initially responded to cardiopulmonary resuscitation (CPR), 78% were dead within 4 days, all on ventilators on the ICU. Data from Taiwan have shown similarly poor outcomes.[39] Of 24 patients on dialysis having a cardiac arrest, 75% were initially resuscitated but only 46% survived 24 h, 8% survived 1 month, and none survived to hospital discharge. This contrasts strikingly with data from New Mexico where 11 of 56 patients with cardiac arrest (20%) left hospital alive, but this is probably an atypical outcome.[40] Patients need to understand the likely outcome of attempted resuscitation. Data from many non-renal studies have shown an enormously exaggerated impression of the success of CPR. In one dialysis population of 449 patients, 87%

wanted CPR if they had a cardiac arrest on dialysis, and patients were more likely to be actively keen on resuscitation if they had seen a cardiac arrest on television![41] In a Japanese study only 5% of patients had discussed CPR with their doctors, and 29% with their families, but 42% did want to have attempted resuscitation if they had a cardiac arrest, and 12% even if they had become terminally ill with cancer or severely demented.[42] There are clearly wide gulfs between patients and medical staff in their attitudes to CPR and understanding of the likely outcomes, but also certainly a differential expectation about quality of life on dialysis and what the future holds.

Infection, especially septicaemia, is a common cause of death in ESRD, and has been associated in particular with older age (in some studies), diabetes, temporary vascular access, low serum albumin, and dialyser reuse.[43] The single most important action to minimize this risk is avoiding the use of temporary (non-tunnelled) vascular access.

## 15.5 Stopping dialysis

Cessation of dialysis is an increasingly common cause of death, but not a simple phenomenon to define clearly. Stopping dialysis is not the same as never starting—or conservative care in ESRD (see later), although of course in this case patients still ultimately die with or from uraemia. Patients may stop dialysis because of gradually increasing ill-health, because of severe intercurrent illness, or as an imminently pre-morbid decision when death is closely inevitable. Rarely patients stop dialysis in the absence of physical decline, usually when they have repeated dialysis-related technical problems, but occasionally simply as a result of boredom, exhaustion, or depression and rarely as an active suicide attempt. One single-centre study suggested that 66% of patients had deterioration in a chronic disease, 22% an acute intercurrent problem, 9% had failure to thrive, and only 1.5% of patients a technical dialysis-related problem and 1.5% to have failed a trial of dialysis.[44] In this study 26% of these patients had had a previous stroke and 23% dementia. Registry data may not accurately reflect cessation of dialysis since patients may be classified as dying from cardiac causes or a sudden death rather than dialysis withdrawal. Holley analysed 212 deaths from a single centre and found that in as many as 26% of cases dialysis had been discontinued before death.[45] Only 6 of these 56 patients, however, had been labelled as dying from uraemia or from cessation of dialysis. Holley suggested, therefore, that stopping dialysis was not a surrogate of dialysis withdrawal.

Mailloux *et al.* identified that 18.5% of all deaths in dialysis patients in New York State between 1970 and 1988 were from dialysis withdrawal, the same proportion as dying from a cardiac cause.[46] In this series withdrawal was commoner after the first 4 years of dialysis, and in those over 61 years old. Bajwa *et al.* documented that 17% of 76 patients died from dialysis withdrawal over a 3-year period, and again these patients were older, but also more likely to be divorced, widowed, living in a nursing home, or with increased co-morbidity and decreased physical functioning.[47] These authors also noted that withdrawal almost inevitably followed a relentless series of dialysis-related problems. Neu reported a similar overall picture.[48] Dialysis withdrawal occurred in 22% of all their deaths, and was more common in the elderly and nursing-home residents, although 39% of these patients had no new medical problems at the time the decision was made to stop dialysis. This is not a universal finding; for example, Roberts and Kjellstrand found that only 1.5% of patients stopping dialysis had no technical problems or new health problems—the vast majority did have.[49] Very similar results were reported from Newcastle, UK, with 17% of all deaths resulting from cessation of dialysis between 1964 and 1993 associated with increasing age, diabetes, and multiple medical problems.[50] The suggestion of dialysis withdrawal was initially raised by the physician in 57% of deaths, by the patient in 24%, and by the family in 22%.

Discontinuation of dialysis may of course be perceived as a relief from suffering in the patient's eye, or as a failure by the medical and nursing team. It is very important that discussions do occur with patients about this topic, and that they involve nursing staff, counsellors, social workers, and the family. Some patients feel empowered when planning to stop dialysis as it gives them back control over their illness and life.

In patients established on haemodialysis the time to death after ceasing dialysis is a median of 8–9 days in almost all studies.[51] A significant minority of patients survive over 10 days, and a few as long as 1 month. Patients stopping dialysis because of general ill-health, who were essentially dying from something else, had a median survival of only 2 days.[45] Qualitative studies on the nature of these deaths by interviews with the patients and their families have revealed that most patients were thought to have had a 'very good' or 'good' death (38% and 47% of patients respectively), and only 15% a 'bad' death after dialysis withdrawal.[52] Patients' deaths were better when they occurred at home or in a hospice as opposed to a hospital. Pain and agitation were the commonest problems encountered at the time of death, occurring in 42% and 30% of patients during their last day of life.[44] Death from withdrawal of dialysis may be increasing. In Albuquerque, new Mexico, 20% of patients died from dialysis withdrawal over the whole period 1976–1996, but 44% of all patients dying in the decade 1990–1996.[53]

## 15.6 Death in children with renal failure

Death is uncommon in children with ESRD. Between 1972 and 1992, 22 of 291 children with ESRD from Florida died.[54] The overall risk of death was 80 times the general paediatric population. Death, not surprisingly, is not due to cardiac or vascular disease. Children die from infections and bleeding complications, including cerebrovascular haemorrhage and post-operatively. There is no difference in the mortality in children dialysed by haemodialysis or peritoneal dialysis, and there has been no change in the last 30 years. Infections were predominantly fungal or Gram-negative bacteria, and fatal infections usually occurred in the first year on dialysis. A Dutch study suggested an overall standardized mortality rate of 31 for children with ESRD, and in this study the commonest causes of death were cerebrovascular events (both haemorrhage and infarction associated with hypertension: 24%) and infections (21%).[55]

## 15.7 Conservative care in ESRD

In many countries now, conservative care is increasingly discussed with patients, and actively managed. Hirsch *et al.* in 1994 found that one-quarter of all patients referred to the nephrology service were not offered dialysis, mostly because of co-morbidities and poor functional state.[56] Joly *et al.*, in their study of French octogenarians, identified 37 out of 144 patients who were not offered dialysis, usually as a result of a medical decision.[15] These patients were more socially isolated, referred later, had lower Karnofsky scores, and more diabetes than those offered dialysis. These patient died from uraemia (34%), pulmonary oedema or cardiac failure (24%), sudden death (8%), infections (5%), and cancer (5%). Main studied 11 patients from the north of England who did not start dialysis over a 12-month period.[57] Only one of the 11 had had renal pre-ESRD care, six were over 80 years old, six were thought likely to die very soon with or without dialysis, all 11 had significant co-morbidities, and four were incompetent to make the decision. Most of these 11 patients died, however, *with* and not *from* their renal failure.[57] Sekkarie and Moss tried to establish the reasons for lack of referral in some cases—25% of physicians did not or would not consult a nephrologist when deciding a patients should not receive dialysis, and 60% used age as a criterion for not referring.[58]

## 15.8  Summary

Death rates are increased in patients with kidney disease, both by modifiable and non-modifiable factors. For most patients it should be possible to increase life expectancy by careful attention to the modifiable factors. It should also be eminently possible to provide patients with a 'good' death.

### Case study

Mr JH was diagnosed with type II diabetes aged 65. His father had also been diabetic and had died age 62 from an acute myocardial infarction. JH developed microalbuminuria 1 year after initial diagnosis, and subsequently overt proteinuria. Over the next 5 years his GFR fell from 45 ml/min to 12 ml/min, at which point he began dialysis. He developed peripheral vascular disease, necessitating below-knee amputation, and angina. He switched from peritoneal dialysis to haemodialysis after membrane failure. At this point he was keen to discuss his likely prognosis, and what sort of life expectancy he could expect. This questioning led to a discussion of the options in the event of a cardiac arrest, and he decided not to be resuscitated should this happen Over the next year he had numerous admissions for peripheral vascular disease, access-related complications, and coronary ischaemia. He then began expressing his frustration about dialysis and the quality of his life, and the possibility of stopping dialysis was raised. His family were very opposed to this idea. Three weeks after these discussion were begun he was found dead in his bed at home one Monday morning.

## Appendix: End-of-life care, the terminal phase (by J. Chambers)

> Death is one of the attributes you were created with; death is part of you. Your life's continued task is to build your death.
>
> Montaigne, 1533–92

The care of patients with ESRD who are approaching the end of their life, often due to the failure of other organs and systems, is as important as the active management of their diseases at other stages. The emphasis of care, however, changes. The emphasis of active management is the prolongation of life and prevention, or reduction, of future complications of the disease. The emphasis of management at the end of life is relief of symptoms, maintenance of comfort, and attention to psychosocial and spiritual concerns. Patients who die following withdrawal from chronic dialysis present both a unique opportunity and an enormous challenge to those caring for them. The opportunity is afforded by the certain knowledge of death in a defined time, while the challenge and privilege is to ensure and enable there to be as much quality and dignity in the dying as is possible. For many, the decision to withdraw from dialysis follows weeks or months of increasing suffering as, despite dialysis, their co-morbid conditions continue their inexorable course. For others, a new event, such as the diagnosis of cancer, leads to a changed situation. The causes of death and the timescale to death for those who opt for conservative management and do not start on dialysis are more varied and less predictable.

### Quality in end-of-life care

What constitutes a 'good death' will differ from person to person. For some it will always be necessary to 'Rage, rage against the dying of the light'.[59] Others aspire to the peaceful death so often described in death notices. Perhaps what is most important is to try to ascertain and then endeavour to fulfil the person's wishes. Several studies have looked at the patient's perspective of quality in end-of-life care; these help us to define the key areas of concern. One such study[60] used qualitative face-to-face interviews with three groups of participants to determine their views on end-of-life issues. Forty-eight of a group of 126 were patients on dialysis. The participants identified five domains for end-of-life care: receiving adequate pain and symptom management, avoiding inappropriate prolongation of dying, achieving a sense of control, relieving burden, and strengthening relationships with loved ones. It not only behoves us to take notice of our patient's wishes as a duty of care but we can also use the identification of their concerns as a framework to help us clarify their own goals for treatment. Singer *et al.* additionally describe using this framework to teach doctors in training, thus instilling good practice from early on in a medical career.[60]

Additional resources for designing and planning end-of-life care include; a report from the UK organisation Age Concern[61] which identifies 12 principles of a good death (see Box) and frameworks produced in the US by an expert committee of the Institute of Medicine Committee[62] and the American Geriatric Society.[63] A practical UK initiative has been the introduction of an integrated care pathway for the care of the dying.[64] It presupposes recognition that the patient is dying and aims to ensure that all aspects important in caring for the dying are attended to along with the discontinuation of unnecessary interventions. Many of the areas addressed in the pathway mirror those identified in Singer's study; management of physical symptoms, the focus of nursing interventions on comfort not routine observations, removal of non-essential drugs, and anticipatory prescribing of drugs which might be needed for terminal care. In addition it encompasses communication with respect to insight of patient and family, and religious and spiritual support.

Knowledge of certain death in the immediate future provides the opportunity to discuss future care wishes, including place of care, in a more specific way than an advance directive, as it focuses on what a patient wishes rather than interventions he or she does not want. It also allows for exploration of hopes, fears, and anxieties. Singer *et al.*'s study reminds us of the importance of strengthening relationships with loved ones; this, for example, may be a realistic hope for someone who is dying. Which of us has not been moved by the marriage of someone close to their death when they knew they were dying? This had meaning for the person who was dying and could afford comfort to the bereaved.

## Recognition of the terminal phase

The terminal phase is more predictable for those who withdraw from dialysis than for many other groups of people; indeed cessation of dialysis is followed by certain death. However, many patients withdraw from dialysis as they die from their co-morbid conditions, perhaps only missing one dialysis session, in effect dying from these conditions rather than from renal failure. Recognition of the preterminal state is very important to enable proper emphasis to be made on the quality of life and relief of suffering. I would argue that for a significant proportion of chronic dialysis patients, an increase in unpleasant symptoms, particularly pain, often indicates that prognosis may be measured in months or weeks. It is important that at this time there is good symptom control including, where indicated, collaboration with local palliative care services. If the patient does not die, then a better quality of life may have been achieved, and if death occurs, then a reduction in suffering prior to it and the focus of care on those areas described above will have taken place.

## Pain and other symptom management at the end of life

Many patients will withdraw from dialysis, in part, because of the burden of symptoms they are experiencing. We know that the incidence of distressing symptoms is high and likely to be higher in those coming towards the end of life. Faisinger *et al.*[65] report significant symptom distress

## Twelve principles of a good death

♦ To know when death is coming, and to understand what can be expected.

♦ To be able to retain control of what happens.

♦ To be afforded dignity and privacy.

♦ To have control over pain relief and other symptom control.

♦ To have choice and control over where death occurs (at home or elsewhere).

♦ To have access to information and expertise of whatever kind is necessary.

♦ To have access to any spiritual or emotional support required.

♦ To have access to hospice care in any location, not only in hospital.

♦ To have control over who is present and who shares the end.

♦ To be able to issue advance directives which ensure wishes are respected.

♦ To have time to say goodbye, and control over other aspects of timing.

♦ To be able to leave when it is time to go, and not to have life prolonged pointlessly.

with respect to pain, reduced mobility, and pruritus occurring in more than a quarter of 531 dialysis patients who completed the Edmonton Symptom Assessment system. Symptoms relating to the dialysis procedure will cease on withdrawal but those of the co-morbid condition are likely to continue and those associated with uraemia and fluid overload may become worse. The key to symptom management is anticipatory prescribing and attention to route of administration using the easiest and least invasive.

**Pain** may not be a feature of dying following withdrawal of dialysis, but it is likely to continue for those in whom it is already present and new discomforts can occur from joints and skin pressure with reduced mobility. Data from family questionnaires[66] after death suggest that 73% of patients experienced pain in the last week of life, with 36% describing it as often extremely severe. Fear of a painful death is also a real concern of patients and families; acknowledgement of this is an important part of its management. Analgesia should be available for all patients; those who have pain should have it administered regularly and by the principles of the WHO analgesic ladder (see Chapter 8). Those without pain should have rapid access to it if needed. Where the oral route is lost, paracetamol and NSAIDs may be administered rectally, as can some strong opioids. Where the parenteral route is needed, the least painful administration is by the subcutaneous route, either intermittently with a butterfly needle retained *in situ* or by continuous infusion with a portable pump. Drugs and doses are described in the suggested guidelines for pain management in Chapter 8. In addition, end-of-life guidelines modified from those used for non-renal patients, are appended (p. 262). As patients can experience unpleasant toxicity, such as myoclonus, hallucinations, and agitation from the metabolites of morphine at this time it is the author's practice to use either fentanyl or alfentanil, if the subcutaneous route is needed.

**Shortness of breath** is very common in the last days of life, whatever the cause of dying. The incidence is likely to be increased in those ceasing dialysis because of fluid retention and symptomatic acidosis with air hunger. Occasionally the former is best relieved by ultrafiltration. The general management strategies for dyspnoea causing patient distress include non-pharmacological methods, such as ensuring a comfortable position, a fan with cool air directed on the face, oxygen and the reassuring presence of family or staff. In addition strong opioids, used in doses between 50% and 100% of those needed for pain relief, can be given as needed or regularly, orally, or by subcutaneous injection or infusion. A benzodiazepine such as midazolam, given subcutaneously, either separately or in combination with opioids, fentanyl or alfentanil, can also contribute to relief, particularly if there is accompanying agitation or severe distress.

**Retained respiratory tract secretions** may contribute to distress, particularly to those close to the patient. Management depends on anticipation; antisecretory drugs may reduce further production but cannot dry secretions already present. Hyoscine butylbromide, hyoscine hydro-bromide, and glycopyrronium are all used in this situation; hyoscine butylbromide is less likely to cause sedation than hyoscine hydrobromide, as it does not cross the blood–brain barrier and has a reduced incidence of paradoxical agitation. Each can be given by subcutaneous injection or infusion in combination with other drugs if needed.

**Terminal restlessness and agitation** occur in a significant proportion of all terminal illnesses, but may be increased in those dying from renal failure because of uraemia-induced neurological instability. Before resorting to pharmacological interventions it is important to deal with psycho-logical and spiritual issues, exclude physical causes such as pain, review current medication, as well as attending to the environment to maximize cognition. Pharmacological management may include sedation with benzodiazepines such as midazolam or antipsychotic medication such as haloperidol. The use of stat subcutaneous doses of midazolam enables the clinician to monitor response and choose an appropriate dose for continuous subcutaneous infusion if needed.

If **nausea and vomiting** are present prior to the terminal episode, antiemetics may be con-tinued in a syringe driver if the patient becomes unable to swallow. As-required medication should be available to those not on regular medication (see Chapter 8). Other symptoms of progressive uraemia may include thirst, itching, and hiccoughs; these should be actively man-aged. Thirst can frequently be relieved by good mouth care and sucking ice chips in conjunction with review of medication and liberation of oral intake for comfort. Measures decribed in Chapter 7 for other common symptoms are equally applicable here.

Comfort care of the patient is paramount; this includes discontinuation of unnecessary observations and non-palliative medication, concentration on mouth and skin care, and attention as needed to bowels and bladder if the patient is still passing urine.

Open communication about dying, with attendance to the patient's wishes will help avoid inappropriate prolongation of dying and may help the patient feel a sense of control. Relieving burden is two-fold: the burden of physical care and the burden of decision-making by proxies. Release from these concerns, and relief of physical suffering, may then allow time for strengthening of relationships. In discussion about place of care the patient's wishes often take into account his or her desire not to be a burden on their family. Accurate information about care and support that is available will facilitate decision-making. In the UK the decision to cease life-sustaining treatments is taken by the doctor in conjunction with the patient, if competent, thus relieving the family of extra burden at that time. Support of the patient's religious and spiritual needs, while essential throughout illness, attains a special importance at the end of life.

Thus it can be seen that there is much that is active that can be done to enable the person who is dying to achieve comfort and dignity. By doing so, support is given also to the family and the professional staff caring for them. It helps patients and family to see the same level of medical commitment continue through the terminal phase as was present prior to it; what changes is the goal of that care. Staff can take pride in and gain satisfaction from fulfilling their vocation to 'cure sometimes, to help often, to comfort always.[67]

# References

1. Holland, D.C., Lam, M. (2000). Predictors of hospitalisation and death among pre-dialysis patients: a retrospective study. *Nephrol. Dial. Transpl.*, **15**: 650–8.

2. United States Renal Data System (2002). *USRDS Annual Data Report*. http://www.USRDS.org (accessed April 2003).

3. Australia and New Zealand Dialysis and Transplant Registry (2002). *2002 Annual Report*. http://www.anzdata.org.au (accessed April 2003).

4. Brazilian Kidney Transplant Registry 1997 (1998). http://www.unifesp.br/dis/gamba/97/rghd97i.htm (accessed April 2003).

5. Salamone, M. (2000). Italian Registry of Dialysis and Transplantation. http://www.sin-ridt.org/-sin-ridt/sin-ridt.org.htm (accessed March 2003).

6. Mailloux, L.U., Belluci, A.G., Wilkes, B.M. (1991). Mortality in dialysis patients: analysis of the causes of death. *Am. J. Kidney Dis.*, **18**: 326–31.

7. McKenzie, J.K., Moss, A.H., Feest, T.G., Stocking, C.B., Siegler, M. (1998). Dialysis decision making in Canada, the United Kingdom and the United States. *Am. J. Kidney Dis.*, **31**: 12–18.

8. Charra, B., Chazot, C., Calemard, E., Laurent, G. (1993). Survival on renal replacement therapy. *Lancet*, **341**: 415–18.

9. Nishizawa, Y., Shoji, T., Maekawa, K., Nagasue, K. (2003). Intima media thickness of carotid artery predicts cardiovascular mortality in haemodialysis patients. *Am. J. Kidney Dis.*, **41**: S76–S79.

10. Goodman, W.G., Goldin, J., Kuizon, B.D., Yoon, C. (2000). Coronary artery calcification in young adults with and stage renal disease who are undergoing dialysis. *New Engl. J. Med.*, **342**: 1478–83.

11. Foley, R.N., Parfey, P.S., Hefferton, D., Singh, I., Simms, A., Barrett, B.J. (1994). Advance prediction of early death in patients starting maintenance dialysis. *Am. J. Kidney Dis.*, **23**: 836–45.

12. Byrne, C., Vernon, P., Cohen, J.J. (1994). Effect of age and diagnosis on survival of older patients beginning chronic dialysis. *J. Am. Med. Assoc.*, **271**: 34–6.

13. Lamping, D.L., Constantinovici, N., Roderick, P., *et al.* (2000). Clinical outcomes, quality of life and costs in the North Thames Dialysis Study of elderly people on dialysis. *Lancet* **356**: 1543–50.

14. Letourneau, I., Ouimet, D., Dumont, M., Pichette, V., Leblanc, M. (2003). Renal replacement therapy in end stage renal disease patients over 75 years old. *Am. J. Nephrol.*, **23**: 71–7.

15. Joly, D., Anglicheau, D., Alberti, C., *et al.* (2003). Octogenarians reaching end stage renal disease: cohort study of decision making and clinical outcomes. *J. Am. Soc. Nephrol.*, **14**: 1012–21.

16. Bleyer, A.J., Tell, G.S., Evans, G.W., Ettinger, W.H., Burkart, J.M. (1996). Survival of patients undergoing renal replacement therapy in one center with special emphasis on racial differences. *Am. J. Kidney Dis.*, **28**: 72–81.

17. Pei, Y.P., Greenwood, C.M., Chery, A.L., Wu, G.G. (2000). Racial differences in survival of patients on dialysis. *Kidney Int.*, **58**: 1293–9.

18. Chertow, G.M., Johanssen, K.L., Lew, N., Lazarus, J.M., Lowrie, E.G. (2000). Vintage, nutritional status and survival in hemodialysis patients. *Kidney Int.*, **57**: 1176–81.

19. Okechukwu, C.N., Lopes, A.A., Stack, A.G., Feng, S., Wolfe, R.A., Port, F.K. (2002). Impact of years of dialysis therapy on mrtality risk and the characteristics of longer term dialysis survivors. *Am. J. Kidney Dis.*, **39**: 533–8.

20. Chandra, S.H., Schultz, J., Lawrence, C., Greenwood, R., Farrington, K. (1999). Is there a rationale for rationing chronic dialysis. *Br. Med. J.*, **318**: 317–28.

21. Walters, G., Warwick, G., Walls, J. (2000). Analysis of patients dying within one year of starting renal replacement therapy. *Am. J. Nephrol.*, **20**: 358–63.

22. Jungers, P., Massy, Z.A., Nguyen-Khoa, T., *et al.* (2001). Longer duration of predialysis nephrological care is associated with improved long term survival of dialysis patients. *Nephrol. Dial. Transpl.*, **16**: 2357–64.

23. Stack, A.G. (2003). Impact of timing of nephrology referral and pre-ESRD care on mortality risk among new ESRD patients in the Unites States. *Am. J. Kidney. Dis.*, **41**: 310–18.

24. Stoves, J., Bartlett, C.N., Newstead, C.G. (2001). Specialist follow-up of patients before end stage renal failure and its relationship to survival on dialysis. *Postgrad. Med. J.*, **77**: 586–8.

25. Winkelmayer, W.C., Owen, W.F., Levin, R., Avorn, J. (2003). A propensity analysis late versus early nephrologist referral and mortality on dialysis. *J. Am. Soc. Nephrol.*, **14**: 486–92.

26. Van Biesen, W., Wiedmann, M., Lamiere, N. (1998). End stage renal disease treatment: a European perspective. *J. Am. Soc. Nephrol.*, **9**: S55–S62.

27. Roubicek, C., Brunet, P., Huiart, L., Thirion, X., *et al.* (2000). Timing of nephrology referral: influence on mortality and morbidity. *Am. J. Kidney Dis.*, **36**: 208–10.

28. Bloembergen, W.E., Port, F.K., Mauger, E.A., Wolfe, R.A. (1995). A comparison of death between patients treated with hemodialysis and peritoneal dialysis. *J. Am. Soc. Nephrol.*, **6**: 184–91.

29. Murphy, S.W., Foley, R.N., Barrett, B.J., *et al.* (2000). Comparative mortality of hemodialysis and peritoneal dialysis in Canada. *Kidney Int.*, **57**: 1720–6.

30. Foley, R.N., Parfey, P.S., Harnett, J.D., *et al.* (1998). Mode of dialysis therapy and mortality in end stage renal disease. *J. Am. Soc. Nephrol.*, **9**: 267–76.

31. Xue, J.L., Everson, S.E., Constantini, E.G., *et al.* (2002). Peritoneal and hemodialysis: II mortality risk associated with initial patients characteristics. *Kidney Int.*, **61**: 741–6.

32. Collins, A.J., Hao, W., Xia, H., *et al.* (1999). Mortality risks of peritoneal and hemodialysis. *Am. J. Kidney Dis.*, **34**: 1065–74.

33. Bloembergen, W.E., Stannard, D.C., Port, F.K., *et al.* (1996). Relationship between dose of hemodialysis and cause specific mortality. *Kidney Int.*, **50**: 557–65.

34. Eknoyan, G., Beck, G.J., Cheung, A.K., *et al.* (2002). Effect of dialysis dose and membrane flux in maintenance hemodialysis. *New Engl. J. Med.*, **347**: 2010–19.

35. Traynor, J.P., Simpson, K., Geddes, C., Deighan, C.J., Fox, J.G. (2002). Early initiation of dialysis fails to prolong survival in patients with end stage renal failure. *J. Am. Soc. Nephrol.*, **13**: 2125–32.

36. Takeda, K., Harada, A., Okuda, S., *et al.* (1997). Sudden death in chronic dialysis patients. *Nephrol. Dial. Transpl.*, **12**: 952–5.

37. Bleyer, A.J., Russell, G.B., Satto, S.G. (1999). Sudden and cardiac death rates in haemodialysis patients. *Kidney Int.*, **55**: 1553–9.

38. Moss, A.H., Holley, J., Upton, M.B. (1992). Outcomes of cardiopulmonary resuscitation in dialysis patients. *J. Am. Soc. Nephrol.*, **3**: 1238–43.

39. Lai, M-N., Hung, K., Huang, J., Tsai, T.J. (1999). Clinical findings and outcomes of intrahaemodialysis cardiopulmonary resuscitation. *Am. J. Nephrol.*, **19**: 468–73.

40. Tzamaloukas, A.H., Murata, G.H., Avasthi, P.S. (1991). Outcome of cardiopulmonary resuscitation in patients on chronic dialysis. *ASAIO J.*, **37**: M369–M370.

41. Moss, A.H., Hozayen, O., King, K., Holley, J., Schmidt, R. (2001). Attitudes of patients toward cardiopulmonary resuscitation in the dialysis unit. *Am. J. Kidney Dis.*, **38**: 847–52.

42. Miura, Y., Asai, A., Nagata, S., *et al.* (2001). Dialysis patients preferences regarding cardiopulmonary resuscitation and withdrawal of dialysis in Japan. *Am. J. Kidney Dis.*, **37**: 1216–22.

43. Powe, N.R., Jaar, B., Furth, S.L., Hermann, J., Briggs, W. (1999). Septicaemia in dialysis patients: incidence, risk factors and prognosis. *Kidney Int.*, **55**: 1081–90.

44. Cohen, L.M., Germain, M.J., Poppel, D.M., Woods, A.L., Kjellstrand, C.M. (2000). Dialysis discontinuation and palliative care. *Am. J. Kidney Dis.*, **36**: 452–3.

45. Holley, J. (2002). A single centre review of the death notification form: discontinuation dialysis before death is not a surrogate for withdrawal from dialysis. *Am. J. Kidney Dis.*, **10**: 525–30.

46. Mailloux, L.U., Belluci, A.G., Napolitano, B., Mossey, R.T., Wilkes, B.M., Bluestone, P.A. (1993). Death by withdrawal from dialysis : a 20 year clinical experience. *J. Am. Soc. Nephrol.*, **3**: 1631–7.

47. Bajwa, K., Szabo, E., Kjellstrand, C.M. (1996). A prospective study of risk factors and decision making in discontinuation of dialysis. *Arch. Intern. Med.*, **156**: 2571–7.

48. Neu, S., Kjellstrand, C.M. (1986). Stopping long term dialysis. An empirical study of withdrawal of life supporting treatment. *N. Engl. J. Med.*, **314**: 14–20.

49. Roberts, J.C., Kjellstrand, C.M. (1988). Choosing death. Withdrawal from chronic dialysis without medical reason. *Acta Med. Scand.*, **223**: 181–6.

50. Catalano, C., Goodship, T.H.J., Graham, K.A., *et al.* (1996). Withdrawal of renal replacement therapy in Newcastle; 1964–1993. *Nephrol. Dial. Transpl.*, **11**: 133–9.

51. Cohen, L.M., McCue, J.D., Germain, M.J., Kjellstrandm C.M. (1995). Dialysis discontinuation: a 'good' death? *Arch. Intern. Med.*, **155**: 42–7.

52. Cohen, L.M., Germain, M.J., Poppel, D.M., Woods, A.L., Pekow, P.S., Kjellstrand, C.M. (2000). Dying well after discontinuing the life support treatment of dialysis. *Arch. Intern. Med.*, **160**: 2513–18.

53. Bordenave, K., Tzamaloukas, A.H., Conneen, S., Adler, K., Keller, L.K., Murata, G.H. (1998). Twenty one year mortality in a dialysis unit: changing effect of withdrawal from dialysis. *ASAIO J.*, **44**: 194–8.

54. Neiberger, R., Schwalbe, M., Pena, D., Fennell, R. (1995). Cause of death for children on chronic dialysis: a 20 year study. e-Neph: www.eneph.com/feature_archive/outcomes/v24n2978.html (accessed on 29 April 2003).

55. Groothoff, J.W., Gruppen, M.P., Offringa, M., *et al.* (2002). Mortality and cause of death of end stage renal disease in children: a Dutch cohort study. *Kidney Int.*, **61**: 621–9.

56. Hirsch, D.J., West, M.L., Cohen, A.D., Jindal, K.K. (1994). Experience with not offering dialysis to patients with a poor prognosis. *Am. J. Kidney Dis.*, **23**: 463–6.

57. Main, J. (2000). Deciding not to start dialysis—a one year prospective study in Teeside. *J. Nephrol.*, **13**: 136–40.

58. Sekkarie, M.A., Moss, A.H. (1998). Witholding and withdrawing dialysis: the role of physician specialty and education and patient functional status. *Am. J. Kidney Dis.*, **31**: 464–72.

59. From Dylan Thomas 'Do not go gentle into that good night'.

60. Singer, P.A., Martin, D.K., Merrijoy, K. (1999) Quality end-of-life care patients' perspectives. *J. Am. Med. Assoc.*, **281**(2): 163–8.

61. Debate of the Age, Health and Care Study Group (1999). *The Future of Health and Care of Older People: the Best is Yet to Come*. London: Age Concern.

62. Field, M.J., Kassel, C.K. (eds) for the Institute of Medicine (1997). *Approaching Death: Improving Care at the End of Life*. Washington, DC: National Academy Press.

63. Lynn, T. (1997). Measuring quality of care at the end of life: a statement of principles. *J. Am. Geriatr. Soc.*, **45**: 526–7.

64. Ellershaw, J., Foster, A., Murphy, D., Sjea, T., Overill, S. (1997). Developing an integrated care pathway for the dying patient. *Eur. J. Palliat. Care* **4**(6): 203–7.

65. Fainsinger, R.L., Davison, S.N., Brenneis, C. (2003). A supportive care model for dialysis patients. *Palliat. Med.*, **17**: 81–2.

66. Cohen, L.M. (2004) *Planning a Renal Palliative Care Program and its Components*. In: *Supportive care for the renal patient*, ed., E.J. Chambers, M.J. Germain and E. Brown pp. 27–34. Oxford: Oxford University Press.

67. Anon 16th century French. *Guerir quelquefois, soulager souvent, comforter toujours.*

# Guidelines for the care of patients with end-stage renal disease who are in the last days of life in hospital

**The aim of treatment is the comfort of the patient and the support of those close to them.**

Use these guidelines when the whole team, the patient, and family agree that the patient is in the last days of his or her life. It is a guide to treatment and practitioners should exercise their own professional judgement according to the clinical situation.

**Before using these guidelines, the following should be considered:**

- Has there been discussion with the patient, family, and renal team that the focus of care is the comfort of the patient and not the prolongation of life?
- Have the patient and family been asked about their preferred place of care?
- Have all unnecessary investigations, including blood tests and routine monitoring, e.g. blood pressure, been discontinued?
- Have all non-palliative medications been discontinued and is comfort care, particularly care of the mouth and skin, in place?
- **Are the drugs needed for palliation prescribed by a route appropriate for the patient's situation and are they available as needed?**
- Have the patient and family been asked about their spiritual and religious needs at this time?

**For good symptom control prn medication should be prescribed for likely symptoms even when the patient is asymptomatic.** All of the drugs listed below should be given subcutaneously (SC), unless otherwise specified. Intravenous (IV) doses of drugs are similar but tolerance to opioids and midazolam will occur more quickly if the IV route is used.

## Pain

- **All patients should have a strong opioid prescribed, to be available as needed (prn).**
- **Recommendation: fentanyl 25 µg SC prn up to hourly or alfentanil 0.1–0.2 mg SC up to hourly.**

### 1. Patient in pain: already on strong opioid

(a) Opioid-responsive pain:
- Increase present dose by 30% or
- Add up previous day's prn doses and add to the regular dose
- **Plus prn medication, SC fentanyl or alfentanil 1/10th to 1/6th of the 24-h dose.**

---

### Patient has a fentanyl patch

- If the pain is controlled continue with patch
- If pain not controlled continue with patch, titrating additional analgesia with prn or continuous s/c fentanyl or alfentanil

(b) Opioid poorly responsive: ◆ Consider adjuvant; see box or contact local palliative care service.

(2) Patient in pain: opioid naïve

(a) Pain continuous
- Start continuous SC infusion in syringe driver with either fentanyl or alfentanil
- Starting dose depends on size, age, and severity of pain
- **150–300 µg/24 h fentanyl or 0.6–1.2 mg/24 h alfentanil are possible starting doses**
- **Plus prn medication, SC fentanyl or alfentanil 1/10th to 1/6th of the 24-h dose.**

(b) Pain intermittent
- see also box for adjuvant drugs
- prescribe fentanyl 25 µg SC or alfentanil 0.1–0.2 mg SC as needed up to hourly
- after 24 h, or sooner, review medication, if two or more prn doses needed or patient is still in pain, set up SC syringe driver to run over 24 h as above.

---

## Adjuvant drugs for specific indications

- **bowel colic** - consider hyoscine butylbromide
- **joint stiffness, bed sores** - consider rectal paracetamol, or NSAIDS
- **neuropathic pain** - consider clonazepam
- **associated anxiety and distress** - add midazolam

A combination of midazolam and fentanyl or alfentanil can be very effective in agitated patients who are in pain.

---

◆ Fentanyl and alfentanil are suggested as alternative strong opioids to morphine for patients in renal failure as they have no active metabolites with the potential to cause symptomatic and distressing toxicity such as myoclonic jerks and agitation.

◆ 300 µg/24 h SC fentanyl and 2 mg/24 h SC alfentanil are approximately equivalent to 60 mg oral morphine/24 h or 8 mg oral hydromorphone/24 h.

◆ Fentanyl and alfentanil can be mixed with all the common drugs in a syringe driver, though care should be taken with alfentanil and cyclizine as it may crystallize.

**If uncertain, please contact senior medial, nursing or pharmacy staff on your team or your local palliative care service**

For all of the symptoms below all patients should have prn medication prescribed and available should symptoms develop.

At this stage the goal is relief of symptoms and the cause of the symptom may not be relevant.

## Retained respiratory tract secretions

Symptoms absent: hyoscine butylbromide 20 mg SC stat and 2-hourly prn.

Symptoms present: hyoscine butylbromide 40–120 mg/24 h SC + 20 mg 2-hourly prn.

## Terminal restlessness and agitation

Symptom absent: midazolam 2.5 mg–5 mg SC up to hourly prn.

Symptom present: midazolam 2.5 mg SC up to hourly prn. If two or more doses are required consider a syringe driver with 10–20 mg/24 h + prn dose as needed.

## Nausea and vomiting

Symptoms absent:

1. If already taking an effective antiemetic, e.g. metoclopramide, cyclizine, haloperidol or levomepromazine these can be continued in a syringe driver and given over 24 h.

2. If not taking an antiemetic prescribe levomepromazine 5 mg SC prn up to 3 doses/day.

Symptoms present:

Start **levomepromazine** 5 mg SC prn up to 8-hourly or
Start 5–10 mg SC/24 h by continuous infusion, with 5 mg SC available prn.

| Drug | Action | Starting dose with range/24 hrs |
|---|---|---|
| Fentanyl | Analgesic and for Dyspnoea | Opioid naïve 150–300 mcg* |
| Alfentanil | Analgesic and for Dyspnoea | Opioid naïve 0.6–1.2 mg* |
| Cyclizine | Antiemetic | 100–150 mg |
| Haloperidol | Antiemetic | 2.5–5 mg (range 2.5–10) |
| | Antipsychotic | 5 mg (range 5–10 mg) |
| Metoclopramide | Antiemetic | 20–30 mg (range 30–40 mg) |
| Levomepromazine | Antiemetic antipsychotic | 5–15 mg 15–25 mg |
| Midazolam | Sedative | 10–20 mg (range 10–60 mg) |
| Clonazepam | Anxiolytic, | 0.5–1 mg (range 1–2 mg) |
| | for neuropathic pain | " |
| Hyoscine butylbromide | Anticholinergic for colic | 40 mg/24 hrs range 40–160 mg |

*any two of the above drugs can be mixed together except cyclizine and hyoscine butylbromide which may crystallise

*care needed with alfentanil and cyclizine as it may crystallise. If an antiemetic is needed with hyoscine butylbromide or alfentanil, levomepromazine or haloperidol may be used

*dose titrated against need

## Shortness of breath

- There are many causes of shortness of breath at the end of life.
- The following may be helpful:
- Position the patient   • cool fan on the face   • oxygen
- The reassuring presence of family or staff.
- Explanation to patient and family.
- Strong opioids such as fentanyl and alfentanil, used at doses of 50–100% of that used for pain can be used prn up to hourly if needed.
- Benzodiazepines, such as midazolam 2.5–5 mg SC can be given up to hourly.
- Cheyne Stokes respiration is usually a terminal event and the patient is often unconscious. It is important to explain this and reassure the relatives that we do not believe the patient is suffering at this time.

**For all drugs see accompanying text and tables in this chapter and chapters 7 and 8**

**If uncertain, please contact senior  medial, nursing or pharmacy staff on your team or your local palliative care service**

# Index